Medical Microbiology

Sixth Edition

Medical Microbiology

C. G. A. Thomas MA, BM,
BCh (Oxon.), FRCP (Lond.), FRCPath

Consultant Microbiologist,
Norfolk and Norwich Hospital
Formerly Radcliffe Travelling Fellow of
University College, Oxford

Baillière Tindall   **London • Philadelphia**
Toronto • Sydney • Tokyo

Baillière Tindall
W. B. Saunders

24–28 Oval Road
London NW1 7DX, England

The Curtis Center, Independence Square West,
Philadelphia, PA 19106–3399, USA

55 Horner Avenue
Toronto, Ontario M8Z 4X6, Canada

Harcourt Brace Jovanovich Group (Australia) Pty Ltd
30–52 Smidmore St, Marrickville, NSW 2204, Australia

Harcourt Brace Jovanovich (Japan) Inc.
Ichibancho Central Building, 22–1 Ichibancho
Chiyoda-ku, Tokyo 102, Japan

First published 1964
Fifth edition 1983
Sixth edition 1988
Reprinted 1990

This book is printed on acid-free paper

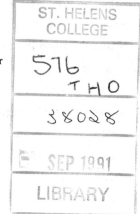

Typeset by Setrite Typesetters Ltd, Hong Kong
Printed in Great Britain at the University Press, Cambridge

British Library Cataloguing in Publication Data

Thomas, C.G.A. (Cyril Geoffrey Arthur)
    Medical microbiology.—6th ed.
    1. Medicine. Microbiology
    I. Title
    616'.01

ISBN 0-7020-1270-X

Contents

Preface

Let thy Studies be free as thy Thoughts and Con-
templations, but fly not upon the wings of Imagination;
Joyn Sense unto Reason, and Experiment unto Specu-
lation, and so give life unto Embryon Truths, and
Verities yet in their Chaos.
    Sir Thomas Browne of Norwich, 1605—1682

The aim of this book is to provide a concise general account of
microbiology with emphasis on those aspects which are relevant
to the day-to-day practice of medicine. Details of technique and
systematic microbiology are the province of the specialist microbiologist and have therefore been given little attention.

When supplemented by lectures and a practical course the
book will provide medical students with a basic knowledge of
medical microbiology, but it is most desirable that they should
also find time to read more widely. It is hoped that the book will
also prove useful to those who wish to refresh their minds before
their final examinations, to medical graduates working in fields
other than microbiology and to nurses, technicians and other
workers in the health services.

The book was originally based on lectures given to medical
students at St Thomas's Hospital, Guy's Hospital and the University of Rochester, New York. It has been extensively modified in
the light of experience gained as a hospital microbiologist in
Norwich. For this edition many sections have been rewritten to
incorporate recent advances and the text as a whole has been
thoroughly pruned to make room for new growth. The index has
been revised and extended to increase its value as a source of
useful information.

My thanks are due to the many people who have helped me
with this edition. In particular I wish to thank my former colleagues Dr Richard G. Tucker and Dr Ruth R. White and my wife
Dr Barbara E. Thomas for their constructive criticism.

C. G. A. Thomas

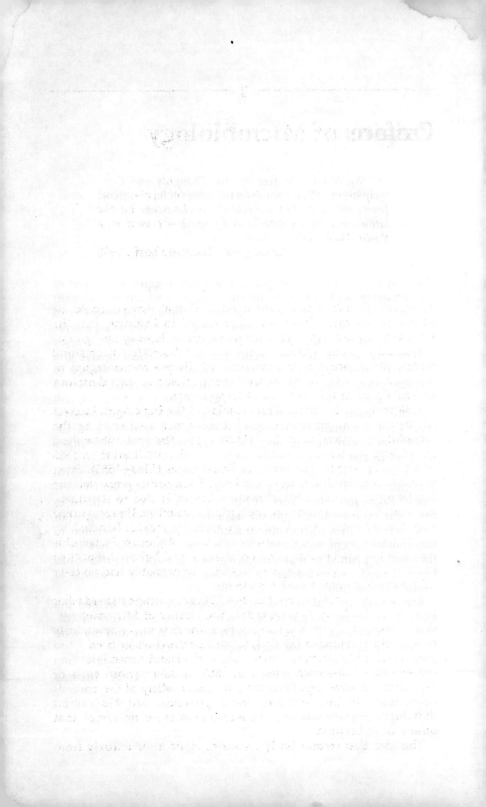

Origins of Microbiology

But what if one should tell such people in future that there are more animals living in the scum on the teeth in a man's mouth, than there are men in a whole kingdom?...

Antony van Leeuwenhoek, 1683

From early times a few people realized that disease could be spread by contact. There is a clear record in Leviticus that the Jews were aware of the contagious nature of leprosy and gonorrhoea, although the ultimate cause was attributed to supernatural forces. The concept of transmission of disease by contagion or infection can have had no general recognition and such doctrines do not figure in the writings of Hippocrates.

Following the intellectual hibernation of the Dark Ages, interest in the cause and transmission of disease was awakened by the devastating epidemics of the Middle Ages. The first outstanding scientific contribution on the subject was the publication in 1546 of *De Contagione* by Hieronymus Fracastorius (1483–1553). From a study of epidemics in Northern Italy, Fracastorius presented the fundamental concept that epidemic disease is due to the transmission of an agent from one individual to another. He recognized that disease could be spread by contact, by articles handled by the patient or through the air from a distance. Although Fracastorius refers to the *seminaria* or germs of disease and believed that they could multiply and propagate their like, he probably had no clear idea that they were living organisms.

Antony van Leeuwenhoek (1632–1723), a draper and haberdasher of Delft in Holland, is accepted as the 'Father of Microbiology'. With lenses of his own making he was the first to see an entirely new world of animalcules. In 1665 he examined water from a tub and found little animals 'more than a thousand times less than the eye of a full-grown louse'. In 1683 he saw various sorts of organisms in scrapings from his own teeth. Many of the animalcules seen by Leeuwenhoek were protozoa, but his careful drawings, descriptions and measurements leave no doubt that others were bacteria.

The idea that certain lowly creatures could arise entirely from dead organic matter was still widely held in the seventeenth century. Such myths were discredited by Francesco Redi (1626–97) who in 1668 showed, for example, that putrefying flesh did not produce maggots if flies were excluded. The problem of spontaneous generation of microscopic creatures was more difficult to resolve. Lazzaro Spallanzani (1729–99) showed in works published in 1765 and 1776 that animalcules failed to appear in infusions if the flasks were boiled long enough and stringent precautions were taken to prevent the entry of air. Spallanzani's work was ahead of its time. Because of subsequent inconclusive experiments by other less able workers and the special problems raised by heat-resistant forms of life (spores), the idea of spontaneous generation of microbes lingered on.

The possible medical significance of animalcules was largely overlooked in the two hundred years following Leeuwenhoek's discoveries. Agostino Bassi was the first person to prove that a microbe could cause disease. He demonstrated in 1835–6 that a disease of silkworms (*muscardine*) was contagious and could be transmitted naturally by direct contact or infected food, or experimentally by means of a pin previously sterilized in a flame. The causative organism was shown to be a fungus. In later writings Bassi argued that the theory of contagion by living organisms was obviously applicable to many human diseases.

By the middle of the nineteenth century there was a general awareness of the existence of various germs or micro-organisms, but their significance was largely obscure until the French chemist Louis Pasteur (1822–95) began his experiments on fermentation. Pasteur proved that the conversion of sugar to alcohol in the production of beer and wine was caused by the activity of living micro-organisms. In this particular fermentation the organisms were yeasts, but in other types of fermentation bacteria or moulds were responsible. Various 'diseases' of wine and beer were due to the intrusion of alien organisms and were preventable if these were excluded. In one of the classics of scientific research Pasteur confirmed what Spallanzani had realized a century earlier: he proved that microbes are not spontaneously generated from dead organic matter.

From diseases of wine and beer Pasteur turned his attention to a silkworm disease (*pébrine*) which was at that time ravaging the silk industry in France. Although he could not identify the causative organism (a protozoon) he showed that the disease could be eradicated by assuming a microbial cause. Turning now to diseases of animals and man, Pasteur made a series of observations which pointed clearly to the view that specific micro-organisms cause specific diseases.

The complete establishment of the germ theory of disease

depended on the work of Robert Koch (1843–1910) in Germany. In 1876 he proved that *Bacillus anthracis* was the cause of anthrax. He infected mice with the blood of sheep which had died of anthrax, transferred infection twenty times from mouse to mouse, each time demonstrating the organism in their blood, isolated the organism in pure culture and used such a culture to transmit the disease. In 1882 Koch made the momentous announcement that a major human disease, tuberculosis, was caused by a micro-organism, *Mycobacterium tuberculosis*.

Koch's outstanding contribution was to perfect a simple method of obtaining bacteria in pure culture. The principle was demonstrated in London in 1881, when he showed that isolated colonies could be obtained by streaking material on gelatin-coated slides. Gelatin was not wholly satisfactory and was soon replaced by agar, which proved to be an almost perfect basis for solid media. Petri became one of the immortals by seeing the advantage of a dish with a lid on it.

Koch laid down the principles of proof required before a particular microbe could be accepted as the cause of a disease. These principles had been deduced earlier on theoretical grounds by Henle, but Koch provided the experimental proof and they are rightly referred to as 'Koch's postulates'. They are three in number: (1) the microbe must be found in all cases of the disease and its distribution in the body must correspond with that of the lesions; (2) it must be grown outside the body in pure culture for several generations; (3) the cultures must be able to reproduce the disease in susceptible animals, and the microbes must be recoverable from these animals in pure cultures. These are ideal criteria and are not always attainable in practice, e.g. *Mycobacterium leprae* is undoubtedly the cause of leprosy, but it has never been cultured *in vitro*. Koch's postulates have now been fulfilled so many times that the germ theory of disease is established on an unassailable basis. In many diseases the appearance of specific antibodies in the blood provides important additional evidence.

Alexander Ogston, a Scottish surgeon, provided Britain's major contribution to the golden age of bacteriology. In 1880–2 he showed that cocci produced inflammation and suppuration and were the main cause of acute abscesses. He discovered and named staphylococci and distinguished them from streptococci.

Quite early it began to be realized that some microbes were even smaller than bacteria. Ivanowsky (1892) and Beijerinck (1898) showed that mosaic disease of the tobacco plant could be transmitted to healthy plants by means of tissue juices freed from bacteria by filtration. Loeffler and Frosch (1898) reported that foot-and-mouth disease of animals could also be transmitted by bacteria-free filtrates. From such beginnings evidence accumulated for the existence of a vast class of minute organisms known as viruses which we now know to be responsible for many infectious diseases of man, animals, plants and other organisms. Even bacteria do not escape infection, as was shown by Twort (1915) and d'Herelle (1917), who independently discovered the class of viruses known as bacteriophages or simply as phages. Today the precise three-dimensional shape of several viruses is known and the complete sequence of the thousands of nucleotide bases which make up their nucleic acid has been determined.

Intensive investigation of the role of microbes as agents of disease has yielded the richest harvest of useful information ever known to medicine. Many major pestilential diseases have been brought under control and other infectious diseases which were once common are now rare. In 1940 Chain and Florey and their colleagues opened the antibiotic era by showing that penicillin was an effective chemotherapeutic agent. In 1949 Enders and others showed that poliovirus could be readily grown in tissue culture and it soon became clear that viruses could be studied in any well-equipped laboratory. Immunology has grown with our knowledge of microbes and effective vaccines for preventing infectious diseases have been the most obvious end-products. The eradication of smallpox in 1977 through international co-operation was a unique achievement in the history of medicine. Immunology has spread into fields remote from microbes, such as tissue transplantation and immunological tolerance, and is now established as a discipline in its own right, dealing with fundamental problems of biology. Modern developments in biochemistry, genetics and molecular biology depend to an enormous extent on work with microbes. Thus the tremendous achievement of cracking the genetic code was largely based on a study of the chemical and genetic mechanisms of the bacterium *Escherichia coli* and one of its phages. Today it is possible to extract genetic material from a bacterium, virus or animal cell and link it with the genetic material of living *E. coli* where it will replicate. The results of such genetic manipulation of bacteria are already playing an important role in everyday medical practice. Medical graduates with the necessary mental agility will find that the new and thriving disciplines of medical microbiology offer fields of research and discovery every bit as exciting as those open to the early bacteriologists.

General Properties of Bacteria

A desoxyribonucleic acid fraction has been isolated from Type III pneumococci which is capable of transforming unencapsulated R variants derived from Pneumococcus Type II into fully encapsulated Type III cells.

O. T. Avery et al., 1944

Bacteria are microscopic, rigid-walled, unicellular organisms which multiply asexually by binary fission. They are a heterogeneous group possessing in varying degrees properties common both to simple plants and to simple animals.

Microscopes

It is convenient at this stage to consider the types of microscope available for the direct observation of bacteria and other microorganisms. The unit of measurement in bacteriology is the micrometre or μm (1 μm = 10^{-6} m).

The light microscope

The ordinary microscope fitted with an oil-immersion lens is used for the routine examination of stained films of bacteria. The high-power lens is useful for examining living bacteria in wet preparations. With the light microscope the resolving power (i.e. the production of a formed image) is limited to a value of approximately half the wavelength of light. Since the wavelength of visible light is about 0.5 μm the strongest lenses cannot resolve images of objects less than about 0.25 μm. Particles down to about 0.075 μm may be visible as dots of indeterminate shape. Even the best microscopes are working near their limits when very small bacteria are being studied and finer structural details are beyond the range of these instruments.

Ultraviolet microscopy

By using shorter ultraviolet rays and the camera in place of the eye, particles as small as 0.075 μm can be resolved.

Dark-ground illumination

This is a method of increasing the effective resolving power of the ordinary microscope. A special condenser is used to reflect a powerful source of light obliquely on to a wet preparation of the material being examined. Very small particles scatter the light and can be seen as brilliant images moving against a dark background. It is possible by this method to see very small or very thin microbes, such as certain spirochaetes.

Phase-contrast microscopy

By special optical arrangements the ordinary microscope can be modified so that differences in the phase of light waves which have passed through substances of different refractive indices are appreciated as differences in intensity. The method is of value in studying fine detail in unstained living bacteria, protozoa, etc.

The electron microscope

In principle this apparatus resembles the light microscope. A beam of electrons replaces the conventional light source and focusing is brought about by magnetic fields instead of glass lenses. The material under investigation is examined in a high vacuum. The electrons behave as rays of very short wavelength and will resolve objects as small as 0.001 μm. Minute structural details of bacteria can be examined in ultra-thin sections but the main application has been in the study of viruses.

The *scanning electron microscope* offers even greater effective resolution than the transmission electron microscope. A flying spot of electrons is used to scan the object and the emergent electrons are collected and displayed on an oscilloscope. Three-dimensional images of extraordinary clarity can be obtained.

Classification and nomenclature

On the basis of their morphology, staining reactions, nutrition, metabolism, antigenic structure, chemical composition and genetic homology bacteria have been classified into orders, families, genera and species. Within a species, bacteria differing from each other in minor respects are variously designated groups, types or varieties; some properties may be characteristic of particular strains. There is often disagreement about what weight should be attached to different properties, and the classification of bacteria is not nearly so clear-cut and final as it is in the case of higher plants and animals.

Continuing efforts are being made to find new properties that would facilitate bacterial classification. Chromatography has been used to identify metabolic end-products, the amino acid composition of bacterial cell walls, and substances obtained by pyrolysis of whole organisms. The base composition of bacterial deoxyribonucleic acid (DNA) can be used as a measure of genetic homology. The extent to which single-stranded DNA obtained from one organism will hybridize with single-stranded DNA from other organisms is a measure of their relatedness. The proportion of guanine plus cytosine to total nucleotide bases (G + C content) is characteristic for different groups of bacteria, e.g. the G + C content of *Staphylococcus aureus* is 31—36% and of *Escherichia coli* is 50—52%. This substantial difference confirms that these two organisms are not closely related. However, a similarity of G + C content does not necessarily mean that two organisms are genetically similar.

Numerical (Adansonian) classification provides an almost unbiased method of classifying bacteria. A large number of characters, preferably hundreds, is determined for each strain of bacterium and, giving each character *equal* weight, the similarity between pairs of strains is expressed as a coefficient. When all the strains have been compared they can be arranged in groups according to their similarity coefficients. A computer is used for the calculations.

As far as possible each distinct kind of bacterium is assigned a name indicating its genus and species. The generic name is often conventionally abbreviated. Thus we have *Staphylococcus aureus* (*Staph. aureus*) or *Mycobacterium tuberculosis* (*M. tuberculosis*). In the colloquial language of the hospital older names are frequently used in parallel with the newer scientific names, e.g. *M. tuberculosis* is commonly referred to as the tubercle bacillus. This use of the term 'bacillus', meaning any rod-shaped organism, should not be confused with the special use of the word *Bacillus* which denotes a particular genus of spore-bearing rods.

Shape

Three fundamental morphological forms are recognized: spherical (coccus), straight rod (bacillus) and curved or spiral rod (vibrio, campylobacter, spirillum and spirochaete). Within these three general categories there is great diversity.

Cocci may be arranged like bunches of grapes (*Staphylococcus*). They may be slightly oval or pointed at the ends and arranged in chains (*Streptococcus*) or in pairs (*Streptococcus pneumoniae*). They may be in pairs with the adjacent sides flattened (*Neisseria*) or in groups of four (*Micrococcus tetragenus*) or in cubical packets of eight (*Sarcina*).

Bacilli are usually obvious rods, but in some genera (*Brucella* and *Haemophilus*) the organisms take the form of short coccobacilli. Other bacilli show a tendency to form threads (*Proteus*) or grow in chains (*Bacillus*) or produce club-shaped organisms (*Corynebacterium*). Some bacilli are spindle-shaped (*Fusobacterium*). Some bacteria (*Actinomyces* and *Nocardia*) grow in the form of branching filaments.

Spiral forms include rods with just enough curvature to give the organism a curved or comma shape (*Vibrio* and *Campylobacter*), longer rigid rods with several curves or spirals (*Spirillum*) and long flexible organisms with several or many spirals (spirochaetes).

Size

Typical cocci are about 1 μm in diameter. Most bacilli are 2–5 μm long and 0.5–1.0 μm wide. Many of the important spirochaetes are 5–20 μm long and only 0.1–0.2 μm wide.

The individual cells in a culture often vary greatly in size, but in a particular species they tend to have a characteristic average size, e.g. *Bacillus anthracis* is larger than most other pathogenic bacteria. With all species the average size of the cells varies with the conditions. Thus rapidly dividing cells are smaller than those of a culture that has just started to grow, and cells that have been exposed to penicillin are usually larger than normal.

Staining reactions

Gram's method

This is the most important staining procedure used in medical bacteriology, but despite an immense amount of work the mechanism is still uncertain.

Technique

The following method is reliable for staining ordinary films:

1   Fix the dry film by passing three times through a flame.

2 Stain with crystal violet (or methyl violet) for 15 seconds and pour off the excess.

3 Flood with Lugol's iodine, leave for 30 seconds and pour off the excess.

4 Flood with acetone for not more than 2−5 seconds and wash with water immediately. Alternatively, ethanol can be used for decolorization: wash with ethanol until no more colour comes away and then wash with water.

5 Counterstain with dilute carbol fuchsin for 20 seconds (or neutral red for 1−2 minutes).

6 Wash with water and blot dry.

Results

Bacteria can be divided into two classes:

Gram-positive organisms retain the violet stain following treatment with acetone or ethanol and are a deep *violet*.

Gram-negative organisms lose the violet stain in the decolorization process, but take up the counterstain and are *pink*.

Gram-positive species vary in the tenacity with which they retain the violet stain and some may be largely decolorized. Moreover, in any culture of gram-positive species there are likely to be old or dead cells which are gram-negative. Since gram-negative bacteria do not give false positive reactions it is usually safe to assume that organisms giving a doubtful reaction are gram-positive.

In most species the individual cells stain more or less uniformly, but in some species, e.g. *Corynebacterium diphtheriae,* they tend to show alternate bands of light and dark. Bipolar staining, i.e. when a bacillus stains more intensely at the ends than in the middle, is fairly common but is especially marked in *Yersinia pestis* (Fig. 44A, p. 290).

Differential qualities

The gram reaction is one manifestation of fundamental differences in the properties of the species we recognize as gram-positive and gram-negative. Bearing in mind that the differences are sometimes of degree only and that there are important exceptions, it may be noted that: (1) the composition of their cell walls is different; (2) gram-positive organisms have less synthetic ability and so more complex nutritional requirements; (3) exotoxins are produced mainly by gram-positive organisms, whereas endotoxins are constituents of most gram-negative organisms; (4) gram-positive organisms are more resistant to mechanical damage; (5) the two groups show different spectra of susceptibility to chemotherapeutic agents, disinfectants, dyes, simple chemicals and enzymes.

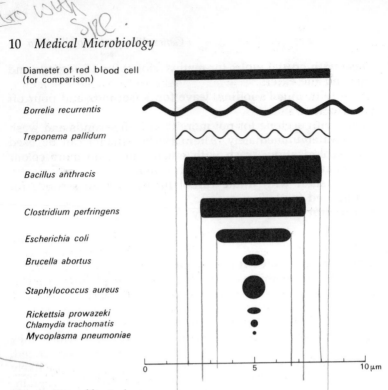

Fig. 1   Size of bacteria.

Value in identification

Most bacteria can usefully be divided into four categories depending on whether they are cocci or rod-shaped (including curved and spiral rods) and whether they are gram-positive or gram-negative. The reactions of different genera can be summarized as follows:

1 All cocci are gram-positive except for the genus *Neisseria* (and *Branhamella* and *Veillonella*).
2 All rod-shaped bacteria are gram-negative except for the genera *Bacillus, Clostridium, Corynebacterium* and *Mycobacterium* (and the less important genera *Lactobacillus, Actinomyces* and *Nocardia, Erysipelothrix* and *Listeria*).

Ziehl-Neelsen (ZN) stain for acid-fast bacilli

Organisms of the genus *Mycobacterium* are difficult to stain by Gram's method, but take up hot carbol fuchsin and hold it so firmly that they resist decolorization with strong mineral acids. A suitable method is as follows:

1 Cover the heat-fixed film with strong carbol fuchsin, heat with a flame until it steams (but not boils), and keep it steaming for 5–10 minutes, replenishing the stain if necessary.
2 Wash with water.
3 Flood with acid alcohol (3% HCl in 95% ethanol) and leave for 5–10 minutes (much longer does no harm).
4 Wash with water. If the film shows more than the faintest pink, decolorization (3) must be repeated.
5 Counterstain with Loeffler's methylene blue (or malachite green) for 15–30 seconds.
6 Wash with water and blot dry.

M. tuberculosis and other acid-fast bacilli show up as bright red rods. In a modification of the ZN method a fluorescent dye (auramine) is substituted for carbol fuchsin and the slide is illuminated by ultraviolet light. Large numbers of slides can be rapidly scanned for fluorescent bacilli using the lower powers of the microscope.

Other stains

Special methods are available for staining flagella, capsules, spores, spirochaetes and the metachromatic granules of *C. diphtheriae*; for identifying particular chemical compounds; for identifying antigens (fluorescent antibody techniques); and for staining bacteria in tissue sections.

Structure

Bacteria consist essentially of cell wall and protoplast, i.e. that part of the organism enclosed by the cell wall.

Protoplast

With few exceptions bacteria are stained deeply and evenly by basic dyes. Basophilia is due to large amounts of ribonucleic acid (RNA) which is distributed uniformly through the cytoplasm, mainly in the form of *ribosomes*, particulate structures concerned with protein synthesis. There is no obvious differentiation into cytoplasm and nucleus, but there is much evidence for the genetic control of metabolism by deoxyribonucleic acid (DNA), and using appropriate techniques nuclear structures can be seen microscopically.

Bacteria may contain cytoplasmic inclusions and the presence of these may be useful diagnostically, e.g. polymetaphosphate granules in corynebacteria are responsible for *metachromasia*.

Bounding the bacterial cytoplasm is the *cytoplasmic membrane*, a fine lipoprotein sheet which contains some of the cell's respiratory enzymes and is also responsible for much of the selective permeability of bacteria. Transport of many small molecular weight substances across the cytoplasmic membrane is actively facilitated by carrier proteins (permeases), and an outstanding feature of bacteria is their high internal concentration of osmotically active substances. Few direct measurements of internal osmotic pressure have been made, but values of about 5 atmospheres have been reported with *E. coli*, a gram-negative organism, and 20 atmospheres with *Staph. aureus*, which is gram-positive.

Cell wall

The cell wall accounts for up to 20% of the total dry weight of the cell and much of the cell's metabolic capabilities are devoted to its manufacture. It is a rigid structure which retains its shape in the face of drastic chemical and physical treatments.

Mucopeptides (also known as glycopeptides, peptidoglycans and mureins) form the most characteristic chemical component of the wall: they are complex polymers of amino sugars, cross-linked by peptide chains of relatively few specific amino acids. Not only are mucopeptides responsible for much of the strength of the wall, they are remarkable for the number of components, such as muramic acid, diaminopimelic acid and the D-isomers of glutamic acid, alanine and aspartic acid, which are unique to bacteria and related organisms, such as rickettsiae and chlamydiae. In some gram-positive bacteria the mucopeptide comprises almost all the wall substance, but in others there may be additional polysaccharides and teichoic acids (polyribitol or polyglycerol phosphates). Gram-negative bacteria have relatively little mucopeptide in their walls, and the main constituents are polysaccharides and lipoproteins.

The cell wall is freely permeable to a wide variety of solutes and it is generally considered to be metabolically inert. Its main function is a mechanical one, enabling the delicate cytoplasmic membrane to withstand the high internal osmotic pressure found in bacteria. The supporting action of the wall is clearly seen when the mucopeptide is destroyed by mucopolysaccharidases, e.g. lysozyme, or prevented from forming, e.g. by penicillin. In these circumstances the bacteria swell and burst; the turbid culture clears and is said to have *lysed*. By damaging or removing the wall in the presence of high concentrations of some material that does not penetrate the membrane easily, e.g. sucrose, it is possible to obtain osmotically sensitive spheres known as *spheroplasts*. If the structures are completely lacking in cell wall material they are

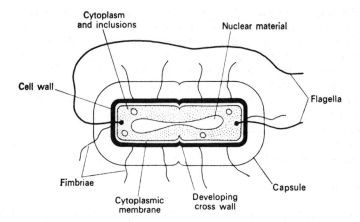

Fig. 2 Structure of a bacterial cell.

known as *protoplasts*. Spheroplasts, but not protoplasts, may regenerate cell walls and divide.

Other structures

Flagella

These are long, delicate, whip-like processes attached to the bacterial cell (Fig. 41B, p. 272; Fig. 43B, p. 287). They are too fine to be seen with the ordinary microscope. They are composed of protein. Some species do not possess flagella. Others may have a single flagellum or several flagella arising from the sides of the organism or from one or both ends.

Flagella are organs of motility. They were once thought to flail like whips but there is now evidence that they rotate, clockwise or anticlockwise. It is important to distinguish *true motility*, a progression of the bacterium relative to other organisms, from *Brownian movement*, a jerky movement due to molecular bombardment, and *streaming movements* of all bacteria in one direction due to currents in the fluid.

The chief motile bacteria include most varieties of *E. coli*, nearly all species of *Salmonella, Proteus, Pseudomonas, Vibrio* and *Campylobacter*, and some species of *Bacillus* and *Clostridium*. Spirochaetes and 'gliding bacteria' are also motile, but this is a function of the entire cell since they do not possess flagella.

The chief non-motile bacteria include all species of *Shigella, Brucella, Haemophilus* and *Mycobacterium*, nearly all species of *Corynebacterium*, and all cocci of medical importance. Organisms with obvious capsules do not produce flagella and are non-motile, e.g. *Klebsiella pneumoniae, Clostridium perfringens* and *Bacillus anthracis*. Non-motile variants of motile species are sometimes encountered.

Motile bacteria possess chemosensors and show positive and negative chemotaxis, i.e. they move towards some chemicals, mostly sugars and amino acids, and are repelled by others, mostly harmful substances and bacterial excretory products. In terms of their pathogenicity and power of invading the tissues, motile bacteria show no advantage over those which do not possess flagella.

Fimbriae (pili)

These are short, very thin, thread-like processes attached in large numbers to the cell walls of certain bacteria. They can be seen only with the electron microscope. Fimbriae are mostly found in gram-negative bacteria such as *E. coli, Shigella flexneri*, salmonellae and *Neisseria gonorrhoeae*.

Sex pili

These are highly specialized hair-like structures found in *E. coli* and related bacteria. They play an important role in the transfer of genetic material across the cell membrane in conjugation.

Capsules

Some bacteria are surrounded by a thick gelatinous layer outside the cell wall (Fig. 33C, p. 231; Fig. 41C, p. 272). Capsules of this type can be stained by special methods, but their presence in ordinary films can often be inferred from the appearance of a halo around each bacterium or by noting that the bodies of bacteria are kept apart from their neighbours.

Str. pneumoniae and *K. pneumoniae* form capsules in the tissues and in cultures. The capsular material is responsible for the mucoid colonies of these organisms. *B. anthracis, Cl. perfringens* and *Y. pestis* form obvious capsules in the tissues but not in ordinary cultures. Many species, including *Neisseria meningitidis, Streptococcus pyogenes, Bordetella pertussis* and *Haemophilus influenzae*, have very thin capsules. These can rarely be seen by ordinary microscopic methods and their presence is mainly inferred from chemical and immunological evidence that the organism is coated with certain antigens.

Spores

Some bacteria have the ability to pass into a highly resistant resting stage by the production of thick-walled spores. Spore formation is a characteristic feature of two genera: *Bacillus*, the spore-bearing aerobes, and *Clostridium*, the spore-bearing anaerobes (Fig. 35B, p. 246; Fig. 36, p. 248).

Sporulation depends on the depletion of some particular nutrient at a time when conditions for growth are otherwise favourable. It usually occurs in the later stages of an artificial culture. It does not occur in the tissues. An ingrowth of the cytoplasmic membrane cuts off a portion of the cell's cytoplasm and nuclear material, the spore primordium or *forespore*, which later develops a thick cortex and a tough spore coat. The mature spore is a round or oval body which stains with difficulty. It is at first contained in the cell, but finally the rest of the bacterium disintegrates and the spore is set free (Fig. 3).

Germination of the spore into a fresh vegetative cell occurs when the spore finds itself in a suitable warm, moist environment in which certain trigger nutrients are present. Each spore germinates into a single bacillus, so the process as a whole is not reproductive.

The most important property of spores is their extreme resistance to desiccation, heat and disinfectants and the fact that they can remain viable and a potential source of danger for long periods. The resistance of spores dictates the use of stringent methods of sterilization in medical practice and in the food industry.

Growth and multiplication

When a bacterium has grown to a critical size there is division of nuclear material, formation of a transverse septum which divides

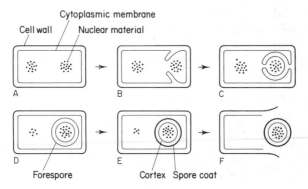

Fig. 3 Spore formation. A, Vegetative cell. B, Ingrowth of cytoplasmic membrane. C, Developing forespore. D, Forespore completely cut off in the cell cytoplasm. E, Development of cortex and spore coat. F, Liberation of spore.

the cytoplasm and finally ingrowth of the cell wall. The daughter cells may separate almost at once or may adhere in pairs, chains, clumps or filaments.

Growth phases

When a few quiescent organisms are introduced into a batch of liquid medium which meets their requirements for growth and multiplication the culture passes through four growth phases (Fig. 4):

1 *Lag phase.* During this period, which may last 1–4 hours, the cells do not multiply. There is a steady increase in cell size accompanied by great metabolic activity.
2 *Logarithmic phase.* In this period the cells multiply at maximum rate and the logarithm of the total number of cells increases linearly with time. Each species has a characteristic *mean generation time* which may vary from 20–30 minutes for rapidly growing species to as long as 24 hours for very slow growing species such as *M. tuberculosis.* After a few hours the log phase is brought to an end chiefly because of accumulation of end-products which inhibit growth. The final cell population is often 10^8 to 10^{10} organisms/ml. Cells in the log phase are younger, smaller, more active physiologically and more virulent than they are in other phases. They are also more susceptible to antibacterial agents such as penicillin.
3 *Stationary phase.* For several hours the small amount of multiplication which takes place is balanced by death of cells and the total population remains constant.

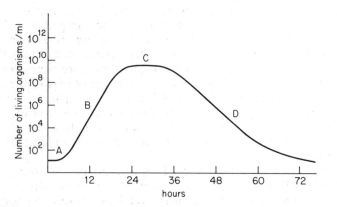

Fig. 4 Bacterial growth curve. A, Lag phase. B, Logarithmic phase. C, Stationary phase. D, Decline phase.

4 *Decline phase.* In this period there is progressive death of cells. After days or months the culture may become sterile.

Conditions for growth

Bacteria require water, inorganic salts, sources of carbon and nitrogen, growth factors in some cases, and a source of energy. They vary in their gaseous requirements. In addition their growth depends on the oxidation-reduction potential, the hydrogen ion concentration and the temperature.

Water

Desiccation kills bacteria, but in some circumstances they may survive for long periods in a state of suspended animation. A common method of preserving laboratory cultures is to dry the organisms *in vacuo* from the frozen state (freeze-drying or lyophilization) and store *in vacuo*.

Inorganic salts

These are required for osmotic regulation and to provide trace elements essential for certain enzyme systems. All bacteria require phosphate. Sulphate is essential if there is no other source of sulphur. Various metallic ions including Na, K, Mg, Ca, Fe, Mn, Zn, Cu, Co and Mo are also required.

Carbon, nitrogen, growth factors and energy

Bacteria show a wide spectrum of nutritional types. Two main groups can be distinguished, autotrophs and heterotrophs.

Autotrophs can live in an entirely inorganic environment. They are free-living organisms of no direct medical importance. They obtain carbon from carbon dioxide and nitrogen from ammonia, nitrites and nitrates. A few are *photosynthetic* and obtain their energy from light by means of a chlorophyll. Most are *chemosynthetic* and obtain their energy by oxidizing substances such as ammonia, nitrite, ferrous iron, sulphides, sulphur and hydrogen. Autotrophs have remarkable synthetic ability. On their simple diet they can manufacture all the complicated proteins, carbohydrates, lipids, nucleic acids, enzymes and coenzymes needed for growth and metabolism.

Heterotrophs require preformed organic matter for energy and synthesis. All bacteria of medical importance come into this category. At the bottom of the scale are heterotrophs with great synthetic ability and very simple nutritional requirements. Thus *E. coli* can obtain its nitrogen from ammonium salts but requires a complex source of carbon such as glucose. Most strains of *K. pneumoniae* can utilize citrate as a sole source of carbon. In general heterotrophs obtain their carbon, nitrogen and energy from organic compounds such as carbohydrates and amino acids. Many pathogenic species cannot synthesize certain key substances such as vitamins, purines and pyrimidines. These organisms will grow only when small amounts of such *growth factors* are supplied ready-made. At the top of the scale some of the more parasitic and pathogenic species require a highly complicated diet. Thus some streptococci require 17 amino acids, nine B vitamins, the purines adenine and guanine, the pyrimidines cytosine, thymine and uracil, and a carbohydrate for energy.

Gaseous requirements

Carbon dioxide. All bacteria require CO_2 for metabolism, but often it can be generated in sufficient amount by the culture itself. *Brucella abortus* and *Capnocytophaga ochracea* require much more than they find in air and 5−10% CO_2 is used for primary isolation. Growth of nearly all organisms, especially *N. gonorrhoeae*, *N. meningitidis*, streptococci, *Campylobacter jejuni* and *Bacteroides*, is improved by the presence of additional CO_2.

Oxygen. Bacteria can be classified into three groups on their oxygen requirements:

1 *Strict or obligate aerobes* will grow only in the *presence* of oxygen, e.g. *M. tuberculosis* and *Pseudomonas aeruginosa.*
2 *Anaerobes* will grow only in the *absence* of oxygen or, if oxygen is present, only if the environment has a sufficiently *low* oxidation-reduction potential, i.e. an environment with strong reducing powers. Anaerobes include nearly all species of *Clostridium,* anaerobic streptococci and anaerobic staphylococci, the genus *Veillonella,* the *Bacteroides* group, and some lacto-bacilli, diphtheroids (*Propionibacterium acnes*) and spirochaetes.
3 *Facultative anaerobes* will grow under either aerobic or anaerobic conditions. Nearly all organisms of medical importance, except those mentioned in 1 and 2, come into this category.

In practice there is a spectrum of microbial sensitivity to oxygen with tolerance ranging from *microaerophilic organisms,* such as *Campylobacter jejuni, A. israeli,* some strains of streptococci and most mycoplasmas, which grow best at reduced oxygen tensions to some strict anaerobes which are killed by exposure to oxygen. Extreme sensitivity to oxygen is associated with a lack of superoxide dis-mutase. This enzyme removes the highly toxic superoxide free radical which is formed by metalloflavoproteins in the presence of oxygen. Oxygen at pressures greater than atmospheric (*hyperbaric oxygen*) has been used in the treatment of anaerobic infections, notably gas gangrene.

Nitrogen. Gaseous nitrogen is not required by bacteria of medical importance. Nitrogen-fixing bacteria are important in agriculture.

Oxidation-reduction (redox) potential

A low redox potential in cultures or in the tissues is the fundamental condition required for the germination of spores of the genus *Clostridium* and for the growth of anaerobes generally. Absence of molecular oxygen is an important factor in producing a low redox potential.

Hydrogen ion concentration

Most bacteria of medical importance grow best at a neutral or slightly alkaline reaction (pH 7.2–7.6). Growth is usually poor below pH 6.0 or above pH 7.8 and ceases below pH 5.0 or above pH 9.0. Notable exceptions are *Vibrio cholerae* which grows best in a strongly alkaline solution (pH 8.0–9.0) and *Lactobacillus acidophilus* which flourishes in a highly acid environment (pH 4.0).

Temperature

Bacteria pathogenic for man usually grow best at body temperature, 37°C. The optimum growth temperature is occasionally higher, e.g. *Campylobacter jejuni* (43°C) and *Mycobacterium avium* (40°C), or lower, e.g. *Yersinia pestis* (30°C) and *Mycobacterium ulcerans* (32°C). Many pathogens will multiply over a range of 20–43°C, but some species such as *N. gonorrhoeae* will grow only in a narrow range around 37°C. The optimum temperature for most saprophytes is lower, usually 20–30°C. A few species such as *Ps. aeruginosa* will multiply at or near refrigerator temperature (4°C) and have been known to contaminate stored blood.

Organisms encountered in medical bacteriology are *mesophilic* in their temperature requirements. Some *psychrophilic* (cold-loving) species found in fish, brine and soil will multiply at 0°C or even lower and some *thermophilic* species found in hot springs and manure heaps will multiply at temperatures as high as 55–80°C. In hydrothermal vents where water is under great pressure certain species can grow at temperatures above 100°C!

Metabolism

The main metabolic pathways utilized by bacteria are the same as those utilized by other forms of life. As a group, however, bacteria have explored the metabolic side paths with extraordinary success and the range of substrates they can utilize and the types of end-products they produce show great diversity. The rate at which bacteria accomplish their metabolic processes is unusually rapid. This is mainly because their large surface area relative to their volume facilitates the exchange of nutrients and end-products.

Carbohydrates are a major source of energy for bacteria of medical importance. Some, such as streptococci and lactobacilli, break down glucose by glycolysis to produce lactate as the main end-product (homofermentative types). Others produce varying amounts of other end-products (heterofermentative types). Many bacteria can carry out the intermediate reactions of the tricarboxylic acid cycle and various reactions with pyruvate and two-carbon fragments. These reactions serve synthetic as well as catabolic processes and act as a bridge between carbohydrate metabolism and the metabolism of protein and fatty acids.

The degree to which a substrate such as glucose is utilized varies. In *aerobic respiration* the hydrogen derived from oxidative processes is finally transferred to molecular oxygen by means of the cytochrome systems. Glucose is completely broken down to carbon dioxide and water and maximum energy is liberated. In *fermentation* the hydrogen is transferred to other hydrogen acceptors or is liberated as hydrogen gas. Breakdown proceeds to an intermediate compound and a relatively small proportion of the total energy is liberated. Depending on their use of these two types of oxidation bacteria fall into three broad groups:

1 Obligate aerobes possess cytochromes and carry out aerobic respiration.
2 Streptococci, lactobacilli and, with rare exceptions, obligate anaerobes do not have cytochromes and can only carry out fermentations.
3 The great majority of organisms have cytochrome systems which they can use when oxygen is available, but adopt a fermentative process when oxygen is limited or absent.

Bacteriocins (colicins, pyocins, etc.)

Many bacteria produce bacteriocins, complex bactericidal substances active against related bacteria. All bacteriocins contain protein. Susceptible organisms may belong to the same or to a closely related genus. Thus *E. coli* and other intestinal bacilli produce colicins active against other coliform organisms. Colicins adsorb to receptors on the bacterial surface. The pattern of sensitivity to various colicins is characteristic for a particular strain. The specificity of colicin action resembles that of phages, and some colicins may in fact be defective phages that can kill bacteria but not grow in them. Colicin-typing is used in epidemiological studies to identify strains of *Shigella sonnei* and *E. coli.* Pyocins are used for typing *Ps. aeruginosa.*

Rickettsiae and chlamydiae

The rickettsiae, a group of organisms which cause typhus fever and related diseases, and the chlamydiae, which cause trachoma, inclusion conjunctivitis, genital infection, lymphogranuloma venereum and psittacosis, are *obligate intracellular bacteria.* Thus the composition of their cell walls, possession of both DNA and RNA, sensitivity to chemotherapeutic agents and multiplication by binary fission are all typical of ordinary bacteria. Like other bacteria they possess their own enzyme systems, but these are not sufficiently comprehensive to give them an entirely independent metabolism.

L-forms

Some bacteria can change into minute living organisms of spherical or indefinite shape, barely visible with the ordinary microscope but capable of growth on artifical media. These L-forms (L for Lister Institute) arise spontaneously in cultures of *Streptobacillus moniliformis* and can be induced in other species of bacteria by various agents including penicillin. They differ from normal bacteria in their failure to synthesize cell wall. In certain circumstances L-forms may revert to the normal bacterial form. There is no clear distinction between L-forms and spheroplasts (p. 12).

The importance of L-forms in human infections is uncertain. L-forms are resistant to penicillin although their parent forms may be sensitive. It is possible that L-forms could develop during therapy with drugs such as penicillin, which interfere with normal cell wall formation, and then revert to bacteria when therapy is discontinued.

Bacterial genetics and variation

The properties of a living organism are determined by its ability to carry out certain metabolic reactions which in turn depend on its capacity to synthesize certain enzymes. These characteristics are ultimately controlled by the genetic material of the cell, i.e. DNA. In a bacterium such as *E. coli* the DNA is in the form of a single circular chromosome, a giant thread-like molecule consisting of two polynucleotide chains wound around a common long axis to form a double-stranded helix. The chromosome normally forms a closed loop about 1 mm in circumference and is intricately folded to fit into the nuclear region of the cell. Along the length of the chromosome various segments of the DNA represent individual genes. There are some 3000–6000 genes in *E. coli*. The location of many of the genes on the chromosome has been determined and chromosome maps have been prepared. The genetic information in the chromosome depends on the sequence of the four DNA nucleotide bases: adenine, guanine, thymine and cytosine. These are arranged in pairs along the double helix like rungs in a twisted rope ladder. Adenine on one chain pairs with thymine on the other chain; similarly, guanine pairs with cytosine. The full sequence of 4700 kilobases which make up the genome of *E. coli* is known.

The translation of this information into the manufacture of enzymes depends on a triplet code, each individual amino acid being coded for by a sequence of three pairs of nucleotide bases on the double helix. The triplet code corresponding to each of the twenty amino acids which normally make up protein is known. All living creatures use the same code except for certain ciliates, e.g. *Paramecium*, in which the code is very slightly different. The sequence of these base triplets in the chain determines the sequence of amino acids in a particular polypeptide chain. In the translation of the genetic code into proteins the base sequence of the DNA is first transcribed into a complementary sequence of bases in messenger RNA (mRNA). The newly synthesized mRNA migrates to the ribosomes where it serves as a template for the assembly of amino acids into polypeptide chains. This is not a direct process but is accomplished through intermediate molecules of transfer RNA (tRNA) which possess a sequence of bases complementary to those of the mRNA. There are specific tRNA molecules for each amino acid.

Bacteria usually breed true, i.e. in the process of reproduction there is replication of the DNA and an identical set of genes is passed on to each daughter cell. However, the rate of bacterial reproduction is so rapid and bacterial populations are so vast that changes in properties (variations) are readily detected. The properties of a bacterium at a particular time (its *phenotype*) depend on its genetic constitution (its *genotype*) and environmental factors. Variations are therefore of two types.

Genotypic variation

This is a heritable variation due to changes in genetic constitution. Completely new properties may arise by mutation, but in addition bacteria can acquire new heritable properties by transfer from other organisms.

Mutation

The progeny of a single bacterial cell are not genetically homogeneous but contain a definite proportion of cells which differ from the parent in some heritable property. If 10^8 *E. coli* all derived from a single colony are spread on a plate of nutrient medium containing streptomycin it might be found that 10 colonies develop. Subcultures from these colonies would all be capable of growing on streptomycin medium. In other words, 1 in 10^7 of the *E. coli* are variants resistant to streptomycin. Variants of this kind are spontaneous mutants and the environment is important only in that it favours or *selects* the mutants. In ordinary circumstances a streptomycin-resistant mutant has no advantage over the rest of the organisms, so its presence is overshadowed and it remains undetected. In the presence of streptomycin the new property greatly enhances the fitness of the organism to survive and multiply. In time the mutant strain would probably replace the parent.

The mutation rate varies with different properties and different bacteria, but it is commonly between 1 in 10^7 and 1 in 10^{10}. These rates are for a single property. The total number of mutants, involving a variety of properties, is far greater. Mutagenic agents, such as X-rays, ultraviolet light and alkylating agents, cause a general increase in the rates of mutation. Every mutation is due to a change in the structure of a gene. In chemical terms this means an alteration in the base sequence of the DNA double helix. This may be due to substitution of one base pair for another, deletion of bases or insertion of new bases.

Smooth-rough (S→R) variation is one of the most obvious and important types of mutation shown by pathogenic bacteria. The variation involves a change of colonial appearance from smooth to rough, a loss of surface components (somatic and capsular antigens) and a loss or diminution of virulence. It commonly occurs when bacteria are grown for long periods on artificial media. The variation can often be reversed by passaging the culture through susceptible animals. S→R variation is best shown by salmonellae, shigellae and pneumococci, but analogous changes

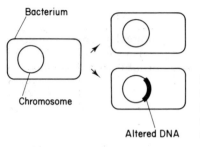

Bacterium

Chromosome

Altered DNA

Fig. 5   Mutation. The DNA
of the bacterial chromosome
undergoes a change in base
sequence during the course
of cell division.

occur in most genera, although the colonial changes are not always
so obvious.

Other types of mutations may involve morphology (size of cell,
ability to form spores, capsules and flagella), colonial appearance
(size, shape, pigmentation), biochemical activity (nutritional
requirements, fermentative power, enzymic activity), antigenic
properties (flagellar variation, loss of antigens), ability to produce
toxins, sensitivity to phage and drug sensitivity.

Chemicals that are carcinogenic for man damage DNA and are
mutagenic for bacteria. Bacterial mutagenicity tests therefore
provide a rapid method of screening for carcinogens. Thus if
mutants of *Salmonella typhimurium* that have lost the ability to
synthesize histidine are exposed to mutagens they undergo additional mutations that can have the effect of repairing the original
defect. These back mutations can be detected by the ability of the
bacteria to grow on a histidine-free medium.

Extrachromosomal inheritance and conjugation

Many bacteria possess genetic elements that replicate and function
independently of the main chromosome. These extrachromosomal
genetic elements, known as *plasmids*, have been extensively studied
in *E. coli* and *Staph. aureus*. They consist of closed circular molecules of double-stranded DNA, commonly 1–2% of the size of
the chromosome. They range in size from 2 kilobases (i.e. 2000
nucleotide bases) with a circumference of 0.7 μm to over 300
kilobases with a circumference of 100 μm (1 kb corresponds to a
molecular weight of about 1.5 Mdaltons). The information they
carry is often in the form of transposable genetic elements or
transposons ('jumping genes'). These are segments of DNA, usually
containing several genes, which have the property of being readily
transferable into the DNA of bacterial chromosomes, plasmids
and infecting phages. Genetic recombination resulting from the
transfer of transposon DNA can occur in conjugation, transformation and transduction. Plasmids may be lost by cells during

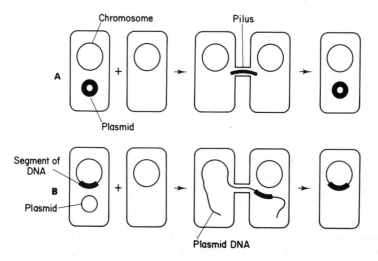

Fig. 6 Conjugation. A, The DNA of a plasmid (e.g. a drug-resistance plasmid) is transferred through a pilus to another bacterium and becomes a plasmid in the new host. B, The plasmid (e.g. a fertility plasmid) attaches itself to the bacterial chromosome and allows transfer of chromosomal DNA into the chromosome of another bacterium. The plasmid itself may or may not be transferred.

growth so that some genetic properties of the cells may be unstable characters. Plasmids fall into two classes: those that are transmissible by cellular conjugation and those that are not.

Transmissible plasmids occur in *E. coli* and other intestinal bacilli and their activity results in the formation of fine, hair-like projections (sex pili) from the cell surface. These pili provide the route by which plasmid DNA is passed from one cell to another during conjugation, i.e. the process resembles sexual reproduction. Transmissible plasmids are generally classified according to the property by which they were first recognized, e.g. fertility (F) plasmids, colicinogenic (Col) plasmids and the drug-resistance transfer (R) plasmids. However, there is little essential difference between them: genes responsible for pilus formation are common to members of the different classes and it is often found that one plasmid also has the properties of another.

Fertility plasmids were originally discovered in *E. coli* strain K12. When a culture of this organism possessing the plasmid (F^+ cells) was mixed with an F^- culture, cells of the latter rapidly acquired the F^+ property. A very small number also gained genetic characteristics that were carried by the chromosomes of the F^+ cells. It is now known that in a few F^+ organisms the fertility plasmid attaches to the main chromosome of the cell and thereby facilitates the unidirectional transfer of chromosomal genes to the recipient cell when recombination occurs.

Colicinogenic plasmids possess genes that determine the production of some colicins and frequently the transmission of colicinogeny to other cells. Under certain conditions Col plasmids also behave as fertility plasmids.

Drug-resistance transfer plasmids carry genes that enable the cell to grow in the presence of one or more antibacterial drugs. By conjugation with drug-sensitive organisms, the resistance properties of one type of cell can be spread rapidly through a population of sensitive bacteria. Experiments have shown that drug-resistance transfer occurs in natural populations such as the coliform organisms in the intestinal contents.

Other plasmids carry genes which enable the organism to ferment sugars, resist the bactericidal action of serum, produce toxins or surface antigens and adhere to the surface of animal cells.

Non-transmissible plasmids are found in many organisms including *Staph. aureus* where they account for resistance to antibacterial drugs, and in *E. coli* where some R plasmids and Col plasmids are non-transmissible by conjugation. Although direct transmission of these plasmids from cell to cell is not possible, transfer of their genes to another cell can often be effected by a transducing phage.

Not all antibacterial drug-resistance properties of cells can be attributed to genes carried by plasmids. Drug-resistance genes may also be chromosomally determined, in which case transfer, if it occurs at all, is mediated by a transducing phage or by F^+ plasmid-facilitated chromosome transfer.

Transformation

With a number of species it is possible to transfer properties to an organism by means of purified DNA obtained from another culture of the same bacterium. The DNA of the donor strain is incorporated in the recipient strain where it functions genetically. Thus rough (R) non-capsulated pneumococci of one antigenic type can be transformed into smooth (S) capsulated strains of a different antigenic type by means of DNA of the desired S type. Transformation of pneumococci was first described by Griffith in 1928 though at the time the mechanism was a complete mystery. Drug resistance and other properties can also be transferred by means of free DNA. Reciprocal transformation can also be affected between pneumococci and some strains of streptococci.

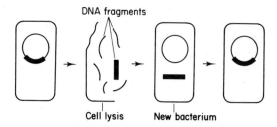

Fig. 7 Transformation. The DNA of the bacterial chromosome is liberated by cell lysis and a particular fragment is taken up by a new bacterium and incorporated in its chromosome.

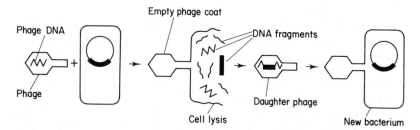

Fig. 8 Transduction. A phage infects a bacterium and a daughter phage picks up a fragment of bacterial chromosomal DNA and transfers it to a new bacterium.

Transduction

This occurs when a phage incorporates part of the genetic material of a host bacterium and carries it to another bacterium. Thus resistance to various antibiotics can be transduced in certain sensitive strains of *Staph. aureus*. Certain antigenic and biochemical properties can be transduced between closely related strains of salmonellae.

Recombinant-DNA techniques (genetic engineering)

It is convenient to group together various techniques by which molecular biologists bring about genetic changes in bacteria. Such changes could not happen naturally. In principle it is possible to take a gene, i.e. a length of DNA, from a bacterium, virus or animal cell and introduce it into the genetic apparatus of a living bacterium where it will replicate and instruct the cell to produce a specific protein. In practice subtle and complicated manipulations

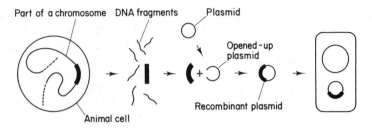

Fig. 9 Recombinant-DNA techniques. A series of enzymes has been used to split the DNA from an animal cell into fragments and insert the required fragment into a plasmid. The plasmid has then been introduced into a bacterium.

are required to select, or synthesize from mRNA, the desired DNA sequence together with the necessary regulatory signals for transcription and translation. It is also essential to introduce the DNA into the bacterium in some way that will ensure that it can be replicated, that its structural sequence is expressed as protein and that the protein is produced in useful amounts. The new bacteria are known as *recombinants* and the methods used to create them are referred to collectively as *recombinant-DNA techniques* or simply as *cloning*.

Potential applications of recombinant-DNA techniques are almost limitless. Achievements of medical interest include the design and creation of novel strains of *E. coli* capable of manufacturing such non-bacterial proteins as the envelope antigen of hepatitis B virus, the haemagglutinin of influenza virus, growth hormone, insulin, interferon and the blood-clotting protein, factor VIII. It is also possible to produce reagents (DNA probes) which can be used to detect the nucleic acid of specific pathogens in clinical specimens.

Phenotypic variation

This is a non-heritable variation representing a temporary adjustment to the environment, and normally involves the cell population as a whole.

Organisms show variations of size, shape, staining reactions, metabolism and susceptibility to drugs at different phases of their growth cycle. Different media may affect morphology and colonial appearances or inhibit formation of structures such as flagella and spores. The environment may affect biochemical properties. *Staph. aureus* makes its golden pigment most abundantly at room temperature. *C. diphtheriae* produces toxin in response to deprivation of iron. Organisms produce certain *inducible* enzymes only when they are exposed to the specific substrate, e.g. penicillinase (β-lactamase) induction occurs when certain strains of *Staph. aureus* are exposed to penicillin. Conversely, organisms may fail to synthesize certain enzymes on a biosynthetic pathway when the end-product of that pathway is present in the culture medium (*enzyme repression*). In all these examples reversion to the normal type occurs as soon as the environmental stimulus is removed.

DNA probes

A DNA probe is a fragment of single-stranded DNA that can hybridize with other pieces of single-stranded DNA (or the corresponding RNA) which possess identical complementary nucleotide sequences. Because all microbes have some unique sequences it is possible to prepare probes for detecting virtually any microbe.

Preparing a probe is usually a long and tedious process. In outline, an appropriate segment of the organism's DNA (the future probe) is removed from the rest of the DNA by means of restriction endonucleases and is inserted into a plasmid. The plasmid is introduced into a strain of *E. coli* which produces multiple copies of the plasmid from which large quantities of the probe can be separated. The probe is labelled with a radioactive isotope or an enzyme and is then denatured to produce single-stranded DNA. Probes are usually obtained from commercial sources or research laboratories.

Once a probe is available, hybridization reactions are simple to perform in ordinary clinical laboratories. Samples of the specimens to be tested are commonly dotted on a nitrocellulose filter ('dot-blot' hybridization). In the 'Southern blot' technique separated DNA fragments from a restriction enzyme digest are transferred to the filter from a gel. The filter is treated to denature the DNA to single strands and the labelled probe is added to initiate the hybridization reaction. After washing to remove excess probe, the filter is tested for evidence of probe binding. Radioactive probes can be detected by autoradiography. Non-radioactive probes such as those labelled with biotin offer many advantages. The protein avidin has a high affinity for biotin and biotin-labelled probes can be readily detected by exposing the filter to avidin coupled to a suitable enzyme. On addition of a chromogenic substrate a colour change is produced.

DNA probes are being increasingly used to supplement or replace traditional methods of diagnosing infection based on isolation of organisms and detection of specific antigens and antibodies. Probe techniques are often cheaper, simpler and more reliable.

Bacteria and cancer

It has been suggested that bacteria play a role in the aetiology of some forms of cancer. For instance, patients who have undergone partial gastrectomy have an increased incidence of gastric cancer. In these patients the stomach is colonized by bacteria which can convert ingested nitrates, nitrites and secondary amines into highly carcinogenic nitrosamines. The incidence of cancer of the large bowel is high in countries such as the UK and the USA and low in parts of Africa and India. These differences may be related to dietary habits which influence the composition of the intestinal flora. Among the metabolic activities of some intestinal bacteria is the degradation of bile salts with the production of carcinogens.

General Properties of Viruses

A virus is bad news wrapped in protein.
P. B. Medawar

Viruses are small infective agents which can grow and reproduce only in living cells. Although some of the smallest viruses consist of little more than nucleic acid and a protein coat, show no independent metabolism and may even be obtainable in crystalline form, for all practical purposes viruses behave as living organisms. They have the power to enter specific living cells within which they multiply and cause signs of disease. Later they escape from the cell and are transmitted to fresh cells which they infect. Viruses are antigenic and in intact animal hosts the production of specific antibodies is closely correlated with the development of immunity. Finally, viruses frequently show mutations or variations of their biological properties of a sort shown by other living organisms.

Classification and nomenclature

The Linnaean (binomial) system of nomenclature has so far not proved satisfactory for the classification of viruses and in the main each virus is named according to the disease for which it is responsible. All viruses contain nucleic acid and it has been shown that the type of nucleic acid is characteristic for particular viruses. It can be deoxyribonucleic acid (DNA) or ribonucleic acid (RNA). Viruses that have been adequately studied can therefore be assigned to one or other of two fundamental classes: DNA viruses and RNA viruses. Within these two classes certain broad groups of viruses are recognized, mainly on the basis of their morphology and structure.

DNA viruses

Poxviruses: smallpox (variola), vaccinia and various animal poxviruses; molluscum contagiosum virus.
   Herpesviruses: herpes simplex virus, B virus, pseudorabies virus, Epstein-Barr virus; varicella-zoster virus; cytomegalovirus.

Adenoviruses: viruses causing respiratory diseases and conjunctivitis.

Papovaviruses: human papillomavirus; animal viruses including papilloma, polyoma and vacuolating viruses.

Parvoviruses: human parvovirus (B19); adeno-associated viruses.

Other viruses: hepatitis B virus.

RNA viruses

Picornaviruses: polio, coxsackie, echo, hepatitis A and other enteroviruses; rhinoviruses; encephalomyocarditis viruses; foot-and-mouth disease virus.

Reoviruses: viruses causing mild respiratory and intestinal diseases.

Orbiviruses: arboviruses (arthropod-borne viruses), e.g. Colorado tick fever virus.

Rotaviruses: viruses causing infantile gastroenteritis.

Orthomyxoviruses: influenza viruses; swine influenza virus.

Paramyxoviruses: parainfluenza, mumps and Newcastle disease viruses; measles virus; respiratory syncytial virus.

Togaviruses: arboviruses causing encephalitis, e.g. western equine encephalitis, and tropical fevers, e.g. yellow fever; rubella virus.

Bunyaviruses: arboviruses, e.g. Bunyamwera and California subgroups of viruses; sandfly fever, Rift Valley fever, Crimean (Congo) haemorrhagic fever and hantaviruses.

Rhabdoviruses: rabies virus and vesicular stomatitis virus.

Coronaviruses: viruses causing cold-like illnesses.

Arenaviruses: lymphocytic choriomeningitis virus, Lassa fever virus, Junin virus, Machupo virus.

Retroviruses: human immunodeficiency viruses; human T-cell lymphotropic viruses; animal tumour viruses.

Other viruses: Marburg and Ebola viruses.

Miscellaneous viruses

Presumed viral agents ('slow viruses') causing kuru and similar conditions; other viruses infecting man, animals, insects, plants and bacteria (bacteriophages).

Size

The size of most viruses has now been determined. Three main methods have been used: (1) filtration through membrane filters of known pore size ('ultrafiltration'); (2) determination of the sedimentation rate in the ultracentrifuge; (3) direct measurement by electron microscopy.

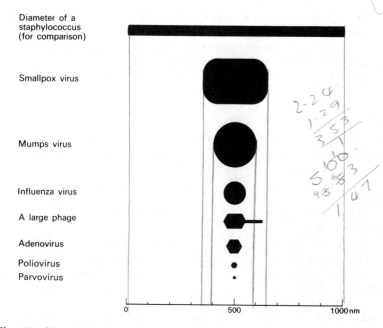

Diameter of a
staphylococcus
(for comparison)

Smallpox virus

Mumps virus

Influenza virus

A large phage

Adenovirus

Poliovirus
Parvovirus

0   500   1000nm

Fig. 10 Size of viruses.

The dimensions found for a virus depend to some extent on the method of measurement. The unit of measurement is the nanometre or nm (1 nm = 10^{-9} m). As a rough guide very small viruses such as polio, coxsackie, and echoviruses have a diameter of 20–30 nm; medium-sized viruses such as adenovirus, influenza and measles are 75–150 nm; large viruses such as variola and vaccinia are 200–300 nm. These figures can be compared with the measurements of chlamydiae and rickettsiae (300–500 nm) and staphylococci (1000 nm).

Shape and structure

Much of our information is derived from the use of the electron microscope. Contrast can be improved by *shadow-casting,* in which atoms of a heavy metal such as gold or chromium are allowed to fall on the specimen at an oblique angle. The best way of revealing fine detail is to use *negative staining,* in which the particles are surrounded by an electron-dense material such as potassium phosphotungstate. For study of viruses in tissues the material is usually fixed in glutaraldehyde and mounted in methacrylate plastic. Ultra-thin (20–50 nm) sections are cut with special knives. Interpretation of electron micrographs is not easy since the virus is examined in a high vacuum and is thereby completely dehydrated and liable to be flattened and distorted.

The fine structure of a virus is beyond the range of the electron microscope and most viruses appear as simple fuzzy balls. By computer analysis of X-ray diffraction patterns of crystallized samples of virus it is possible to work out viral structure in atomic detail. In 1985 a cold virus (human rhinovirus 14) and poliovirus became the first animal viruses to have their precise three-dimensional shape determined.

Most animal viruses are roughly spherical, but careful analysis has shown that many of them are in fact regular polyhedra. Influenza virus may take the form of filaments. Enveloped viruses tend to be amorphous. Typical poxviruses such as variola and vaccinia are shaped like bricks with rounded corners (Fig. 12C) but certain others such as the viruses of orf and milker's nodes are oval structures (Fig. 49, p. 329). Rhabdoviruses such as rabies virus are bullet-shaped (Fig. 51, p. 358). Bacterial viruses (bacteriophages) are commonly tadpole-shaped with a polyhedral head and a straight tail (Fig. 55, p. 372).

In animal viruses each infective particle or *virion* (Fig. 11) consists of a *nucleocapsid*, i.e. a nucleic acid *core* surrounded by a protein shell or *capsid*. In addition, the infectivity of some viruses is dependent upon the nucleocapsid being enclosed within a lipoprotein *envelope*.

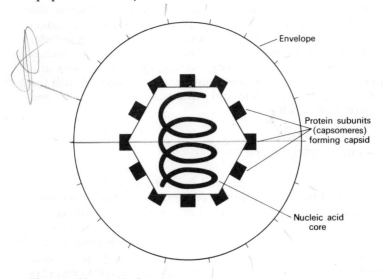

Envelope

Protein subunits (capsomeres) forming capsid

Nucleic acid core

Fig. 11 Structure of a virion.

Nucleocapsid

The surface of the capsid is formed by protein subunits or *capsomeres* arranged symmetrically with regard to each other. According to the way the capsomeres are arranged the capsid itself has one of two symmetrical forms.

Icosahedral symmetry (Fig. 12A). The capsomeres are so arranged that the capsid has the symmetrical properties of an icosahedron, a regular solid with 20 faces in which each face is an equilateral triangle. The precise geometric structure permits the close packing of virions in a regular manner so that a viral 'crystal' may form within an infected cell or in a concentrated suspension of the virus *in vitro*. Icosahedral symmetry is found in herpesviruses, adenoviruses, papovaviruses, parvoviruses, picornaviruses, reoviruses and togaviruses.

Helical symmetry (Fig. 12B). An alternative capsid structure permitting the protein subunits a similar spatial relationship to each other is a helical arrangement of capsomeres. The nucleic acid chain follows the helix. This is possible only with highly flexible single-stranded molecules. Thus orthomyxoviruses, paramyxoviruses, bunyaviruses, rhabdoviruses and retroviruses which have this capsid structure all possess single-stranded RNA.

Envelope

In some viruses the nucleocapsid has an envelope. During intracellular growth of enveloped viruses virus-specific proteins are inserted into the lipoprotein membranes of the host cell. Nucleocapsids migrate to the modified membrane which evaginates so that the mature virion is eventually released from the cell by budding. Animal viruses possessing envelopes include

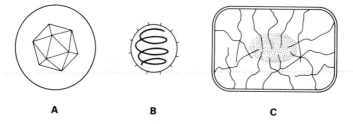

A **B** **C**

Fig. 12 Symmetry of viral capsid. A, Icosahedral symmetry (herpes simplex virus). B, Helical symmetry (influenza virus). C, Complex symmetry (vaccinia virus).

poxviruses, herpesviruses, orthomyxoviruses, paramyxoviruses, togaviruses, bunyaviruses, rhabdoviruses, coronaviruses, arenaviruses and retroviruses. The infectivity of enveloped viruses is destroyed by fat solvents, e.g. ether.

Complex viruses

Some viruses, in particular the poxviruses, have a more complex structure and do not fit into the scheme outlined above. Thus in vaccinia virus the region between the core and the envelope contains a complex arrangement of membranes and tube-like structures (Fig. 12C, p. 35).

Chemical composition

All viruses contain protein and nucleic acid. Nearly all viruses known to infect man can be classified as either DNA or RNA viruses but there is still uncertainty about a few of them. Most phages are DNA viruses.

The nucleic acid of a virus can be single-stranded or double-stranded. Double-stranded DNA is found in all DNA viruses except parvoviruses which have single-stranded DNA. Single-stranded RNA is found in all RNA viruses except reoviruses, orbiviruses and rotaviruses which have double-stranded RNA. The nucleic acid of DNA viruses consists of a single, giant thread-like molecule. In RNA viruses the nucleic acid may consist of a single molecule, e.g. picornaviruses, or several separate segments of RNA, e.g. orthomyxoviruses. The size of the nucleic acid molecules determines the number of genes carried by a virus, e.g. the RNA of poliovirus has a molecular weight of 2.6×10^6 corresponding to about 5 genes; the DNA of vaccinia virus has a molecular weight of 160×10^6 corresponding to about 160 genes. With some viruses the base sequence of the viral nucleic acid has been worked out in detail by restriction endonuclease mapping, e.g. the full sequence of 250 kilobases which make up Epstein-Barr virus DNA is known.

The chemical complexity of viruses varies with their size. Very small viruses such as the picornaviruses probably contain protein and nucleic acid as their sole constituents; enveloped viruses such as influenza virus contain not only protein and RNA but also protein, lipid and carbohydrate derived from the envelope; vaccinia virus contains protein, DNA, lipids, neutral fat, carbohydrate, and may contain various smaller molecules such as biotin, riboflavin and flavin adenine dinucleotide, although it is possible that these are contaminants from the host cells.

As a rule, purified viruses are devoid of enzymes, an exception being the neuraminidase present in the envelope of ortho-myxoviruses and some paramyxoviruses. Other important exceptions occur in those *negative strand* RNA viruses (orthomyxovirus, paramyxoviruses, bunyaviruses and rhabdoviruses) in which the RNA is unable to function directly as messenger RNA (mRNA). The virions of these viruses contain a transcriptase enzyme, an RNA-dependent RNA polymerase, or in the case of retroviruses, a reverse transcriptase which forms virus-specific DNA from which mRNA can be transcribed. Catalase, phosphatase and lipase activity has so far been inseparable from preparations of vaccinia virus.

Entry into host cells

The essential component of a virus is its nucleic acid. The sur-rounding coat of protein and sometimes other materials can be regarded as a mechanism to protect the nucleic acid and facilitate its attachment to and entry into a new host cell. With certain viruses such as polio and some togaviruses it is possible to obtain protein-free nucleic acid preparations which by themselves are capable of infecting cells. In the case of phage the DNA in the head of the phage is injected into the bacterium but the protein components remain outside.

The outer structures of the virion enable it to attach to specific receptors on the host cell wall. Thus influenza and allied viruses attach themselves to mucoprotein receptors. These are then destroyed by a viral enzyme (neuraminidase) and in the process the virus is released and passes into the cell. Viruses gain entry into the cell by endocytosis (pinocytosis), the mechanism by which large molecules normally enter. The virus enters a small pit on the surface of the cell, the pit is pinched off to form a vesicle and the vesicle carries the virus into the interior of the cell. Here the vesicles fuse with vacuoles known as endosomes which in turn fuse with enzyme-containing vacuoles known as lysosomes. Finally, the viral nucleic acid escapes from the lysosomes into the cytoplasm.

Metabolism

Viruses differ fundamentally from all other forms of life. Extracellular viral particles are completely inert, but when they infect living cells the viral nucleic acid replicates and directs the synthesis of enzymes and structural viral proteins using the metabolic machinery of the host cell.

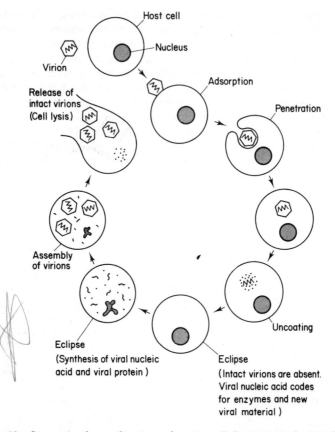

Fig. 13   Stages in the replication of a virus. Poliovirus is depicted here. The cycle varies slightly with different classes of virus, e.g. enveloped viruses are released by budding through the cell membrane and not by cell lysis.

Reproduction

Viruses will grow and reproduce only in living cells, i.e. they are obligatory intracellular parasites. After a virus has entered a cell it becomes increasingly difficult to detect infective virus. During this *eclipse phase* the virus is present as smaller non-infective subunits which multiply inside the cell. The subunits are later reassembled to form new complete viruses. The separate antigenic components of some viruses are synthesized independently in separate parts of the cell, some in the nucleus and some in the cytoplasm, e.g. in herpesviruses the viral DNA is replicated in the nucleus, viral proteins are synthesized in the cytoplasm and assembly occurs within the nucleus. In cells infected simultaneously with two very similar but distinct viruses it is sometimes found that a small proportion of the new viruses produced are hybrids possessing some of the properties of both the original strains. This process is known as *genetic recombination*. In these experiments characteristics can sometimes be donated by virions which have previously been completely inactivated by heat or ultraviolet light. Recombination offers a rapid and effective means of producing live vaccine viruses to specification, e.g. combining the low virulence of one virus with the infective and antigenic properties of another.

Effect on host cells

The effects produced by growth of a virus in a cell vary greatly.

Cell degeneration. This is the most common effect. Visible changes rarely occur during the eclipse phase. With some viruses, such as poliovirus, mature fully infectious virions accumulate in the cytoplasm of the cell until many thousands are present. The cell then dies and undergoes sudden disruption (cytolysis) and virions are released. With enveloped viruses, such as influenza and herpes, which are liberated from the cell by budding through the cell membrane, the release of virus is more drawn out. The cell remains alive and intact and for a while appears relatively normal although it is releasing virus. Ultimately the cell dies. Cell degeneration is the main feature of the *cytopathic effect* (CPE) seen when viruses are grown in tissue culture (Fig. 18, p. 54).

Cell fusion. As well as producing degenerative effects, some viruses, such as measles and herpes simplex, cause the infected cells to fuse with their neighbours, producing giant cells and syncytia. One striking example of the cell-fusion effect is the ability of some viruses, in particular parainfluenza virus type 1, to produce heterokaryons, e.g. hybrid cells of two different species such as human cells and chick cells.

Cell proliferation. A few viruses, such as the papovaviruses, produce tumours. In tissue cultures of certain animal cells infected with such viruses some of the cells are transformed into malignant cells which will produce tumours when transplanted into the host animal. The cells do not contain or release infectious virus, but possess new antigens. If transformed cells are fused with uninfected cells of a line normally susceptible to the virus, it is sometimes possible to recover infectious virus from the hybrid cells.

Lysis. Phages typically show their presence by an explosive disruption of their host bacterium.

Latent infections. Sometimes viruses cause no obvious signs of cell disturbances. These latent infections come to light only when conditions change.

Inclusion bodies. Presumptive histological evidence that a cell is infected by a virus is given by finding characteristic round, oval or irregular intracellular structures known as inclusion bodies. In many viral infections the inclusion bodies consist of masses of virions (*elementary bodies* of the histologist) set in a matrix of cellular material. With other viruses they may represent degenerative changes.

The part of the cell in which inclusions occur is characteristic for different viruses. Nuclear inclusions are produced by herpesviruses, adenoviruses and yellow fever virus. Cytoplasmic inclusions are produced by vaccinia, molluscum contagiosum and rabies viruses. Measles virus produces both nuclear and cytoplasmic inclusions. Inclusions of most viruses are acidophilic in their staining reactions. Not all viruses produce inclusion bodies.

Effect on intact host

Under natural conditions there is usually an interval of days or weeks between infection and the appearance of signs and symptoms of illness. This is known as the *incubation period*. In this period the virus undergoes several cycles of infection, eclipse and release in different parts of the body. The tissues affected in the intact host are not necessarily those in which the virus will grow *in vitro*, e.g. poliovirus grows well in monkey kidney tissue culture, but in poliomyelitis the kidneys are not affected.

Antigens and immunity

All viruses are antigenic, i.e. when animals are naturally infected with a virus or are injected with virus-containing material they produce specific antibodies. Antibodies to antigens on the surface of the virion often render it non-infective (virus neutralization). Such antibodies are important in the development of immunity, though recovery from viral diseases mainly depends on cell-mediated mechanisms. Viral antigens and the methods used to detect them are considered in detail elsewhere (Chapters 8 and 9).

Haemagglutination

The chance observation that influenza virus grown in the chick embryo had the property of clumping chick red cells led to a valuable *in vitro* method for recognizing and titrating viruses. The precise physical conditions and the species of red cells needed vary with different viruses, but a large number of them have been shown to cause haemagglutination, e.g. orthomyxoviruses, paramyxoviruses, poxviruses, adenoviruses, coxsackieviruses, echoviruses and togaviruses.

Viral haemagglutination results from a linking together of the red cells by the viral particles or, in the case of poxviruses, from the action of soluble substances (lipoproteins) produced by the viruses. The process does not involve antibodies and should not be confused with the usual types of red cell agglutination met with in haematology.

The mechanism of viral haemagglutination is most clearly understood in the case of orthomyxoviruses and certain paramyxoviruses. Influenza, parainfluenza and mumps viruses agglutinate fowl, guinea-pig and human red cells. Under ideal conditions visible clumping occurs within a few seconds. The viral particles become attached to mucoprotein receptors on the red cells and form bridges between the cells. Following adsorption to red cells the virus is spontaneously released. This is due to a viral enzyme, neuraminidase, which inactivates the receptor by splitting off small molecular weight compounds. Red cells which have released virus are no longer agglutinated by further virus, but they may be agglutinable by other myxoviruses. The virus itself is unaltered and the adsorption-release cycle can be repeated with fresh cells. Haemagglutination is inhibited by sera containing neutralizing antibodies and by mucoproteins present in serum and other biological fluids. In serological tests the mucoprotein inhibitors can be removed from the test sytem by means of a *receptor destroying enzyme* (RDE) present in culture filtrates of *Vibrio cholerae*.

Orthomyxoviruses and paramyxoviruses can also be detected by sensitive *haemadsorption* techniques, e.g. the clumping of red cells on the surface of virus-infected monkey kidney cell cultures.

Toxic effects

Viruses do not produce soluble toxins, but very high concentrations of some viruses have a direct toxic or lethal effect on living cells. The toxicity is usually a property of the intact virion and can be neutralized by specific antiserum. It does not depend on viral multiplication. Some viruses induce formation of a toxic product distinct from the virus itself. Toxicity has been demonstrated in influenza, mumps, eastern and western equine encephalitis and adenoviruses.

Interference phenomenon

Although two distinct viruses can sometimes grow simultaneously in an intact host or even in a single cell, it has often been found that infection with one virus will prevent or *interfere* with subsequent infection by another virus. Thus intraperitoneal injection of monkeys with a neurotropic strain of yellow fever virus protects them from an otherwise fatal outcome when they are injected simultaneously or in the next few hours with a highly virulent strain of yellow fever virus. It also gives them protection against the antigenically unrelated virus of Rift Valley fever. Many other examples are known. In some cases interference can be produced by a virus that has been rendered noninfective by heat or ultraviolet light.

Interference is not due to the production of antibodies, since it can occur between antigenically unrelated viruses and in tissue culture and phage-bacterium systems where no antibodies are produced. Moreover, interference is usually established very rapidly, within a few seconds in some experiments. Interference is essentially due to something going on inside the cell and its persistence depends on the continued presence of the interfering virus.

Viral interference can be demonstrated in artificial infections in man, but whether the phenomenon is responsible for any significant degree of immunity under natural circumstances is not known. Some human viruses can persist in cells for a long time without causing much damage and it is possible that such viruses prevent infection by more dangerous viruses.

Interferon

Light was shed on the mechanism of interference by the observation that chick embryo cells exposed to inactivated influenza virus liberated a soluble antiviral substance called *interferon* which when added to normal embryo cells rendered them incapable of supporting the growth not only of active influenza virus and certain related viruses but also of some completely unrelated viruses, such as vaccinia. Many viruses have subsequently been shown to induce production of interferon in tissue culture and in intact animals.

Interferon production is thought to be a fundamental cellular response to the presence of foreign nucleic acid. Double-stranded RNA invariably induces interferon but single-stranded RNA and double-stranded DNA are ineffective. One of the most powerful inducers of interferon is the synthetic polynucleotide known as poly I:C. This is an analogue of double-stranded RNA. Few viruses contain double-stranded RNA but those that do, such as reoviruses, probably induce interferon immediately they enter the cell. Other RNA viruses produce double-stranded RNA during replication. It is not clear how DNA viruses induce interferon.

Viruses and double-stranded RNA are not the only agents that induce interferon. It is also produced in the course of immune reactions, notably when sensitized T-lymphocytes are exposed to the appropriate antigen. Interferon can also be induced by a wide range of non-viral agents including protozoa, bacteria, bacterial endotoxin, polysaccharides and fungal products. The activity of some of these agents depends on the presence of traces of double-stranded RNA. In some viral infections, notably acute fulminant viral hepatitis, interferon production is grossly defective.

The interferons produced by cells of different species differ slightly in their chemical and antigenic properties and are largely species-specific in their action, e.g. chick interferon shows powerful antiviral action in chick cells but not in mouse cells; human interferon shows powerful action only in human cells. Three main types of human interferon are distinguished on the basis of antigenic specificities: alpha (leucocyte or lymphoblastoid), beta (fibroblast) and gamma (immune). A typical interferon is a glycoprotein with a molecular weight of about 20 000 daltons. It is a potent biological substance and trace quantities can inhibit viral multiplication. Interferon has no direct action on the virus and does not interfere with the attachment of the virus to the cell nor with the subsequent processes of penetration or uncoating of the nucleic acid core. It binds to specific receptor sites on the cell surface and initiates enzyme reactions which stop the production of viral protein by the synthetic machinery of the host cell. It also produces changes in cell membranes which hinder the escape of the virions. Interferon stimulates immune reactions and is important in controlling the numbers and activity of macrophages and lymphocytes. It also has growth inhibitory properties, particularly against malignant cells, and may have a future as an anti-cancer agent.

Variation

Laboratory studies have drawn attention to the frequency with which viruses show variation in properties such as host range, tissue tropism, virulence, antigenic composition, heat stability and resistance to inhibitory substances. This variation which is based on mutation is most obvious when it concerns host range and virulence. When first isolated some viruses have a very narrow host range which makes them difficult to study. By repeated passage through different host systems, often using routes of infection which are not available to the virus in natural circumstances, it is possible to obtain strains which have become *adapted* to growth in animals, developing eggs and tissue culture. These adapted strains of viruses are often more amenable to study in the laboratory and are of great practical use when the mutation diminishes virulence without greatly affecting antigenic specificity. Live attenuated strains of this kind have been used very successfully as vaccines, e.g. yellow fever virus attenuated by growth in tissue culture. Strains suitable for vaccines have also been obtained by genetic recombination and by the action of mutagens on virus suspensions. Of particular interest are the temperature-sensitive mutants of some respiratory viruses which can grow in the cooler, upper parts of the respiratory tract and thus induce immunity, but cannot survive and cause disease in the lungs.

The existence of naturally occurring families of very closely related but not identical viruses such as smallpox, alastrim (a mild version of smallpox), cowpox, vaccinia and other poxviruses is almost certainly an expression of variation that has occurred naturally. Similarly the sudden world-wide outbreak of a viral disease, such as Asian influenza in 1957, represents the appearance of a variant against which the population possesses little or no immunity.

Differences in the properties of subtypes or strains of a particular virus are associated with differences in the base sequence of their nucleic acids. Techniques such as nucleic acid hybridization, restriction endonuclease mapping and the use of monoclonal antibodies have shown that mutation can occur at a very high frequency, particularly in RNA viruses. Thus antigenic variation is common in many viruses besides influenza virus, e.g. human immunodeficiency virus (AIDS virus), rabies, measles and picornaviruses.

Cultivation of Organisms

Medical microbiology is a cottage industry.

Contemporary comment

Growth of bacteria

Isolation of pure cultures

For proper examination bacteria must be obtained in *pure culture*. Very rarely this may be achieved by inoculating a liquid medium, but it is usually impossible to be certain that only one kind of bacterium is present. If the original inoculum contains even a very few bacteria of a different kind a *mixed culture* will result.

The classical method of obtaining organisms in pure culture is by *plating out* on a solid medium (Fig. 14). A small quantity of material (pus, sputum, etc.) is streaked out with a sterile wire loop on to the surface of the medium in a culture plate (Petri dish). By periodically sterilizing the loop in a flame and streaking from previous streaks on to uninoculated areas progressively smaller inocula are deposited on different areas of the medium. When the plate is incubated a crop of colonies appear. Each colony represents the progeny of a single cell or a very small group of cells. It is usually possible to judge from the appearance of the colonies whether one, two or more kinds of bacteria are

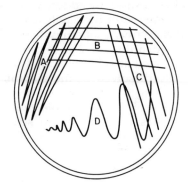

Fig. 14 Method of inoculating an agar plate ('plating out').

present. Isolated colonies can be picked off and the characteristics of the pure cultures can be studied in fresh media.

When small numbers of bacteria are present in the original material the chances of isolating them are greater if they are allowed to multiply in a liquid medium before plating out. Thus, in taking blood cultures, the blood is always inoculated into broth which is incubated for 24 hours or more before subcultures are made on to solid media.

Composition of media

Chemically defined (synthetic) media prepared from pure chemical substances (amino acids, growth factors, salts, etc.) are used for special purposes such as studying the nutritional requirements of bacteria and performing bio-assays.

Media used in routine diagnostic bacteriology usually contain a mixture of naturally occurring biological substances and their partial breakdown products. Peptone, meat extract and salt provide the basis of most media. Peptone is a complex mixture of water-soluble products obtained by enzymic digestion of meat. Whole blood, heated blood, serum, yeast extract, glucose and glycerol may be added to increase the nutritive value.

In addition to their nutrient ingredients many media incorporate substances which, in the presence of a mixed growth, encourage growth of wanted organisms and inhibit growth of unwanted organisms (*selective media*, including some known as *enrichment media*) or make it possible to distinguish one kind of organism from another (*differential media*).

The complete medium is adjusted to the required pH, commonly 7.0−7.2, sterilized by autoclaving, steaming or filtration and stored in containers sealed against contamination. Cotton-wool plugs trap airborne bacteria in their layers and are an effective barrier.

Media in solid form are usually prepared by adding agar to the desired nutrient medium. Agar consists of inert polysaccharides extracted from seaweeds. It has no nutrient properties for ordinary bacteria. It is added in sufficient quantities, 1−2%, to convert the medium into a stiff gel. Agar gels melt at about 95°C and solidify at 40−45°C. The agar is normally dissolved in the medium by boiling. Heat-sensitive substances such as blood can be added when the medium has cooled to 50−55°C. The complete medium is poured into sterile culture plates and allowed to set. Agar media remain firm at ordinary incubator temperatures (37°C).

Many different growth media are available and the precise ones used vary greatly in different laboratories.

Media for general purposes

Nutrient broth usually consists of peptone, meat extract and sodium chloride. Freshly prepared infusions or enzymic digests of meat are used to prepare broths suitable for growth of exacting organisms.

Nutrient agar consists of nutrient broth plus agar.

Blood agar consists of nutrient agar with 5–10% of citrated, oxalated or defibrinated blood (usually horse blood). Most bacteria of medical importance will grow on this medium and the presence of intact red cells allows the haemolytic properties of organisms to be recognized.

Heated blood agar ('chocolate' agar) consists of blood agar that has been heated until it has a chocolate colour. This process increases the nutritive value of the medium for delicate organisms.

Cooked meat medium consists of minced meat suspended in broth. It has excellent nutritive properties and supports the growth of a large number of organisms including strict anaerobes. It is a valuable medium for preserving cultures of delicate organisms.

Cystine-lactose-electrolyte-deficient (CLED) medium is a non-inhibitory differential medium mainly used for urine culture. It contains cystine to allow growth of certain cystine-dependent organisms, lactose and bromthymol blue which together confer differential properties, and it is electrolyte-deficient to prevent swarming by *Proteus. Escherichia coli* and other lactose fermenters produce *yellow* colonies. *Proteus* and other non-lactose fermenters produce *blue* colonies.

MacConkey agar (see below) is the most important differential medium for general purposes such as examination of urine, wound swabs, etc.

Bacterial transport medium is used to encourage survival of delicate organisms such as *Neisseria gonorrhoeae* and the protozoon *Trichomonas vaginalis* when there is delay in transporting specimens to the laboratory. The medium commonly contains salts, sodium thioglycollate to provide anaerobic conditions, methylene blue to check that these conditions are maintained, and sufficient agar (about 0.3%) to render the medium semi-solid. The specimen is taken with charcoal-coated swabs which are free of inhibitory substances found in cotton-wool. The swabs are inserted into the medium and snapped off. The caps of the bottles are screwed on tightly.

Media for intestinal organisms

MacConkey agar contains peptone as the main source of nutriment, bile salts which have a weak suppressive effect on non-intestinal bacteria, and lactose and neutral red which together confer differential properties on the medium. *E. coli* ferments lactose and produces *pink* colonies whereas salmonellae and shigellae (intestinal pathogens) do not ferment lactose and produce *colourless* colonies. Other lactose fermenters, e.g. *Streptococcus faecalis* and *Staphylococcus aureus*, and non-lactose fermenters, e.g. *Proteus* and *Pseudomonas aeruginosa*, grow on MacConkey medium. *Streptococcus pyogenes* is inhibited.

Deoxycholate citrate agar (DCA) is similar to MacConkey medium but contains additional salts which confer powerful selective properties on the medium. Salmonellae and shigellae grow freely and produce colourless colonies. *E. coli* is usually suppressed but *Proteus* and *Ps. aeruginosa* may grow. Suppressed organisms are not necessarily dead and the purity of non-lactose-fermenting colonies must be checked by plating out on MacConkey medium. DCA is the medium of choice for routine examination of faeces.

Tetrathionate broth and *selenite F broth* are liquid enrichment media with selective properties for salmonellae. The media should be heavily inoculated with faeces and plated out on MacConkey medium after overnight incubation. Neither medium encourages growth of shigellae but these organisms sometimes survive.

Media for mycobacteria

Dorset egg medium consists of whole egg mixed with water and coagulated by heat (80°C). It does not contain agar.

Löwenstein-Jensen medium consists of Dorset medium with the addition of salts, asparagine, glycerol (which stimulates growth of the human type of tubercle bacillus) and malachite green (which helps to keep down contaminants). It does not contain agar. It is the medium most frequently used in routine work.

Dubos medium is a liquid medium containing salts, casein hydrolysate, bovine albumin and a surface-active agent.

Media for Corynebacterium diphtheriae

Loeffler medium consists of serum mixed with a little glucose broth and coagulated by heat (80°C). It does not contain agar. Although *C. diphtheriae* will grow on many media the characteristic morphology of the organism is best seen on Loeffler medium.

Tellurite medium consists of a blood agar medium containing a trace of potassium tellurite which inhibits many of the commensal organisms of the nose and throat. *C. diphtheriae* grows well and produces black colonies.

Media for other pathogens

Selective media containing antibiotics and other agents are used to isolate many other groups of organisms, e.g. neisseriae (p. 241), vibrios (p. 287), *Yersinia enterocolitica* (p. 292), *Bordetella pertussis* (p. 298) and campylobacters (p. 302).

Media for biochemical tests

Sugar media. Determination of 'fermentation reactions' (strictly, degradation of sugars is either fermentative or oxidative) is often an important step in identifying bacteria. Various carbohydrates, sugar alcohols, glucosides, etc. ('sugars') are dispensed as 1% solutions in peptone water in tubes or small bottles together with an indicator and a small inverted tube (Durham tube) which rests in the medium. After inoculation the set of sugar media is incubated for a suitable period, commonly 24 hours, but many days with some organisms, and a note is made of three features: *opacity* of the medium (to confirm that the organism has grown), formation of *acid* (change of colour of the indicator) and production of *gas* (bubbles in the Durham tube).

Coliform organisms grow well in ordinary sugar media. Some organisms are more exacting in their requirements. *C. diphtheriae* is best studied in liquid media containing added serum. *N. gonorrhoeae* and *N. meningitidis* grow poorly in liquid media and fermentation reactions are carried out on serum agar media.

Other media are used to detect special biochemical properties such as ability to liquefy gelatin or hydrolyse urea. Patterns of fermentation and other tests can be examined with commercially prepared sets of substrates packaged in small plastic containers. Thus the API 20 E strip is widely used to identify enterobacteria and other gram-negative rods. It consists of 20 microtubes containing dehydrated substrates. The tubes are inoculated with a bacterial suspension and the strip is incubated for 24 hours. Metabolic products and enzymic reactions are revealed by colour reactions and the organism is identified by reference to tables or a computer database. Similar strips are available for identifying other groups of organisms.

Culture of anaerobic organisms

Strict anaerobes are usually grown on ordinary media under conditions in which free oxygen is excluded. This is normally achieved by means of an *anaerobic jar* (Fig. 15, p. 50). Plates and liquid cultures (caps of screw-capped bottles are loosened) are placed in the jar. The jar is closed and most of the air is evacuated by

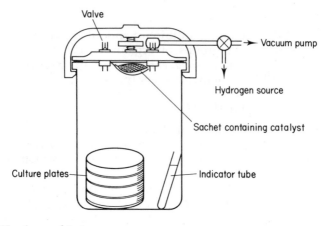

Fig. 15   Anaerobic jar.

means of a pump. Hydrogen together with 5–10% carbon dioxide is then allowed to flow into the jar. Alternatively, hydrogen and carbon dioxide can be generated by adding water to commercially available sachets which are placed in the jar before closure. Under the influence of a catalyst attached to the underside of the lid the hydrogen combines non-explosively with the residual oxygen. The most convenient catalyst consists of pellets of alumina coated with finely divided palladium. It is active at room temperature. The jar is then placed in the incubator. As a check that anaerobic conditions have been achieved the jar should contain an indicator of anaerobiosis, either a chemical that changes colour on reduction, e.g. methylene blue (blue = oxidized, colourless = reduced), or a biological indicator, e.g. a nutrient medium inoculated with a strict aerobe such as *Ps. aeruginosa* which will fail to grow if oxygen is completely absent.

In large laboratories there are advantages in using an *anaerobic cabinet* which functions as a combined work station and incubator. Glove ports and air-locks are used to pass swabs and culture plates into and out of the cabinet. Plates can be inoculated, incubated, inspected and subcultured without exposure to oxygen.

Anaerobes can be grown in *shake cultures*. Tubes of freshly melted agar medium are cooled to 50°C and inoculated. The inoculum is dispersed by rolling the tube between the hands and the medium is allowed to solidify. The tubes are incubated in air. Strict anaerobes grow only in the depths of the medium where no oxygen is available and microaerophilic organisms grow in a narrow zone just below the surface. Facultative anaerobes grow throughout the medium and strict aerobes grow only on the surface (Fig. 16).

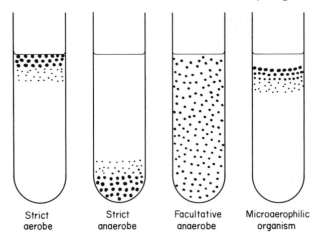

| Strict aerobe | Strict anaerobe | Facultative anaerobe | Microaerophilic organism |

Fig. 16 Growth of bacteria in agar shake cultures.

Anaerobes will grow under aerobic conditions in liquid media if these contain sufficient reducing substances. Cooked meat medium is the most important medium of this type. Addition to liquid media of sodium thioglycollate, ascorbic acid, a couple of dried peas or even an iron nail is also effective.

Carbon dioxide requirements

Some bacteria such as *Brucella abortus* and *N. gonorrhoeae* require 5–10% carbon dioxide for growth, especially on primary isolation. This can be achieved by putting the plates and tubes in a tin or jar together with a lighted candle and shutting the lid firmly. Carbon dioxide from a cylinder or generated in the tin from hydrochloric acid and sodium bicarbonate can also be used. Purpose-built carbon dioxide incubators are available and can be used with advantage for all routine aerobic cultures except sensitivity tests which may give unreliable results in the presence of extra carbon dioxide. Gas mixtures used for growing anaerobes and microaerophilic organisms should contain added carbon dioxide.

Animal inoculation

Although nearly all bacteria of medical importance can be cultivated on inanimate media (*Treponema pallidum* and *Mycobacterium leprae* are notable exceptions) the final identification of an organism may depend on its ability to produce characteristic disease in animals (pathogenicity and virulence tests). Since some animals are highly susceptible to small numbers of some pathogenic bacteria animal inoculation can also be used as a method of isolation. Thus guinea-pigs are occasionally used for the isolation and identification of *M. tuberculosis* and for virulence tests on *C. diphtheriae*. Inoculation of *Tr. pallidum* into the testes of rabbits is used to prepare suspensions of this spirochaete for the treponemal immobilization test.

Growth of viruses

Living cells are essential. They are provided in three main ways: the intact animal, the developing hen's egg and tissue culture.

The intact animal

Early work on human viruses was carried out by showing that bacteria-free filtrates produced disease in animals. The narrow host range of many viruses greatly limited the scope of this work and for a long time man and sometimes primates were the only known hosts susceptible to some viruses. By using special routes of infection (intranasal, intracerebral, etc.) and animals of a special species or special age, a wider host-range could sometimes be established. Thus coxsackieviruses were unknown until the experiment was made of injecting material into suckling mice. Because of its small size and availability the mouse is the most generally useful laboratory animal.

The developing egg

The developing chick embryo offers a cheap, neatly packed, self-sustaining and normally sterile living system which will support the growth of many different viruses. The embryo and its associated membranes provide a diversity of tissues and environments each of which may offer special advantages for the growth of a particular virus or for carrying out a particular type of experiment. Thus smallpox, vaccinia and herpes viruses grow readily in the cells of the chorio-allantoic membrane and with a suitable inoculum produce discrete and usually characteristic pocks which are visible to the naked eye and can be easily counted. Influenza and mumps viruses can be isolated by growth in the amniotic cavity: these viruses also grow well in the allantoic cavity. The yolk sac is suitable for growth of rickettsiae.

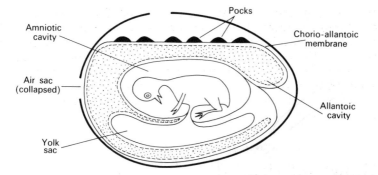

Fig. 17 Pock formation on the chorio-allantoic membrane. Pocks produced by vaccinia virus 3 days after infection of a 10–12 days old chick embryo. A hole has been made in the air sac to allow the chorio-allantoic membrane to collapse.

Tissue culture

Whenever possible viruses are grown in tissue culture. Antibiotics will prevent the growth of bacteria even in the presence of heavily contaminated material and most viruses produce characteristic degenerative changes (*cytopathic effects* or *CPE*) which can be prevented by the addition of specific antibodies (Fig. 18, p. 54).

Types of cells

The cells used in tissue culture can be obtained from almost any normal, malignant or fetal tissue of man or lower animals. Cultures can be either *primary cultures* freshly prepared from the tissues or *subcultures* maintained in the laboratory. Most cultures die out after a few subcultures, but there are now many *continuous cell lines* which have been propagated for years. Tissue culture cells can be preserved by storing in liquid nitrogen. For the study of human viruses primate cells have a broader spectrum of susceptibility than cells of lower animals. The following cell cultures are commonly used:

Continuous cell lines. HeLa cell cultures were derived from a human carcinoma of the cervix. They have a limited range of susceptibility, but are suitable for isolating poliovirus, group B coxsackieviruses, adenoviruses and herpes simplex virus. Some strains of HeLa cells are sensitive to respiratory syncytial virus. HEp2 cells are a very sensitive cell line derived from human

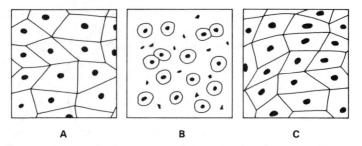

Fig. 18 Cytopathic effect of a virus in tissue culture. A, Control: healthy monolayer of cells in tissue culture. B, Cytopathic effect of virus: cells rounded, degenerate and becoming detached from glass. C, Effect of virus and specific antibody: cytopathic effect prevented.

malignant tissue. The WI38 strain of human embryo lung cells is a suitable substrate for human vaccine production. McCoy cells are of doubtful origin but are probably human synovial cells contaminated with mouse cells. Treatment of McCoy cells with cycloheximide produces non-replicating (stationary phase) cells suitable for isolation of chlamydiae.

Vero cells are a line of monkey kidney cells and are particularly valuable for isolating rubella virus and herpesviruses. RK13 cells are derived from rabbit kidney and have similar properties.

Primary cell cultures. Monkey kidney cell cultures are normally prepared in a central laboratory and sent by post to laboratories requiring them. Their range of sensitivity is greater than that of continuous cell lines, and they can be used to isolate poliovirus, group B coxsackieviruses, many types of echovirus, influenza and parainfluenza viruses, vaccinia virus and M strains of rhinovirus.

Human amnion cell cultures, prepared from amnion obtained at Caesarean section, have a wide range of sensitivity. They can be used to isolate poliovirus, group B coxsackievirus, certain echoviruses which grow poorly in monkey kidney cells, varicella-zoster virus and rubella virus.

Human diploid cell cultures. These cultures, derived from human embryonic tissues such as lung, can be propagated for about 50 subcultures. They are sensitive to H strains of rhinovirus and to cytomegalovirus.

Types of media

Viral transport medium. Many viruses survive for only a short time outside the body unless special precautions are taken. All swabs should be broken off into a bottle of viral transport medium. Post-mortem tissues, biopsy specimens and cerebrospinal fluid can be added directly to this medium. The bottles should be rapidly transported to the laboratory where the contents are used to inoculate tissue cultures. Until this is done the bottles should be kept at 4°C, or at −70°C if procedures cannot be started on the same day. Viral transport medium consists essentially of a balanced salt solution, sodium bicarbonate and a protein such as bovine serum albumin which helps to stabilize labile viruses. Viruses do not multiply in the medium.

Growth media. A solution of glucose, balanced salts, sodium bicarbonate, amino acids and vitamins together with added protein such as calf serum will provide a complete medium which will support cellular multiplication. It is usual to add to the medium penicillin and streptomycin to inhibit bacteria, amphotericin B to inhibit fungi and phenol red to check that the pH is kept within the physiological range. The culture is usually maintained at 37°C and the medium is renewed from time to time.

Maintenance media. A complex chemically defined medium resembling a growth medium but with a reduced amount of added protein will keep tissue culture cells alive but allow little or no multiplication. Media of this kind are used to maintain tissue cultures until they are required for virus isolation.

Techniques

Freshly obtained animal tissue is cut up into small fragments and washed repeatedly with a balanced salt solution. The fragments (or stock laboratory cultures) are then treated with dilute trypsin. This breaks down clumps of cells to yield a suspension largely composed of single cells. In the *monolayer technique* the cells are allowed to settle in a suitable medium. They adhere to the glass and after incubation for a few days they multiply and produce a continuous sheet of cells one layer thick. Cultures of this type are very satisfactory for demonstrating the cytopathic effect of viruses and are widely used for routine purposes. A valuable modification of the technique is to infect the monolayer with a dilute inoculum of virus and then cover the entire sheet of cells with a layer of nutrient agar. This confines the infection to the immediate neighbourhood of the cells exposed to each infective particle. As the virus multiplies it produces a discrete *plaque* of tissue degeneration from which a pure strain or *clone* of virus may be recovered. The plaque technique is the equivalent of 'plating out' in bacteriology.

Sources and Transmission of Infection

Coughs and sneezes spread diseases.
World War II poster

Organisms capable of causing disease in man are derived from three sources:

1 Human beings (the most important source).
2 Lower animals (much less important).
3 Inanimate nature (relatively unimportant).

The relative importance of the three sources depends primarily on the fact that different organisms are adapted to particular natural habitats. Thus human pathogenic micro-organisms prefer human tissues and some will grow and multiply only in these tissues. Animals in close contact with man may become infected with human pathogens, but this is unusual. Similarly, lower animals have their own sets of pathogens, most of which are subtly different from those causing disease in man. A few animal pathogens are quite successful in causing human disease, but on the whole they prefer their specific animal hosts and the majority will infect animals only. Finally, there are large numbers of organisms living in water, soil and decaying animal and vegetable matter; most of these are unfitted to survive and multiply in animal tissues and only a tiny minority can adopt a commensal or pathogenic way of life.

Human sources

The individual's own organisms

The normal human infant is sterile at birth but rapidly acquires a complex bacterial flora. These organisms, derived from other human beings, vary from time to time throughout life. In ordinary circumstances they are harmless, but occasionally they may gain access to tissues normally denied to them and produce disease.

Bacteroides, Escherichia coli and other organisms are harmless commensals of the bowel, but acting together can cause peritonitis if the bowel wall is mechanically damaged. *E. coli* is also the commonest cause of urinary tract infection. *Haemophilus influenzae, Streptococcus pneumoniae* and viridans streptococci live harmlessly in the upper respiratory tract, but can cause bronchitis, bronchopneumonia, sinusitis, otitis media, etc., if the mucous membranes are damaged by respiratory syncytial virus or the viruses of influenza, measles and the common cold. On rare occasions viridans streptococci may gain access to the blood, settle on a damaged heart valve and cause infective endocarditis. Injuries and operation wounds offer opportunities for endogenous bacterial infection.

Patients incubating a disease

During the incubation period of an infectious disease the organisms multiply in the tissues but cause no clinical evidence of infection. At some stage the prospective patient may therefore be healthy but highly infectious. Thus in hepatitis A the faeces are a source of infection for about two weeks before the onset of jaundice (Fig. 52, p. 364). In hepatitis B the blood is infectious for more than a month (Fig. 54, p. 367). In rubella (Fig. 50, p. 355), mumps and poliomyelitis the upper respiratory tract is a source of infection for a few days before the onset of symptoms. In infections of the throat caused by *Corynebacterium diphtheriae* and *Streptococcus pyogenes* the period is shorter. Patients who are infectious while incubating a disease are sometimes referred to as *precocious carriers.*

Patients with overt disease

A patient suffering from an acute or chronic infectious disease frequently liberates large numbers of the causative organisms into the environment. Depending on the type of disease, organisms may be present in faeces and urine, droplets and discharges from the mouth, nose, ears and eyes, and in discharges of pus from internal organs, wounds, ulcers, sores and other lesions of the skin.

In many acute diseases the organisms are rapidly killed and there may be only a short time during which the patient is infectious. Other pathogens such as *Mycobacterium tuberculosis, Treponema pallidum* and *Neisseria gonorrhoeae* tend to produce chronic disease in which the organisms are conveyed to the exterior for much longer periods. Herpes simplex virus persists in the tissues in a latent form for the rest of the patient's life, occasionally awakening to produce the infectious 'cold sores' of this disease.

Not all infected patients are a source of infection for others. Sometimes the pathogen defeats its own ends by attacking a deep-seated organ such as the meninges from which egress to another host is impossible. Or the pathogen may be so virulent that it rapidly kills the host and thereby exterminates itself.

Convalescent carriers

In many infectious diseses the causative organisms are not eliminated at the time of clinical recovery. Thus, following diphtheria or streptococcal sore throat, the organisms may persist in the throat; following typhoid fever, dysentery or poliomyelitis the patient may continue to excrete the organisms in the faeces. Such patients are known as *convalescent carriers* or *convalescent excreters*. The number of persons who continue to harbour and excrete the organisms becomes smaller with time, but it is not unusual to find that 5−10% are still carriers after two months. Sometimes the carrier state persists indefinitely. An arbitrary but useful distinction can be made between *temporary excreters* (*temporary carriers*) who excrete the organisms for less than a year and *chronic carriers* who excrete the organisms for more than a year. Chronic carriers are particularly common following typhoid fever (Fig. 19; see also p. 279). In some diseases clinical cure is associated with complete elimination of the organism. Thus convalescent carriers were never found following smallpox.

Contact carriers

Persons in contact with a patient suffering from an infectious disease may acquire the organisms and harbour them without suffering from any apparent disease. Such persons are known as *contact carriers* or *symptomless excreters*. The carrier state may be temporary or chronic. The interactions between host and parasite range from very mild forms of disease to relationships which can best be regarded as commensalism. Thus, in outbreaks of poliomyelitis, cases of overt disease are greatly outnumbered by cases of inapparent or subclinical infection which can be recognized only because the individual produces specific antibodies. These cases are nevertheless infectious to others. The carriage of *Staphylococcus aureus* in the nose and skin of over half the general population and an even higher proportion of hospital workers is undeniably a most important source of disease but is hardly a disease in itself. Other diseases in which contact carriers are common include diphtheria, streptococcal sore throat, meningo-

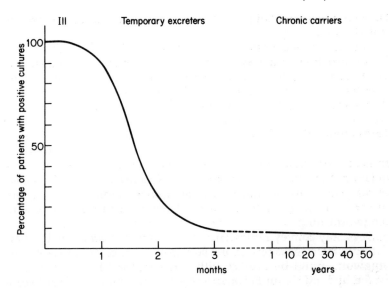

Fig. 19 Persistence of *Salmonella typhi* in the faeces of patients following typhoid fever.

coccal meningitis, dysentery and hepatitis B. Since contact carriers usually go unrecognized they constitute a special hazard for the rest of the uninfected population.

Animal sources

Infectious diseases which primarily affect animals but which may be transmitted naturally to man are called *zoonoses*. The following are a few of the many diseases which may be acquired from animals.

Cows may excrete *Mycobacterium bovis*, *Brucella abortus* and *Coxiella burneti* in their milk, *Campylobacter jejuni* in their faeces and *Leptospira interrogans* (especially serotype *hardjo*) in their urine. These organisms, together with salmonellae, may also contaminate the carcass. *Bacillus anthracis* may contaminate the carcass and spores may survive on hides, bone-meal, etc. The viruses of cowpox and milker's nodes may be present in lesions on the udder. Cows are often infected with ringworm fungi and sometimes with the beef tapeworm, *Taenia saginata*.

Pigs may be infected with *Brucella suis*, *Streptococcus suis*, salmonellae and *B. anthracis*. *Erysipelothrix rhusiopathiae*, the cause of swine erysipelas, may infect wounds and abrasions in man causing erysipeloid. Pigs may be infected with the protozoon *Balantidium coli,* the pork tapeworm *Taenia solium* and the nematode *Trichinella spiralis.*

Goats in the Mediterranean region may excrete *Brucella melitensis* in their milk. They may be infected with *B. anthracis* and *C. burneti.*

Sheep may have anthrax. They are the natural source of orf (contagious pustular dermatitis) and louping-ill viruses and the sheep liver fluke, *Fasciola hepatica.* They may be infected with *C. burneti.* Sheep suffering from enzootic abortion excrete large numbers of *Chlamydia psittaci.*

Horses in some parts of the world suffer from glanders (*Pseudomonas mallei*). In common with other farmyard animals they excrete *Clostridium tetani* in their faeces. They are often infected with ringworm fungi.

Dogs may convey rabies virus and *Pasteurella multocida* by their bites, *L. interrogans* (especially serogroup Canicola) in their urine, ringworm fungi by contact with their skin and hair and the ova of the hydatid worm *Echinococcus granulosus* and the roundworm *Toxocara canis* in their faeces.

Foxes spread rabies virus and are an important host of the hydatid worm *E. multilocularis.*

Cats can be a source of ringworm fungi, *P. multocida* and the as yet unidentified agent of cat-scratch fever. They excrete oocysts of the protozoon *Toxoplasma gondii* in their faeces.

Rats may be infected with plague (*Yersinia pestis*) and murine typhus (*Rickettsia typhi*), both of which are transferred to man by fleas. *L. interrogans* (especially serogroup Icterohaemorrhagiae) may be excreted in their urine and enter man through cuts and abrasions. Rat-bite fever may be due to *Spirillum minus* or *Streptobacillus moniliformis.* Rats commonly excrete salmonellae in their faeces. They are the main host for *T. spiralis.* Laboratory rats may be infected wiith hantavirus.

Mice are commonly infected with salmonellae. They are the natural host of *R. akari* the cause of rickettsialpox and of the virus of lymphocytic choriomeningitis. Field mice are the host of Machupo virus which causes Bolivian haemorrhagic fever.

Various wild rodents are the source of tularaemia (*Francisella tularensis*). They are often infected with hantavirus. A rat-like rodent is the reservoir of Lassa fever virus.

Monkeys are the host of yellow fever virus and also dengue virus in some areas. These diseases are conveyed to man by mosquitoes. Monkeypox has been transmitted to man on very rare occasions. B virus and Marburg virus are serious hazards for laboratory workers handling infected tissues.

Chickens, turkeys and *ducks* often excrete salmonellae in their faeces. These organisms frequently contaminate the meat. Duck eggs are liable to contain salmonellae. The organisms enter the egg before the shell is deposited. Poultry are an important source of campylobacters.

Parrots, pigeons and *other birds* may excrete the organisms of psittacosis and ornithosis (*Chlamydia psittaci*) in their faeces.

Tortoises, terrapins, turtles and *lizards* may excrete salmonellae.

Fish may be infected with *E. rhusiopathiae, Mycobacterium marinum, Vibrio parahaemolyticus* and the fish tapeworm, *Diphyllobothrium latum*.

Various domestic and wild animals are the natural hosts of *Listeria monocytogenes, Yersinia enterocolitica, Y. pseudotuberculosis, Pasteurella haemolytica* and *P. ureae*. They are often infected with the protozoon *Cryptosporidium*. Wild animals are hosts for *Borrelia burgdorferi* causing Lyme disease, rickettsiae causing various types of typhus fever, arboviruses causing encephalitis and febrile illnesses, and various protozoa such as trypanosomes. These diseases are transmitted by arthropod vectors.

Inanimate sources

Pseudomonas aeruginosa, Proteus and many species of *Clostridium* are capable of free-living existence in the soil where they obtain nourishment from decaying animal and vegetable matter. They are also common intestinal commensals of man and animals and may be returned to the soil in the faeces. These organisms show little tendency to produce disease spontaneously. *Ps. aeruginosa* and *Proteus* may infect burns, wounds and the urinary tract (particularly if some abnormality is already present). In the special conditions present in hospitals growth of free-living gram-negative bacilli in moist surroundings can be a major hazard (p. 195). *Cl. tetani* and *Cl. perfringens* only produce tetanus and gas gangrene when they chance to enter tissues which offer anaerobic conditions, e.g. a deep wound contaminated with soil. *Legionella pneumophila* can grow in soil and water and may contaminate the water of humidifiers and air-conditioning systems. *Listeria monocytogenes, Nocardia madurae* and the fungi *Cryptococcus neoformans, Microsporum gypseum, Histoplasma capsulatum, Coccidioides immitis* and *Sporothrix schenki* may be found in soil.

Portals of entry

Transmission of the infecting agent to the new host is sometimes by direct contact but is more often an indirect process involving various vehicles of infection. These include: air, dust, water, milk and food; articles such as clothing and bedding contaminated by a patient, sometimes referred to as *fomites*; medical, surgical and dental instruments, appliances, dressings, and fluids administered parenterally; and various arthropod vectors. The organisms may enter the host by one of four portals of entry:

1　*Transplacental infection.*
2　*Inhalation* and infection through the respiratory tract.
3　*Ingestion* and infection through the alimentary tract.
4　*Inoculation* through skin and mucous membranes.

Some organisms can infect a host through several different portals, e.g. *M. tuberculosis* will cause disease if it is inhaled, ingested or introduced by inoculation. Usually organisms produce infection only if they enter through a particular portal, e.g. salmonellae gain access through the intestinal tract but do not infect wounds; *Staph. aureus* readily infects wounds but is unlikely to set up infection if ingested. The portal of entry does not necessarily show any pathological changes and may be remote from the part of the body which ultimately bears the brunt of the disease. Thus poliovirus enters the host through the pharynx and intestinal tract, but the clinical effects of poliomyelitis are largely confined to the central nervous system.

Transplacental infection

The placenta is an effective barrier and infection of the developing fetus is uncommon. However, if the mother has syphilis, *Tr. pallidum* is extremely liable to cross the placenta with resulting miscarriage or birth of an infant with congenital syphilis. Rubella virus is also very dangerous and infections in the first three months of pregnancy frequently produce congenital abnormalities in the fetus. Cytomegalovirus infection *in utero* is the most common viral cause of mental retardation. Other organisms which occasionally infect the fetus include human immunodeficiency virus (AIDS virus), hepatitis B virus, *Listeria monocytogenes* and the protozoon *Toxoplasma gondii*.

Inhalation and respiratory tract infection

Many common infectious diseases are acquired by breathing contaminated air, the organisms being trapped by the moist surfaces of the nasopharynx and lower respiratory tract. This is the usual mechanism of transmission of such diseases as streptococcal sore throat, diphtheria, meningococcal meningitis, whooping cough, pulmonary tuberculosis, pneumonic plague, measles, influenza and the common cold. The source of the organisms is usually the infected secretions of the respiratory tract of another individual.

Direct transfer

The transfer of infected secretions by kissing or the use of infected cups and cutlery, etc., is undoubtedly a mechanism by which some respiratory tract infections are spread, but is generally less important than air-borne routes. Kissing plays a major role in the transmission of infectious mononucleosis, herpes simplex and cytomegalovirus infection.

Droplet infection

In normal breathing few or no organisms emerge into the air from the nose or mouth. In quiet conversation the number is usually small; in shouting the number is greater. However, these numbers are small compared with the vast numbers of organisms liberated by coughing and sneezing. Most of these organisms, even in sneezing, are derived from the mouth. Nose-blowing is a prolific source of organisms derived from the nose.

In a vigorous cough an occasional very large particle of mucopus may have sufficient size and momentum to shoot across a room. This is unusual and the vast majority of particles from the respiratory tract are in the form of droplets. It has been estimated that a vigorous cough may liberate five thousand droplets and a vigorous sneeze as many as a million droplets. Their fate depends on their size.

Very small droplets of less than 100 μm in diameter account for the majority of droplets expelled. They evaporate almost instantaneously and remain suspended in the air for many hours as *droplet nuclei* which consist of dried secretions and any organisms they may contain. Ultimately they fall to the ground.

Larger droplets having a diameter of 100 μm or more are fewer. They have an extremely short trajectory and even in vigorous coughing and sneezing very few travel more than 0.5–0.75 m in a horizontal direction. With the weaker expulsive force of talking they travel only a few centimetres horizontally. The droplets rapidly fall towards the ground and contaminate whatever is immediately in front of and below the patient.

The importance of direct air-borne infection is uncertain. Droplets are largely formed from the saliva at the front of the mouth and this area is not necessarily contaminated with organisms causing disease in the tonsils, pharynx and lungs. Most droplet nuclei are sterile and even in patients infected with *M. tuberculosis, Str. pyogenes* or *C. diphtheriae* only a minute proportion of the droplet nuclei contain the pathogen. Larger droplets contain more organisms but their short trajectory limits their ability to cause direct infection. It seems reasonable to suppose that a cough or sneeze at short range directly into the face of a victim is a fairly certain way of transferring infection. Droplet infection is probably of particular importance in the spread of viral disease of the respiratory tract and possibly in the spread of bacteria such as *Neisseria meningitidis* and *Bordetella pertussis* which are rapidly killed by drying. In other diseases the expulsion of droplets may be more important as a source of contamination of the patient and his environment. Inhalation of *L. pneumophila* in aerosols produced by contaminated air-conditioning systems is probably the main mechanism by which man acquires legionnaires' disease.

Dust-borne infection

Many respiratory tract infections are probably acquired by an indirect process involving two stages: (1) the donor contaminates himself and his environment; (2) the organisms are conveyed to the recipient in the form of dust.

Contamination caused by the donor can occur by expulsion of droplets, already considered, and by direct outflow of secretions. Normal people frequently touch their nose and mouth, suck pens and pipes and use their handkerchiefs. If they carry *Staph. aureus* and *Str. pyogenes* in their nose or throat these organisms are also found on the skin of their hands, face and other areas, on their clothing, particularly handkerchiefs, pockets and outer clothing on the front of the body, and on objects with which they have come in contact, e.g. bedding, handbags, books, pens, etc. Contamination by other pathogens probably occurs in a similar manner.

The infected secretions dry on whatever they happen to contaminate. If they are shielded from direct sunlight many important organisms will survive for days or weeks, e.g. *M. tuberculosis, Str. pyogenes, Staph. aureus, C. diphtheriae* and smallpox virus. Dispersal of these organisms into the air in the form of dust depends on movement. Large numbers of dust particles are liberated from the skin and clothing by normal body movements. Dispersal of dust from the general environment occurs in such processes as bed-making, sweeping and dusting (Fig. 28, p. 186; Fig. 29, p. 188). It is believed that the inhalation of such infected dust particles is an important mode of infection for many bacterial diseases of the respiratory tract.

Ingestion (intestinal infections)

Organisms responsible for intestinal disease reach their site of activity by being swallowed, e.g. salmonellae, shigellae, entero-pathogenic strains of *E. coli, Vibrio cholerae*, 'non-cholera vibrios', *Campylobacter jejuni, Yersinia enterocolitica*, rotaviruses, cysts of the protozoa *Entamoeba histolytica* and *Giardia lamblia* and ova of various intestinal helminths such as roundworms and tapeworms. *M. bovis* occasionally enters by this route and may cause intestinal disease. Ingestion is also the method of acquiring non-infective food poisoning caused by preformed toxins of *Staph. aureus, Cl. botulinum* and *Bacillus cereus* and by toxins formed in the gut by *Cl. perfringens*. Organisms which enter by the intestinal tract but cause their main symptoms elsewhere include brucellae, *Coxiella burneti*, hepatitis A virus and other enteroviruses (polio, coxsackie and echoviruses) and *Toxoplasma gondii*.

The faeces of a case or carrier are by far the most important source of the intestinal pathogens. Occasionally the organisms may be excreted in the urine, e.g. in enteric fever. Animals are not infrequently the source of salmonellae.

Direct contamination

Objects may be contaminated by faeces or by the hands. Even scrupulously clean people contaminate their hands during defaecation. When a patient has diarrhoea contamination is more likely. Those in attendance may contaminate their hands by touching the patient, handling bed-pans and changing nappies. In this way a wide range of environmental objects in a home, nursery, ward, school or camp may be contaminated. The recipient may transfer infection to his mouth by means of his fingers, eating utensils, feeding bottles and other objects. Dysentery and *E. coli* infections are frequently spread in this manner.

Food-borne infections

These are commonly caused by a carrier engaged in handling and preparing food, but sometimes the basic foodstuff is itself con-taminated. The routes of infection and the methods of control are considered elsewhere (p. 197).

Milk is a particularly dangerous vehicle because, unless it is refrigerated, it offers an excellent medium for multiplication of certain bacteria. The pathogens that may be present are (a) those derived from the cows, e.g. *M. bovis* (bovine tubercle bacilli), *Br. abortus, Coxiella burneti, Campylobacter jejuni, Yersinia enterocolitica* and *Listeria monocytogenes*; (b) those introduced by farm or dairy workers or by contaminated water or equipment, e.g. *Str. pyogenes.* *C. diphtheriae*, salmonellae, in particular *S. typhi* and *S. paratyphi*, shigellae, *Streptobacillus moniliformis*, hepatitis A virus and poliovirus. The streptococci of bovine mastitis are mostly avirulent for man. Other organisms commonly present, e.g. *Str. lactis*, *E. coli* and lactobacilli, turn milk sour but are harmless. All the pathogens are killed by pasteurization. 'Tuberculin-tested' milk implies that the cows when last tested were tuberculin-negative and that the milk reaches certain standards of purity; such milk is most unlikely to contain *M. bovis*, though this has been known to occur, but there is no guarantee that it is free from other pathogens. Tuberculin-tested milk is safe only if it has also been pasteurized.

There is no accounting for human taste. Most cases of kuru were acquired by cannibalism.

Water-borne infections

These occur by seepage from a privy, cesspit or sewer into a well or water-main, or by direct pollution of a water supply by a carrier. Water may itself convey infection or may contaminate food. Water-borne infection has been responsible for many major epidemics of cholera and typhoid fever in the past. Outbreaks of hepatitis A and infection with *Campylobacter jejuni*, enteropathogenic strains of *E. coli* and the protozoon *Giardia lamblia* still occur. Improvements in methods of sewage disposal, water purification and supply have rendered this route uncommon in most countries. In tropical countries drinking water may convey the helminth *Dracunculus medinensis* and the protozoon *Entamoeba histolytica*.

Inoculation

Simple contact

In the absence of any damage to skin or mucous membranes, simple contact is enough to spread some diseases. The diseases are literally 'contagious'. Thus the venereal or *sexually transmitted diseases* (STD) syphilis and gonorrhoea are spread by contact of genital mucous membranes and only very rarely by other means. Other STD include chancroid, granuloma inguinale, lymphogranuloma venereum (LGV), non-specific genital infection (nongonococcal urethritis, etc., mainly due to chlamydiae), herpes simplex, genital warts, acquired immunodeficiency disease (AIDS), molluscum contagiosum, candidiasis, trichomoniasis and infection with scabies mites (*Sarcoptes scabiei*) and pubic or 'crab' lice

(*Phthirus pubis*). Close physical contact between individuals or through the intermediary of clothing, bedding, towels and utensils is important in the spread of (a) skin infections such as impetigo, boils, warts, herpes simplex, scabies (almost entirely hand-to-hand spread) and ringworm; (b) general diseases which affect the skin such as leprosy, yaws and the rashes of secondary syphilis; and (c) infections of the conjunctiva caused by organisms such as *H. influenzae*, *Moraxella lacunata* and *Chlamydia trachomatis* (TRIC agents).

In some helminth infections such as bilharzia, strongyloidiasis and hookworm disease larval forms of the parasites present in water or moist soil infect man by boring their way through the skin.

Wound infection

This occurs when a break in continuity of skin or mucous membranes exposes the underlying tissues. This may result from accidental injuries, burns, surgical operations and, in the case of the puerperal uterus, the physiological events of childbirth.

Staph. aureus wound infection is one of the most important types of surgical sepsis. Although the organism is frequently carried in the nose or on the skin of patients at the time of admission, the strains responsible for most surgical infections are acquired in hospital. These 'hospital strains', which are commonly resistant to penicillin and other antibiotics, originate in a breeding ground consisting of patients and members of the staff who are either carriers or are infected by the organism. Many healthy nurses and doctors carry hospital strains of *Staph. aureus* in their noses. The organisms may also colonize areas of the skin such as the perineum and the axillae. The entire skin and clothing of carriers is almost invariably contaminated and very slight body movement is often sufficient to liberate profuse clouds of the organisms into the environment.

Patients with staphylococcal infections inevitably contaminate their immediate environment. More widespread air-borne contamination occurs during wound-dressing, bed-making and dusting. Grossly purulent lesions are nursed with elaborate precautions and are usually not such an important source of organisms as cases of staphylococcal pneumonia and septic lesions of the skin. Patients with infected eczema can be prolific dispersers of staphylococci, even when the lesions are quiescent. Such patients are particularly dangerous because they are often ambulant.

Patients may themselves become carriers of hospital strains soon after admission. Such carriers are an additional source of infection for other individuals and are themselves more likely to develop infection following surgery than patients who are non-carriers. The most misguided person of all is a member of the medical or nursing staff who continues working when suffering from overt sepsis. Methods of controlling staphylococcal infections are considered in Chapter 14.

Str. pyogenes is not commonly found on the skin nor is it found in the birth canal before delivery. Infection of wounds and the puerperal uterus may be caused by organisms in the individual's own nose or throat, but in most cases the organisms are derived from someone else, often a doctor, nurse or midwife who is a nasopharyngeal carrier. The organisms are usually conveyed by talking or coughing directly into the wound. Transference of infection to clean wounds from other patients with septic lesions was at one time largely by contamination of hands, clothing and instruments, but nowadays is more commonly the result of air-borne contamination arising from wound-dressing, bed-making, etc.

Cl. perfringens and *Cl. tetani* are introduced at the time the wound is inflicted. The same applies to rabies virus which is acquired from the bite of a rabid animal, usually a dog.

E. coli and *Bacteroides* infections are often endogenous, particularly following abdominal operations. *E. coli* and other coliforms can also be conveyed in dust or by lapses in hygienic precautions.

B. anthracis and leptospirae gain access through minute abrasions.

Injection

Medical injections

Hepatitis B virus is present in the blood of certain individuals and an important mechanism by which it is transmitted to another human being is by injection, e.g. by using needles and syringes contaminated with traces of human blood and improperly sterilized. Human immunodeficiency virus (AIDS virus) can also be transmitted by injection. Drug addicts are at risk in both these diseases.

Apart from deliberate injection of living vaccines, other infections conveyed by injection are rarely encountered. Syphilis, malaria, hepatitis B and AIDS may be transmitted by transfusion of improperly screened blood. Cytomegalovirus infection, infectious mononucleosis and non-A, non-B hepatitis may also result from transfusion, but there are no simple screening tests. Cytomegalovirus seldom survives more than five days in stored blood. Epstein-Barr virus survives for longer periods. Non-A, non-B hepatitis virus, like hepatitis B virus and AIDS virus, is extremely persistent and survives indefinitely in blood. Blood products such as factor VIII and IX concentrates must be heat-treated. Needles contaminated with *M. tuberculosis* from the respiratory tract of the person giving the injection have caused a few unfortunate outbreaks in immunization clinics. Considering the vast numbers of injections that are given, infections caused by pyogenic cocci are remarkably few.

Biting insects

Arthropod vectors include true insects (6 legs) such as flies, fleas, lice and bugs and arachnids (8 legs) such as ticks and mites. They are important in the transmission of diseases caused by rickettsiae, arboviruses, protozoa, some helminths and a few bacteria. The following vectors transmit diseases to man:

Mosquitoes: malaria (*Plasmodium malariae*, etc.); many diseases caused by arboviruses, e.g. yellow fever, dengue, equine encephalitis and St Louis encephalitis; filariasis (e.g. *Wuchereria bancrofti* and *Brugia malayi*).

Sandflies; sandfly fever, leishmaniasis (*Leishmania donovani*, etc.), Oroya fever (*Bartonella bacilliformis*).

Tsetse flies: trypanosomiasis (*Trypanosoma rhodesiense*, etc.)

Other blood-sucking flies: filariasis (e.g. *Mansonella perstans*, *Loa loa* and *Onchocerca volvulus*).

Fleas: bubonic plague (*Y. pestis*), endemic (murine) typhus (*R. typhi*).

Lice: epidemic typhus (*R. prowazeki*), trench fever (*Rochalimaea quintana*), European relapsing fever (*Borrelia recurrentis*).

Bugs: Chagas' disease (*Trypanosoma cruzi*).

Ticks: Rocky Mountain spotted fever (*R. rickettsi*), other forms of tick-borne typhus (*R. conori*, etc.), Lyme disease (*B. burgdorferi*), African relapsing fever (*B. duttoni*), some types of encephalitis caused by arboviruses, e.g. Russian spring-summer encephalitis and louping-ill.

Mites: scrub typhus (*R. tsutsugamushi*), rickettsialpox (*R. akari*).

Insects become infected when they bite a host whose blood contains the particular organisms. They do not behave as passive carriers, as do flies in transmitting salmonellae and shigellae from faeces to food, but act as a host in which the organisms can multiply. There is normally an interval of several days before the insects are capable of transmitting infection.

Lower animals are the natural hosts of most diseases transmitted to man by biting insects. In a few diseases man is the primary host and there is no animal reservoir of infection. Thus epidemic typhus, sandfly fever, European relapsing fever and malaria are transmitted by insects from man to man.

Transplantation

Transplant material such as kidneys, bone marrow and corneal grafts may convey infection from one person to another. The infecting agent is most commonly a virus that has been lying dormant in the tissues of the donor. In the recipient the virus becomes reactivated because of low host resistance brought about by immunosuppressive therapy. Cytomegalovirus is the commonest offender. Transmission of AIDS by grafts has been described. Semen used for artificial insemination and *in vitro* fertilization may convey AIDS and hepatitis B if the donor has not been properly screened.

Virulence of the Parasite

...Distinguishing those that have feathers, and bite,
From those that have whiskers, and scratch.

Lewis Carroll

On the basis of their life-habits organisms may be classified as saprophytes or parasites.

Saprophytism is the mode of life of free-living organisms which obtain their nourishment from soil and water. Saprophytes do not require a living host and only in extremely rare circumstances can any of them establish residence as parasites.

Parasitism implies adaptation to life on or in the bodies of higher organisms. The association may take one of three forms:

1 *Symbiosis* is the ability to live in the tissues of the host with mutual benefit. This relationship does not occur in man or higher animals but is important in other branches of biology, e.g. symbiotic nitrogen-fixing bacteria (*Rhizobium* spp.) in the root-nodules of leguminous plants. The term symbiosis is often used in a less restricted sense to describe an association in which two species live together in a close spatial and physiological relationship particularly when this is specific and permanent, e.g. some types of commensalism.

2 *Commensalism* (literally 'eating at the same table') is the ability to live on the external or internal surfaces of the body without causing disease. It is usually an indifferent relationship as far as the host is concerned, but occasionally the organisms confer some slight benefit, e.g. bacteria in the gut digest significant amounts of non-starch polysaccharides and are a source of certain vitamins. Common harmless commensals are sometimes referred to as saprophytes. Pathogenic organisms may occasionally be carried as temporary commensals.

3 *Pathogenicity* is the capacity of an organism to produce disease. All pathogens are endowed with *virulence,* a measure of their degree of pathogenicity. Virulence is a complex property which depends, among other factors, on *invasiveness,* i.e. ability to penetrate the tissues, overcome the host defences, multiply and disseminate widely, and *toxicity,* the capacity to damage the tissues.

The different categories are not clear-cut and organisms form a continuous series from those with little or no power of producing disease to those which almost invariably produce disease when they are present in the body. No parasite can be entirely non-pathogenic or completely devoid of virulence.

The outcome of the host-parasite relationship depends on a balance between the *virulence of the parasite,* i.e. all the functions of the parasite that favour its survival, growth, multiplication and ability to produce pathological changes in the host tissues, and the *resistance of the host,* i.e. all the inherent and adaptive mechanisms of the host that enable it to withstand the deleterious effects of the parasite. If the parasite is kept in check (balanced parasitism) the result is an asymptomatic infection such as commensalism. If the parasite gets out of control (unbalanced parasitism) the combination of damage to the host plus the adaptive reactions of the host produces the picture that we recognize as infectious disease.

The term *opportunist* is given to normally harmless organisms which take the opportunity afforded by lowered host resistance to act as pathogens. Opportunistic infections are now common: patients with impaired resistance are kept alive much longer; artificial joints and other prostheses provide new sites for bacterial infection (p. 232); antibiotics remove the protective effect of the normal flora (p. 213); immunosuppressive therapy is responsible for many 'new' diseases such as infection by 'non-pathogenic' bacteria and fungi and from reactivation of latent viruses and protozoa (see Index, Immunodeficiency).

Although disease is normally the result of increased virulence of the parasites or decreased resistance of the host these two qualities cannot be considered in isolation. Virulence is demonstrable only by production of disease in a host and resistance can be discerned only if a host is challenged by a parasite. Environmental factors have an important influence on the balance between the two. The parasite itself inevitably interacts with other organisms which may show antagonism or synergism.

Ability to grow in host tissues

If an organism is to establish itself as a parasite it must be able to find an environment suitable for growth. The following factors may contribute to this ability:

1 *Nutritional factors.* The basic foodstuffs needed by pathogens are available in the tissues. Paradoxically, non-pathogens are on the whole less exacting in their nutritional requirements

but are usually unable to grow in the tissues. Some organisms will grow in culture only if nutrients are provided in the correct balanced proportions and it has been suggested that the proportions available in the tissues are suitable for some organisms but not for others.

2 *Temperature.* Organisms are more likely to establish themselves as parasites if the optimal temperature for their growth is the same as the temperature of the host. It is possible to increase or decrease the susceptibility of animals to various bacterial and viral diseases by artificially altering the temperature of the host.

3 *pH.* Most organisms will grow at the pH of normal tissues. It has been suggested that those which establish themselves as parasites are less susceptible to acids and other metabolites which accumulate in areas of inflammation.

4 *Oxidation-reduction potential.* A low redox potential in the host tissues is an essential requirement for the growth of strict anaerobes.

5 *Unknown factors.* The above factors offer no satisfactory explanation for the high degree of host specificity shown by many organisms, e.g. why should leprosy, gonorrhoea and measles be exclusively human diseases? Presumably there must be subtle differences in the physicochemical properties of human tissues and tissues of other animals. Most pathogenic bacteria and viruses not only have a specific host range but also tend to attack particular organs or types of cell. Some bacteria are endowed with stickiness for specific types of cell. Thus virulent strains of *Neisseria gonorrhoeae* and some strains of enterotoxin-producing *Escherichia coli* possess pili (fimbriae) which enable the organisms to adhere to the surface of mucosal cells. *Staphylococcus aureus* and *Streptococcus pyogenes* have receptors for fibronectin, a glue-like glycoprotein found on cell surfaces. In natural environments (but not in cultures) many bacteria are covered with a *glycocalyx,* a tangled mass of long polysaccharide fibres which glue the organisms to inert surfaces, other bacteria and animal and plant cells. Many strains of *Staph. epidermidis* produce slime which adheres to plastics and may be one reason why these organisms are so successful in producing persistent infection of intravascular lines and implanted plastic devices. In viral diseases it is believed that infection depends in the first instance on adsorption of virus on specific chemical receptors on the cell wall. Thus influenza virus attaches to a mucoprotein receptor present on respiratory epithelial cells. Epstein-Barr virus attaches to a receptor for complement component C3d on B-cells. Human immunodeficiency virus attaches to CD4 (T4) antigen on helper T-cells.

Basis of virulence

The harmful effects of micro-organisms can seldom be explained by mechanical interference with body functions but are almost invariably determined by their biochemical properties. The properties which make for virulence vary with different organisms but can be considered under certain general categories.

Antiphagocytic and antilytic properties

Surface components. Resistance to phagocytosis mainly depends on the presence of surface components which make it difficult for the phagocytes to ingest the organism. The subject has been most thoroughly studied in the case of *Str. pneumoniae* but the principles involved have general validity.

Virulent strains of pneumococci possess polysaccharide capsules and resist phagocytosis. Rough mutants which have lost the ability to form capsules have also lost their virulence and are readily engulfed by phagocytes. If the phagocytes in an experimental animal are destroyed it is found that these rough mutants are as virulent as the original strain. In some strains of virulent pneumococci it is possible to remove the capsule by digestion with a specific enzyme without affecting the viability of the organisms. These non-capsulated organisms are also avirulent and susceptible to phagocytosis. Injection of large doses of the specific enzyme will protect against otherwise lethal infections by virulent pneumococci. The polysaccharides of pneumococci can be extracted and purified. They will neutralize the phagocytosis-promoting effect of specific antisera and will restore or enhance virulence in experimental pneumococcal infection.

Most pathogenic bacteria do not possess obvious capsules, but a similar function is served by their surface antigens such as the M proteins of *Str. pyogenes* or the endotoxins of gram-negative bacilli. Phagocytes which are unable to ingest virulent organisms can nevertheless ingest less virulent ones. Thus in guinea-pigs dying of streptococcal peritonitis, the phagocytes are powerless to deal with the streptococci but will rapidly ingest large numbers of *Proteus* injected into the peritoneum.

Many organisms withstand destruction when they have been ingested. The mechanisms are not clear but the surface components of the organisms are important.

The ability of many gram-negative bacteria to withstand the bactericidal and bacterilytic action of serum is probably due to their surface antigens (endotoxins).

Leucocidins. Some organisms such as *Staph. aureus* and *Str. pyogenes* produce complex substances which will kill leucocytes.

Toxins

Toxins are bacterial products or constituents which have a direct harmful action on tissue cells. They fall into two groups:

Exotoxins are produced by living bacteria and *diffuse freely into the surrounding medium*, i.e. they are extracellular toxins. Typical exotoxins are produced mainly by gram-positive organisms. They are highly toxic protein substances which are specific in their action, readily inactivated by heat, highly antigenic, completely neutralized by specific antibodies and convertible into toxoids.

Organisms producing exotoxins include *Corynebacterium diphtheriae, Clostridium tetani, Cl. botulinum, Cl. perfringens, Str. pyogenes, Staph. aureus* and a few gram-negative bacteria including *Shigella dysenteriae, Pseudomonas aeruginosa, Vibrio cholerae* and some strains of *Escherichia coli* and *Campylobacter jejuni.*

Endotoxins do not diffuse into the surrounding medium but *form part of the bacterial cell* from which they are liberated when the cell dies and disintegrates, i.e. they are intracellular toxins. Typical endotoxins are constituents of gram-negative organisms. They are moderately toxic protein-polysaccharide-lipid complexes which are non-specific in their action, relatively heat-stable, weakly antigenic, only partially neutralized by antibodies against the intact organism and not convertible into toxoids.

Organisms producing endotoxins include salmonellae, shigellae, brucellae, neisseriae, *V. cholerae, E. coli* and *Ps. aeruginosa.*

The distinction between exotoxins and endotoxins is not always clear-cut. Exotoxins are often liberated in greatest amounts when some degree of autolysis has occurred. Endotoxins are sometimes found in culture filtrates. In addition there are many atypical toxins. *Yersinia pestis* and *Bordetella pertussis* contain endotoxins which have many properties typical of exotoxins. *Bacillus anthracis* does not readily yield toxins when grown *in vitro* but produces an exotoxin when it is growing in the tissues. Weak endotoxic activity is shown by some gram-positive bacteria, including *Mycobacterium tuberculosis*, as well as by rickettsiae, chlamydiae and some viruses.

The significance of toxins is seen most clearly in the case of organisms which produce powerful exotoxins. Botulism is not an infectious disease at all since *Cl. botulinum* does not invade the body. The symptoms of classical botulism are entirely due to consumption of toxins produced when the organisms multiply in foodstuffs. In tetanus and diphtheria the infection remains highly localized and symptoms are due to toxins which diffuse from the infected area. The paralytic effects of botulism, the spasms and convulsions of tetanus, the haemorrhagic adrenals, degenerative changes in cardiac muscle and muscular paralyses of diphtheria can all be reproduced by injecting animals with minute doses of the appropriate cell-free culture filtrate. *Sh. dysenteriae* produces a very potent haemorrhagic and paralytic exotoxin, but it is formed in extremely small quantities and there is no evidence that it is responsible for the intestinal lesions of dysentery. *V. cholerae* and 'enterotoxigenic' strains of *E. coli* produce enterotoxins which interfere with the regulation of electrolyte transfer when injected into isolated intestinal loops of rabbits and which are responsible for the intestinal symptoms caused by these organisms in man.

Many organisms are both invasive and toxin-producing. *Cl. perfringens* and other gas gangrene organisms, *Str. pyogenes* and *Staph. aureus* produce several toxins, some of which are undoubtedly responsible for the pathological lesions and clinical symptoms found in the disease. But the relationships are nothing like so simple as those found in tetanus and diphtheria. Specific antitoxins have little effect on the course of gas gangrene although the toxic element of infection is very important. Streptococcal antitoxin will prevent the rash of scarlet fever, but it does not prevent other pathogenic effects of the organism. Similarly, staphylococcal antitoxin will neutralize staphylococcal toxins *in vitro*, but has surprisingly little effect on the course of staphylococcal infections.

Many infectious diseases are caused by bacteria which, so far as we know, do not produce exotoxins. However, most bacteria possess toxic materials (endotoxins) as part of the cell and these may manifest themselves when the bacteria undergo dissolution in the body. The endotoxins of gram-negative bacteria have been most clearly defined. They are probably identical with the surface somatic (O) antigens found in virulent organisms. Toxicity resides mainly in the lipopolysaccharide (glycolipid) part of the complex, particularly in a component known as lipid A. Irrespective of the organism from which they are derived, all have the same non-specific toxic effect. Parenteral injection in animals results in pyrexia, hypotension, leucopenia, activation of the complement system, endothelial damage, disseminated intravascular coagulation (DIC), liberation of cachectin (tumour-necrosis factor), haemorrhages and necrosis in the internal organs and death. Endotoxins are responsible for the symptoms of gram-negative bacteraemia.

Minute traces of endotoxin cause a gel to form in amoebocyte lysate of the horseshoe crab, *Limulus polyphemus*. The *Limulus* lysate test can be used for rapid diagnosis of gram-negative bacterial meningitis and gram-negative bacteraemia and for detecting pyrogens (endotoxin) in pharmaceutical products.

Potency of toxins. The exotoxins of *Cl. botulinum, Cl. tetani* and *Sh. dysenteriae* share the distinction of being the most poisonous substances known. It is estimated that 1 mg of purified botulinus or tetanus toxin would be sufficient to kill more than 1000 tons of guinea-pigs. The toxin of *Sh. dysenteriae* is equally potent for rabbits. Diphtheria toxin is three hundred times less toxic, but it is still more than one thousand times as poisonous as strychnine. In contrast 1 mg of a typical endotoxin constitutes a lethal dose for 1–10 mice.

Toxoids are toxins which have been modified so that they lose their toxicity but retain their antigenic properties. The change occurs to some extent during prolonged storage but can be effected more rapidly by moderate heat or by treatment with formalin. Formol toxoids are widely used for immunization of man and animals.

Enzymes

Coagulase is produced by *Staph. aureus.* In the presence of a factor present in plasma and body fluids it converts fibrinogen into a fibrin clot. The fibrin may act as a barrier protecting the organisms from phagocytes.

Fibrinolysin (streptokinase) is produced by *Str. pyogenes.* By activating the precursor of a proteolytic enzyme present in plasma it causes lysis of fibrin clots. It may assist in the spread of organisms in the tissues. Similar substances are produced by some staphylococci and clostridia.

Hyaluronidase is produced by *Cl. perfringens, Cl. septicum* and some strains of *Str. pyogenes, Str. pneumoniae* and *Staph. aureus.* It splits hyaluronic acid, the mucoid polysaccharide intercellular cement substance of the tissues. It may act as a bacterial spreading factor by increasing the permeability of the tissues.

Collagenase is produced by *Cl. perfringens* and *Cl. histolyticum.* It breaks down collagen and probably contributes to the ability of these organisms to spread through tissue barriers and cause disintegration of muscle and other tissues.

Lecithinase is produced by *Cl. perfringens* and *Cl. novyi.* It breaks down lecithin, a constituent of cell membranes, and is an important factor in the toxicity and invasiveness of these organisms.

Deoxyribonuclease is produced by *Str. pyogenes* ('streptodornase'), *Cl. perfringens* and *Cl. septicum.* It breaks down deoxyribonucleic acid (DNA), a viscous constituent of pus and inflammatory exudates, and may facilitate the spread of these organisms in the tissues.

Hypersensitivity (allergy)

Some products and constituents of bacteria, viruses and fungi are relatively harmless for normal people, but are toxic for individuals who are suffering from the relevant disease or who have had the disease in the past. Thus tuberculin, a complex preparation obtained from *M. tuberculosis*, is about one hundred times more lethal for tuberculous guinea-pigs than it is for normal guinea-pigs. Allergy develops in nearly all infectious diseases, but it often does not appear until convalescence and it is by no means certain that it always favours the parasite.

Interference with metabolism of host cells

In viral infections an important part of the metabolism of the host cell is diverted to synthesis of viral material. In bacterial infections competition for nutrient material may sometimes account for damage to the host cell, but at present there is little evidence that this is an important mechanism of toxicity.

Metabolic end-products

Simple end-products of microbial metabolism, e.g. lactic acid, may reach toxic concentrations in the immediate vicinity of invading organisms. The contribution of such substances to microbial toxicity is obscure.

Innate Body Defences

Stimulate the phagocytes.

George Bernard Shaw

Innate or non-acquired defence mechanisms are those which operate regardless of the individual's past experience.

Outer defences

Mechanical barriers

Intact skin is a highly effective barrier against microbial invasion. Mucous membranes are more permeable. Thus virulent *Neisseria meningitidis* and *Streptococcus pneumoniae* can penetrate the mucous membranes of the nasopharynx, *Salmonella typhimurium* penetrates the intestinal mucosa and *Treponema pallidum* and *Neisseria gonorrhoeae* penetrate the genital mucous membranes. Parasitization of the mucous membrane is the first step in many viral infections. Mucus itself forms a mechanical barrier. It also discourages penetration of the cells by viruses such as influenza virus by competing with cell surface receptors for viral neuraminidase. Healthy granulation tissue is remarkably impermeable even though the tissues and the environment are separated by only a thin and delicate layer.

Mechanical removal

Organisms impinging on the mucous membranes of the respiratory tract are trapped in a carpet of mucus which is being continuously conveyed towards the oesophagus by ciliary action. Coughing, sniffing, sneezing, blinking and the flow of tears, sweat, saliva, urine and gastrointestinal secretions also remove organisms.

Germicidal activity

Skin, probably because of the fatty acid content of its secretions, is bactericidal for *Streptococcus pyogenes*. Gram-negative bacilli such as *Escherichia coli, Salmonella typhi, Pseudomonas aeruginosa* and *Proteus* are rapidly killed but the mechanism is obscure. If large numbers of these organisms are placed on healthy skin it may be impossible to recover them an hour later. However, *Klebsiella* may survive for several hours and *Staphylococcus aureus* is highly resistant.

Gastric juice, because of its high acidity, is quickly lethal for most organisms, but *Mycobacterium tuberculosis* is resistant. Ingested organisms may escape destruction because they are lodged in food particles or are protected by diluting or buffering action.

Prostatic secretion contains an antibacterial agent which enters the bladder at the end of micturition. Thus there may be chemical as well as anatomical reasons why urinary infections are about ten times more common in women than men.

Breast milk contains various antibacterial substances including an iron-binding protein which inhibits multiplication of some bacteria, e.g. certain strains of *E. coli*. It also contains an antiviral agent (distinct from antibodies or interferon) which protects babies against rotavirus infection and an agent which kills the protozoon *Giardia lamblia*.

Lysozyme is a mucopolysaccharidase present in the tissues and all body secretions except urine. The enzyme is present in particularly high concentration in tears. It has the ability to lyse and thereby kill some bacteria by breaking down the mucopeptides of their cell walls. Thus colonies of a highly sensitive organism, *Micrococcus lysodeikticus*, are dissolved if treated with tears for a few minutes.

Antibodies, particularly IgA, are present in many secretions. They exert a protective effect, particularly against viruses.

Normal flora

Commensals can cause disease (p. 56), but they also prevent it. Each area of the body surface acquires a characteristic flora well adapted to growth in the particular environment. As in any ecological struggle, e.g. weeds in a field or passengers in a crowded railway carriage, the residents tend to suppress intruders. The mechanisms include competition for space and food supplies and antagonism produced by end-products varying from simple metabolites to complex antibacterial substances such as antibiotics and bacteriocins.

The protective effect of the normal flora is well illustrated by the normal adult vagina. The flora consists almost exclusively of lactobacilli which break down the glycogen of the vaginal epithelium to lactic acid. The high acidity renders the vagina highly resistant to invasion by other organisms. When glycogen is not available (before puberty and after the menopause) the flora is more variable, the reaction of the vaginal secretion tends to be alkaline and invasion by pathogenic organisms is relatively common. Striking evidence for the protective role of the normal flora is provided by diseases such as pseudomembranous colitis, staphylococcal enterocolitis and invasion of the respiratory tract by coliform organisms and yeasts which with rare exceptions occur only when the normal flora has been suppressed by antibiotics (p. 213). The normal flora clearly makes an enormous contribution to 'colonization resistance', i.e. the sum total of local protective mechanisms against pathogenic organisms at particular body sites.

The effects of complete absence of normal flora can be examined experimentally. The developing fetus is sterile. By taking elaborate aseptic precautions it is possible to deliver sterile animal fetuses by Caesarean section and allow them to live and breed in an environment completely free from living organisms. Given a proper diet, these *germ-free animals* are healthy and there is no evidence that the normal flora is an essential source of vitamins or other nutritional factors. If the animals remain in a sterile environment they do not contract infectious disease nor do they produce antibodies against micro-organisms. They are also free from dental caries, although they will develop caries rapidly if fed on a sugar-rich diet and infected with certain streptococci, e.g. *Str. mutans*. Their blood level of immunoglobulins is very low, perhaps only 10% of that found in a normal animal. If they are challenged with micro-organisms they are extremely susceptible to generalized and lethal infection by 'non-pathogenic' organisms such as lacto-bacilli, *Bacillus subtilis* and *Str. faecalis*.

Inner defences

Moderate numbers of organisms regularly gain access to the tissues but rarely cause infection because of the effective clearing action of the body fluids and phagocytic cells.

Body fluids

If serum from a normal person is incubated for a few hours with certain species of bacteria it will kill them (bactericidal action) and may also dissolve them (bacterilysis). These effects are seen most clearly with gram-negative bacteria such as *E. coli* and avirulent strains of *Vibrio cholerae, N. meningitidis, Haemophilus influenzae*, salmonellae and shigellae. Virulent strains of the same species may be insusceptible. Gram-positive organisms are less susceptible to the bactericidal action of normal serum and lysis does not occur. The body fluids also have some power of neutralizing bacterial endotoxins and enzymes and have weak virus neutralizing effects. The substances responsible for these activities include the following:

Lysozyme is an enzyme present in all body fluids.

Complement plays an important role in facilitating phagocytosis and promoting inflammation. It includes components which bind to the surface of bacteria, damage their outer layers, attract phagocytes (polymorphs and macrophages) and help these cells adhere to the coated bacteria (immune adherence). Other components stimulate release of histamine from mast cells (basophils) thereby increasing capillary permeability. The complement system is activated by the *alternative (properdin) pathway* initiated by the direct action of bacteria and their products. The system exerts a non-specific bactericidal effect, particularly against gram-negative bacilli. It also has some antiviral and antiprotozoal activity.

Properdin is a complex system of serum proteins, including two distinct enzymes, which act in conjunction with certain components of complement in the alternative pathway.

β-Lysins are complex heat-stable agents present in normal serum. They are bactericidal for various gram-positive organisms.

Tissue constituents and breakdown products such as protamines, histones, polypeptides and spermine have antibacterial activity, particularly for gram-positive bacteria.

Natural antibodies. The serum of normal individuals contains antibodies active against a wide range of organisms (pathogens and non-pathogens) even though these have not caused overt infection. Thus many gram-negative bacilli are killed or lysed by normal serum due to the combined action of antibodies and complement. These 'natural antibodies' are probably not innate components of the body fluids but represent a specific response to previous subclinical infections and exposure of the tissues to organisms of the normal flora, i.e. natural antibodies are the same as specific antibodies.

Phagocytosis

Phagocytes are body cells which are specialized for the capture, ingestion and destruction of invading micro-organisms. The Russian zoologist Metchnikoff (1884) first recognized that ingestion of foreign particles by leucocytes was analogous to the feeding habits of amoebae and that in the body these cells had assumed a defensive function. Phagocytes are of two types:

1 *Polymorphonuclear leucocytes* ('polymorphs' or neutrophils) are highly motile amoeboid cells present in the blood.
2 *Macrophages* are large mononuclear cells which may be *freely wandering* amoeboid cells in the tissues (histiocytes) and blood (monocytes) or *fixed* reticuloendothelial cells, particularly those lining the blood and lymph sinuses of the liver, spleen, lymph nodes and bone marrow.

Almroth Wright (1903) showed that phagocytes can function efficiently only with the help of plasma constituents known as *opsonins* (from the Greek 'to prepare food'). Washed leucocytes have little or no activity against bacteria suspended in saline, but if a little normal serum is added the bacteria are rapidly ingested. The opsonic function of serum is due to the presence of anti-bodies which combine with the surface antigens of the bacteria and render the organisms more palatable to the phagocytes. The antigen-antibody combination probably exposes a region of the immunoglobulin molecule to which a phagocyte can attach. With avirulent organisms the natural antibodies may suffice, but virulent organisms may be completely resistant to phagocytes unless high levels of specific antibody are available. Phagocytosis is greatly enhanced by complement which is normally present in serum. Both polymorphs and macrophages bear receptors on their surface for the Fc portion of the immunoglobulin molecule and the C3 component of complement.

Phagocytes are more successful in capturing and ingesting organisms if they can trap them against a surface (*surface phago-cytosis*). In the presence of rough surfaces such as filter paper, cloth and fibreglass, phagocytes may be capable of ingesting virulent bacteria in the absence of serum. Fibrin deposits and irregularities in tissue surfaces probably serve the same function *in vivo*. Surface phagocytosis is a much less important defence mechanism than opsonization by antibodies. Thus patients with agammaglobulinaemia are highly susceptible to bacterial infection.

Intrusion of bacteria into the tissues results in an inflammatory reaction. Dilatation and increased permeability of the capillaries facilitates the escape of leucocytes and plasma factors from the blood. In the early stages of infection polymorphs are the most active phagocytes. They migrate to the area in large numbers attracted by certain chemical substances (positive chemotaxis). Persistent demand stimulates the haemopoietic tissues to produce polymorphs and the number in the blood increases (leucocytosis). Deposition of fibrin tends to localize the invaders and helps the polymorphs to trap them. The polymorphs may engulf the organisms rapidly and dispose of them on the spot. Pus consists of poly-morphs ('pus cells') in various stages of disintegration together with the liquefied remains of tissue cells and substances which have been digested by enzymes liberated from the dead cells.

In later stages polymorphs are increasingly replaced by wan-dering macrophages which ingest organisms, damaged polymorphs and tissue debris. In some infections such as tuberculosis and typhoid fever macrophages predominate at an early stage.

The fixed macrophages of the reticuloendothelial system are the ultimate clearing depot. Organisms and infected leucocytes which are not dealt with at the site of infection may enter the lymphatic channels and meet the macrophages lining the sinuses of the lymph nodes or they may gain access to the blood and meet similar cells in the spleen, liver and other organs.

The fate of organisms which enter the blood largely depends on their virulence. When animals are injected intravenously with bacteria which are non-pathogenic or of low virulence, the organisms rapidly and permanently disappear from the blood. Inert particles are dealt with in a similar manner. When highly virulent organisms are injected the initial course of events is much the same, but following partial or apparently complete clearing of the blood, the organisms reappear and multiply rapidly until the animal dies. If, however, the animal possesses specific antibodies against the virulent organisms it may be able to deal with them as effectively as a normal animal deals with avirulent organisms or inert particles.

Organisms which are ingested are usually rapidly killed and digested. The organisms are first segregated in vacuoles. These then fuse with *lysosomes* which are tiny intracellular vacuoles packed with hydrolytic enzymes and antimicrobial cationic pro-teins. However, some species resist destruction for long periods and a few which have a predilection for intracellular growth may even multiply within the phagocytes, e.g. *M. tuberculosis, M. leprae*, brucellae, *Listeria monocytogenes* and *Legionella pneumophila*. The intracellular location of the organisms protects them from antibodies and other antagonistic substances, including chemo-therapeutic agents, in the serum. In such circumstances wandering phagocytes are sometimes an important factor in the transport of organisms to new sites in which they can set up foci of infection.

Various rare immunodeficiency states elegantly illustrate the central role of phagocytes in innate immunity. Thus pyogenic infection is a characteristic feature of such conditions as 'lazy leucocyte syndrome' in which polymorphs fail to respond to normal chemotactic stimuli; Chediak-Higashi disease in which the polymorphs have abnormal lysosomes and show defective chemotaxis and phagocytosis; chronic granulomatous disease in which polymorphs and macrophages take up bacteria but, because of a biochemical defect, fail to kill catalase-positive bacteria. Deficiency of certain components of complement such as C3 may also lead to defective phagocytosis and pyogenic infection.

Disposal of viruses

The body encounters viruses very frequently, but how it disposes of them is obscure. Normal body fluids sometimes possess weak virus neutralizing activity, but the important bactericidal and bacterilytic mechanisms are ineffective against viruses. There is no evidence that polymorphs play any part in the disposal of viruses. Clearance of viruses from the blood is mainly effected by fixed macrophages of the reticuloendothelial system. Wandering macrophages dispose of virus-infected cells.

The role of specific antibodies in providing resistance against viruses is well established but other mechanisms are probably more important in the process of recovery. Thus in the early stages of recovery from viral diseases antibodies are often un-detectable, while in established diseases injection of antibodies usually fails to affect the outcome. Patients with agammaglob-ulinaemia can recover normally from viral infections although they produce no antibodies or only trace amounts. In any case, antibodies do not penetrate cells and cannot inhibit intracellular multiplication.

Small lymphocytes play an important role in the defence against viruses. Thus marked susceptibility to viral infections is a feature of one type of thymic dysplasia in which lymphocyte production is defective although antibody production is normal. In experimental animals and in patients injection of antilymphocyte immunoglobulin increases the susceptibility to viral infections. 'Natural killer' (NK) cells (p. 93) lyse virus-infected cells before viral replication has occurred. Delayed hypersensitivity appears in the course of many viral infections and is mediated by small lymphocytes. However, it comes into effect late in the infectious process and it is difficult to see what part it can play in the early stages of recovery.

Production of interferon may be the most important defence mechanism against viruses. Interferon is usually detectable shortly after infection and long before production of specific antibodies. In general, factors which impair recovery from viral infections depress the interferon response. If mice are injected with anti-bodies against interferon and are then infected with various viruses the illnesses they develop are much more severe than those in controls.

Many viruses will multiply only within narrow ranges of temperature and pH, and an increase in body temperature and a lowering of pH in areas of inflammation are important non-specific defence mechanisms. A raised temperature and a lower pH both increase interferon production.

Factors modifying innate resistance

Genetic factors

These are clearly responsible for the innate resistance of a genus or species to infection by a particular organism, e.g. it is common for an organism to be harmless for one species but highly virulent for another. Genetic factors are also responsible for variation in resistance shown by races, families and individuals. Thus by selective breeding it is possible to obtain strains of mice which are more susceptible or more resistant than the parent stock to infection with *S. typhimurium*, St Louis encephalitis virus or the protozoon *Leishmania donovani*. In man genetic effects cannot easily be dissociated from effects due to nutrition, poverty, overcrowding and other environmental factors. There is evidence that, in the same environment, Negroes, Red Indians and Eskimoes are more susceptible than the white races to *M. tuberculosis*. It is thought that the white races have been exposed to selective elimination of their less resistant members for several thousand years, whereas the other races have been in contact with the organisms for a much shorter period. Reiter's syndrome and multiple sclerosis occur with a higher frequency in people with certain histocompatibility (HLA) antigens. The 20% of the population of the UK who are non-secretors of blood group substances are more susceptible to bacterial meningitis than those who are secretors. Sickle-cell anaemia, an inherited condition, provides protection against *Plasmodium falciparum* malaria but is associated with increased susceptibility to pneumococcal infections. In West Africa the black population is less susceptible than white residents to *P. vivax* malaria. This relative resistance is associated with the absence of Duffy blood group substance in a majority of blacks.

Age

Infants are very susceptible to bacterial infections but relatively insusceptible to the viruses of chickenpox, measles and mumps. Poliomyelitis is more severe in adult life than in early childhood. Susceptibility to bronchitis and pneumonia is increased in old age.

Sex

In the UK most cases of tuberculosis and most of the deaths now occur in old men. Earlier this century cases and deaths were predominantly in children and young adults, particularly women. Following typhoid fever, women carry *S. typhi* in their gall-bladder much more frequently than men. The fungus *Paracoccidioides brasiliensis* infects both sexes equally but overt disease is over ten times more common in men than women.

Hormones

Corticotrophin (adrenocorticotrophic hormone) and corticosteroids inhibit the inflammatory reaction and lower the resistance to bacterial and viral infections. Metabolic derangements due to lack of insulin may be responsible for the susceptibility of diabetics to staphylococcal and tuberculous infections. Oestrogens are necessary for maintaining the resistance of the adult vagina against bacterial invasion.

Fatigue

This has little effect on susceptibility to infections. If animals are exercised to exhaustion on a tread-mill there is occasionally a lighting up of latent infection, but only rarely is there an increase in susceptibility to a fresh infection. In man violent exercise in the early stages of poliomyelitis predisposes to paralysis of those muscles which have been used most actively.

Temperature

Exposure to changes in temperature and sitting in draughts are popularly believed to be the cause of many minor human ills. In fact there is almost no evidence for this in man, but the possibility cannot be ignored since temperature is a determinant in several experimental infections in animals. Thus chickens and frogs are naturally resistant to anthrax, but if chickens are chilled and frogs are warmed they both become susceptible.

Nutrition

In experimental animals gross deficiencies of protein or vitamins A, B and C are usually associated with increased susceptibility to bacterial infections. Paradoxically animals deficient in some of the B vitamins are less susceptible to certain viral infections.

In man it is difficult to distinguish effects of malnutrition from deleterious effects due to overcrowding and unhygienic surroundings. There is evidence from surveys of chronically starved prisoners of war that gross malnutrition increases susceptibility to tuberculosis but has little or no effect on susceptibility to other specific infectious diseases. The incidence of dental caries is reduced. Severe vitamin deficiencies are associated with an increased incidence of superficial infections of skin and mucous membranes. The antibody response of starved individuals is virtually normal but cell-mediated immunity is depressed.

Miscellaneous

Injuries, surgical operations, malignant disease, implanted prostheses and *anatomical abnormalities* frequently determine the onset and localization of infection. Damaged tissues and the presence of *soil* and other *foreign particles* favour growth of clostridia. Silica particles potentiate the effects of *M. tuberculosis* in the lung. *Infection* by one organism often facilitates entry by another, e.g. secondary bacterial infection follows many viral infections. Human immunodeficiency virus (HIV) depresses cell-mediated immunity and leads to the devastating infections characteristic of AIDS. *Irradiation* by X-rays, radioactive isotopes and atomic explosions increases susceptibility by depressing the production of leucocytes and antibodies. Reduction in the numbers of leucocytes also occurs in various *blood diseases* and as a result of exposure to certain *drugs* and *poisons. Immunosuppressive therapy* is used in the treatment of neoplastic and autoimmune disease and in tissue transplantation. Thus steroids, cyclosporin, azathioprine and antilymphocyte immunoglobulin are used to delay or prevent rejection of allografts. Undesirable side effects of such therapy include marked susceptibility to bacterial, viral and fungal infections and an abnormally high incidence of malignant lymphomas. *Acute alcoholism* lowers the efficiency of the inflammatory response.

Enhancement of resistance

Injecting animals with various chemical compounds, inert particles and dead bacteria sometimes produces a temporary, non-specific increase in resistance in a particular organ or in the animal as a whole. Thus certain synthetic polynucleotides non-specifically stimulate antibody production, cellular immunity and interferon production. Naturally occurring myelopeptides present in bone marrow have similar immunity-stimulating properties. Injections of live BCG and killed so-called 'Corynebacterium parvum' have been used to stimulate immunity in patients with malignant disease.

8

Acquired Body Defences

Blood is a special kind of juice.

Goethe

Acquired defence mechanisms are those which depend on specific adaptive reactions to previous contact with micro-organisms or their products.

These defence mechanisms are of two kinds:

1 *Antibody-mediated immunity* ('humoral immunity') which depends on the production of specific antibodies (immunoglobulins).
2 *Cell-mediated immunity* ('cellular immunity') which depends on the development of specifically sensitized cells (T-lymphocytes).

The body's acquired defence reactions against microbial invasion are one aspect of a general physiological mechanism for disposal of complex foreign ('non-self') materials, e.g. antibodies are readily produced against non-microbial antigens such as egg albumin or foreign red blood cells, and sensitized lymphocytes are responsible for the rejection of foreign skin grafts.

The acquired defence reactions differ from the innate reactions in three important respects:

1 They *take time* to develop because antibodies and sensitized lymphocytes do not appear for several days.
2 They are *more powerful* because the antibodies and lymphocytes react specifically against the invading microbes and their products.
3 They leave varying degrees of *acquired immunity* because the body continues to produce antibodies or sensitized lymphocytes for long periods or can produce them at short notice if it meets the same antigen on a subsequent occasion (immunological memory or secondary response).

It will be evident that specificity, immunological memory and the recognition of 'non-self' are the key concepts of immunology.

Antibody-mediated immunity

Behring and Kitasato (1890) showed that if an animal was repeat-edly injected with sublethal doses of tetanus or diphtheria toxin it became resistant to many lethal doses of the toxin and its serum acquired the property of neutralizing the toxin. Further, injection of the serum into normal animals would protect them against the toxin. Shortly afterwards Pfeiffer (1894) showed that the serum and body fluids of animals immunized with *Vibrio cholerae* would kill and dissolve the organisms and that immunity to cholera could be transferred to normal animals by means of the serum. Meanwhile, Ehrlich (1891) showed that substances in the serum were responsible for the immunity that could be produced to toxic substances which had no relation to bacteria, e.g. ricin, a poison derived from the castor oil plant.

These newly acquired properties of the blood and other body fluids are due to *antibodies* produced in response to the stimulus of *antigens*.

An *antigen* is any substance which, when introduced into the tissues of an animal, is capable of provoking an immune response.

An *antibody* is an immunoglobulin which is produced as a result of the introduction of an antigen into the tissues of an animal and which can react specifically with that antigen in some demonstrable way.

The fundamental reaction between an antigen and its specific antibody is that they *combine* with one another. The results of this combination depend on the nature of the antigen and the way it is presented to the antibody, e.g. if the antigen is in solution it is precipitated; if it is part of a cell surface the cell is agglutinated. Antigen-antibody reactions form a major part of the body's acquired defences against microbial invasion.

Cell-mediated immunity

In the early days of immunology it was realized that there were some phenomena which, while clearly of an immunological nature, could not be explained in terms of antibody production. Thus the nature of tuberculin hypersensitivity and its relationship to immunity in tuberculosis was very puzzling. It is now known that many types of specific acquired immune response depend on cell-mediated mechanisms in which small lymphocytes play a key role. These reactions depend on the combination of antigens with specific antigen-binding groups on the surface of sensitized T-lymphocytes. Serum antibodies (immunoglobulins) are not involved.

Cell-mediated mechanisms are the basis of delayed hypersensitivity, contact dermatitis and the rejection of allografts. They are important in overcoming infections caused by viruses, bacteria which have a predilection for intracellular growth, fungi and protozoa. Many autoimmune diseases such as thyroiditis and uveitis depend in part on cell-mediated mechanisms. Small lymphocytes provide a biological mechanism by which the body can deal with antigens which are unable to reach the lymphoid tissues and excite antibody production. Cell-mediated immunity is probably the mechanism by which the body rids itself of mutant cells (potential tumours) arising in the course of normal cell division. If such a mechanism for policing the body for malignant cells did not exist the incidence of cancer would probably be vastly greater.

Role of lymphocytes

Lymphoid tissues include the spleen, lymph nodes and various lymphoid accumulations of which the most important is the gut-associated lymphoid tissue including the tonsils, Peyer's patches and solitary follicles. Small lymphocytes circulate between the blood and the lymphoid tissues.

The part played by lymphocytes in immunological responses can best be explained by assuming that stem cells originating in the bone marrow differentiate into two distinct populations of lymphocytes, T-lymphocytes and B-lymphocytes (Fig. 20, p. 92). Both populations contain antigen-sensitive cells, but whereas most T-lymphocytes circulate in the blood and extravascular fluids and encounter their antigens anywhere in the body, most B-lymphocytes remain in the lymphoid tissues and their antigens have to be brought to them. Many marker tests have now been developed by which T-cells and B-cells can be distinguished and enumerated with reasonable certainty, e.g. sheep red cells form rosettes around T-cells; fluorescent monoclonal antibodies can be used to identify T-cells and B-cells and differentiate them into various subpopulations.

Thymus-dependent T-lymphocytes depend on normal functioning of the thymus in early life. Antigens are first processed by mononuclear phagocytes (macrophages) which release soluble products known as *monokines*, e.g. interleukin-1. These activate T-lymphocytes. The T-lymphocytes transform into lymphoblasts which divide and release chemical mediators known as *lymphokines*, e.g. interleukin-2. These activate the mechanisms responsible for cell-mediated immune processes such as graft rejection, delayed hypersensitivity and cellular immunity.

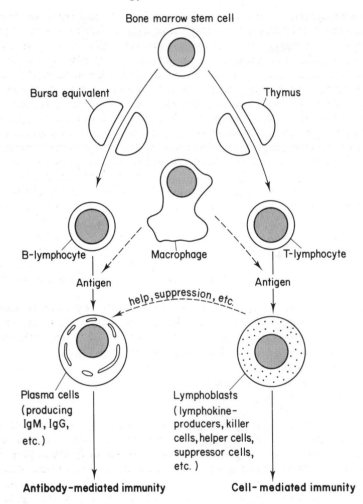

Fig. 20 Role of lymphocytes in humoral and cellular immunity.

T-lymphocytes also produce a population of antigen-sensitive lymphocytes which provide the basis of 'immunological memory'. The interactions of T-lymphocytes with other cells occur only if they share the same major histocompatibility complex (MHC). The phenomenon is known as *MHC restriction*. Thus before T-lymphocytes will kill a virus-infected target cell they must recognize both the foreign viral antigen and the 'self' MHC antigens. T-lymphocytes constitute the major part of the circulating pool of small lymphocytes and have a long life-span, probably several years.

Bursa-equivalent B-lymphocytes proliferate and mature into specialized antibody-producing plasma cells. The presence of an antigen stimulates production of plasma cells manufacturing immunoglobulins with the appropriate specificity. These immunoglobulins are responsible for humoral immunity. Plasma cells have a relatively short life-span, usually only a few days. Other B-lymphocytes become 'memory cells' which are responsible for the secondary response (p. 105). Production of antibodies against most antigens is thymus-dependent and is thought to depend on some form of cooperation between certain T-lymphocytes ('helper cells') and B-lymphocytes. However, only the B-lymphocytes effect the actual synthesis of immunoglobulins. In some circumstances other T-lymphocytes ('suppressor cells') inhibit production of antibodies by B-lymphocytes. B-lymphocytes are mainly restricted to lymphoid tissue. They are called 'bursa-equivalent' lymphocytes because in birds antibody production, but not cell-mediated immunity, depends on cells of a separate organ known as the bursa of Fabricius. The mammalian equivalent of the bursa itself has not been defined but may prove to be haemopoietic tissue in general.

Null cells. A small proportion (1—10%) of lymphocytes are neither B-cells nor T-cells. These 'null' cells include non-specific 'natural killer' (NK) cells which in the absence of antibody are cytolytic for certain tumours and virus-infected cells.

Role of the thymus

The thymus is essential for the development of immunological mechanisms. Its main function is probably to elaborate a factor that induces immunological competence in small lymphocytes. If the thymus is removed from a newborn mouse the animal completely or partially loses the ability to develop delayed hypersensitivity following appropriate sensitization, to reject skin grafts from foreign strains of mice and in some cases from rats as well, and to produce antibodies against certain antigens, although immunoglobulin levels are usually not affected. There is a great diminution in the number of small lymphocytes in the blood, lymph, spleen and lymph nodes and the animal develops a fatal wasting disease 1—4 months later. These effects are greatly diminished if thymectomy is delayed for a few days and in adult mice the effects of thymectomy are negligible. Normal immunological functions can be restored to neonatally thymectomized animals by transplanting normal thymus tissue or by injecting cells from the spleen or lymph nodes of normal mice. Thymus cells themselves are usually ineffective.

The importance of the thymus is also illustrated by 'nude

mice', a breed of hairless mice which do not have a thymus or T-lymphocytes. The animals have defective cell-mediated immunity. They will readily accept grafts of human cancers and can be used to test anti-cancer drugs.

Similar deficiencies of immunity are found in certain rare human congenital diseases. In one type of thymic dysplasia (Di George syndrome) there is a deficiency of T-cell function and, although plasma cells and antibodies are produced normally, lymphocyte production and cellular immunity are impaired. Affected infants are highly susceptible to viral infections. In another type of thymic dysplasia (severe combined immunodeficiency or SCID) the lymphoid stem cells fail to differentiate properly and there is a gross deficiency of both T-cell and B-cell function. The thymus is extremely small, lymphoid tissue and plasma cells are absent and there is virtually no humoral or cellular immunity. Many patients lack the enzyme adenosine deaminase. Affected infants usually die before the age of three, but a few have survived following bone marrow transplantation. If the gene for production of adenosine deaminase could be introduced into bone marrow cells of patients who lack the enzyme, SCID could become the first human disease to be treated by gene therapy.

Antigens

Antigens are characterized by complex molecules with a molecular weight of 10 000 daltons or greater. Most antigens consist of protein or protein combined with other substances. Proteins vary in their antigenic power, e.g. bacterial exotoxins are powerful antigens, but gelatin is almost complete devoid of antigenicity. Other substances possessing the requisite size and complexity to function as antigens are certain highly complicated polysaccharides and polysaccharide-lipid complexes. Antigenicity is not confined to substances of biological origin and some completely synthetic macromolecular polypeptides are antigenic.

Haptens

Haptens or partial antigens are substances which cannot themselves stimulate the production of antibodies but which acquire antigenicity when they are coupled to protein. This may occur artificially when a substance is coupled to a protein in the laboratory or naturally when a substance is combined with protein in the body. Substances are occasionally rendered antigenic if they are attached to large non-protein particles such as collodion. Haptens are of two types:

Complex haptens are substances with large molecules. When they combine with antibody prepared against the complete antigenic complex a *visible precipitate* is produced. The distinction between complex haptens and antigens is not always clear-cut.

Simple haptens are relatively simple chemical substances. When they combine with antibody prepared against the complete antigenic complex there is *no precipitate*. Evidence that combination has taken place is provided by the fact that the antibody is no longer capable of precipitating the complete antigen.

Artificial antigens

Landsteiner made the important observation that if simple non-protein molecules (simple haptens) are coupled with a protein they may largely determine the antigenic properties of the complex as a whole. For this reason haptens are often referred to as *determinant groups (epitopes)*. If such a complex is injected into animals antibodies are produced which react not only with the complete conjugated protein but also with the pure hapten. The antigenic properties of the conjugated protein are sometimes almost completely different from those of the original protein. Spontaneous attachment of a hapten to a body protein may account for specific hypersensitivity to many non-antigenic substances such as drugs and simple chemicals (Chapter 11).

Bacterial antigens

A bacterium typically contains a large number of antigens. As a rule only a small proportion of these are of importance in infection and immunity. In the laboratory detailed antigenic analysis may be necessary for identification of an organism. Bacterial antigens fall into two groups:

1 *Soluble antigens* are products excreted into the environment, e.g. exotoxins, enzymes, haemolysins, etc. Most of them are protein. Superficial cellular antigens, particularly capsules, often dissolve to some extent in the surrounding fluids.
2 *Cellular antigens* are surface structures of the cell. They may be:
a. *Capsular antigens.* These constitute the capsule of the organism. They are often polysaccharide, e.g. *Streptococcus pneumoniae* and *Klebsiella pneumoniae*, but are sometimes polypeptide, e.g. *Bacillus anthracis*, or protein, e.g. *Yersinia pestis*.
b. *Flagellar or H antigens.* H is from the German word *Hauch* which implies the sort of film that forms if one breathes on a cold window pane. H was originally used to describe the thin

swarming growth on solid media of motile (flagellated) strains of *Proteus*, but is now applied to flagellar antigens in general. H antigens are proteins. The flagella of a particular organism often contain several distinct H antigens. Organisms that never have flagella, e.g. *Shigella*, do not have H antigens.

c. *Somatic or O antigens.* These are present in the body of the bacteria. O is from *ohne Hauch* (without a film) and was originally used to describe the growth of non-motile strains of *Proteus* (ordinary colonies), but is now applied to somatic antigens in general. O antigens may be protein, protein-polysaccharide or protein-polysaccharide-lipid. Bacteria usually have several O antigens.

d. *Other antigens.* The *Vi (virulence) antigens* of organisms such as *Salmonella typhi* and the *K (Kapsel) antigens* of *Escherichia coli* are superficial envelope or capsular antigens which sometimes mask the ordinary O antigens. *Fimbrial antigens* are surface antigens present in the fimbriae of gram-negative bacilli: on rare occasions they cause confusion in serological tests.

Viral antigens

Viruses are antigenically less complicated than bacteria. Many of them contain only three or four antigens, sometimes corresponding to known structural features such as the capsid, the envelope or surface projections. Some complicated viruses have more antigens. Thus vaccinia virus contains seven or eight antigens including a complex surface antigen with heat-labile and heat-stable components, a nucleoprotein antigen, a haemagglutinin and a protective antigen stimulating immunity. With many viruses a distinction is made between two types of antigens:

1 *Viral or V antigens* form part of the surface of the intact virion. During viral infections V antigens stimulate production of antibodies which can specifically neutralize the infectivity of the virus. These antibodies are important in immunity.

2 *Soluble or S antigens* are diffusible substances liberated into the surrounding fluids during viral growth. Antibodies against S antigens cannot usually neutralize the virus but they can be detected in other ways, e.g. by complement fixation and gel-diffusion methods. Many viruses are known to produce S antigens including influenza, mumps, herpes, rabies and adenoviruses. Some of these S antigens are complex mixtures, e.g. the S antigen extracted from cells infected with herpes virus consists of at least ten components. S antigens are of two types:

a. *Structural S antigens.* Many S antigens are constituents of the virion, e.g. the soluble nucleoprotein antigens of influenza and mumps viruses. Such S antigens probably represent a part of the virus which has been manufactured in excess during viral multiplication.

b. *Non-structural S antigens.* Other S antigens cannot be found in purified virions and many of them are completely new non-structural proteins formed in the cell as a result of viral infection. Thus by gel-diffusion methods 17 antigens are found in extracts of skin infected with vaccinia virus but only seven of these can be found in disrupted virions. Non-structural S antigens are virus-specific, i.e. their structure is specified by the genes of the virus. Evidence for production of new proteins by virus-infected cells is also provided by biochemical methods. Thus entirely new enzymes are formed when a virus infects a cell.

Human antigens

The antigenic make-up of man is extremely complex. The red cell antigens which determine human blood groups have been extensively studied because of their importance in blood transfusion and rhesus disease. Now that tissue transplantation is an accepted clinical procedure *tissue typing*, commonly performed on lymphocytes, is used to ensure that tissue antigens (histocompatibility antigens) of donor and recipient are matched as closely as possible. The major histocompatibility complex (MHC) of man, also known as the HLA (human leucocyte antigen) system, consists of a group of 'strong' antigens which have a predominant influence in determining whether or not a graft will survive. In autoimmune diseases antibodies are produced against various organ-specific antigens.

Heterophile antigens

Antigens with haptenic groups of very similar or identical structure are widely distributed in nature. Thus the rickettsiae of epidemic typhus share a polysaccharide hapten with certain strains of *Proteus* (the basis of the Weil-Felix reaction). *Treponema pallidum* possesses a lipid complex which is antigenically related to similar complexes in normal human and animal tissues (the basis of the Wassermann reaction and the VDRL test). The virus of infectious mononucleosis (EB virus) shares an antigenic component with sheep red cells (the basis of the Paul-Bunnell test).

Antibodies

Antibodies are a heterogeneous group of globulins mainly found in the plasma. Separation of globulins from other plasma constituents yields a complex mixture of antibodies. Specific antibodies can be obtained in a higher state of purity by recovery from antigen-antibody complexes. Only a monoclonal antibody can properly be regarded as a pure antibody.

Antibodies are indistinguishable from normal plasma globulins in all their ordinary physical and chemical properties. Since antibodies are protein they are also antigenic, i.e. they will stimulate the production of antibodies in another animal (see p. 96).

Most antibodies are gammaglobulins, i.e. they are found in the slowest moving fraction on electrophoresis. However, this fraction is represented by a diffuse band and some antibodies migrate between the β and γ fractions. Similarly, while most antibodies have a molecular weight of about 150 000 daltons and a characteristic sedimentation coefficient of 7S, antibody activity is also often found in a 19S component of molecular weight about 900 000 daltons. Chemical analysis of different antibody fractions shows that these have different properties, e.g. they differ in their carbohydrate content. Finally, immunological methods have shown the existence of distinct classes of antibodies. All the different sorts of antibodies are grouped together under the single functional term immunoglobulin or Ig.

Immunoglobulins

'Immunoglobulin' is the generic term used for all types of proteins with antibody activity, and for certain structurally related proteins with no known antibody activity, e.g. myeloma proteins.

Five classes of immunoglobulins are recognized: IgG, IgA, IgM, IgE and IgD. All have the same basic structure of four linked polypeptide chains: two of the chains have a molecular weight of 50 000 daltons and are known as *heavy chains* and two have a molecular weight of 20 000 daltons and are known as *light chains*. The complete immunoglobulin unit is a Y-shaped molecule which swings open at the 'hinge' on combination with antigen (Fig. 21). The heavy chains differ markedly in each class of immunoglobulin and are responsible for the distinctive physicochemical and antigenic properties of that class. The heavy chains are designated γ, α, μ, ε and δ to match the parent classes IgG, IgA, IgM, IgE and IgD. The light chains, in contrast, are similar in the five classes and are associated with properties common to all the immunoglobulins. The light chains are of two types designated *kappa* (κ) and *lambda* (λ). These are both present in all five classes but are carried on separate immunoglobulin molecules. Each class of immunoglobulin has therefore two types of molecules: type K with κ-chains and type L with λ-chains. Roughly two-thirds of immunoglobulin molecules are type K and one-third type L.

In addition, the classes are themselves heterogeneous and several subclasses and inherited variants or allotypes are recognized. In the disease myelomatosis the immunoglobulins (myeloma proteins) are idiotypic, i.e. unique to a particular patient.

When an individual is immunized against a single antigen the specific antibodies produced usually consist of a mixture of IgG, IgA and IgM. The amount of each produced varies slightly with the nature of the antigen, the stage of immunity and other factors. The different classes have properties which appear to adapt them for different biological functions.

IgG is a 7S globulin of molecular weight 150 000 daltons. Each molecule has two identical combining sites for antigens (Fig. 22A and 22B, p. 100). IgG is the most abundant immunoglobulin and has a serum concentration of 8–16 g/litre. It diffuses into all tissue fluids and secretions except the cerebrospinal fluid, and by an active transporting process it is the only immunoglobulin which can cross the placental barrier from mother to fetus. Most antibodies arising as a result of natural infections or immunization are IgG. IgG is most effective in neutralizing soluble antigens such as exotoxins and very small particulate antigens such as viruses. Four subclasses of human IgG are recognized: IgG1, IgG2, IgG3 and IgG4. They differ in their biological properties, e.g. the IgG antibody response to polysaccharide antigens resides

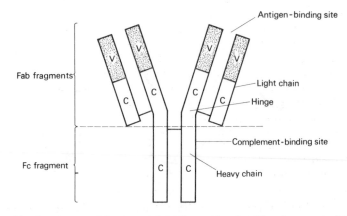

Fig. 21 Structure of immunoglobulin molecule. The heavy and light chains are linked by disulphide bridges and divided into regions of variable (V) and constant (C) amino acid composition.

predominantly within the IgG2 subclass, whereas IgG antibodies to protein antigens are mainly IgG1 and IgG3.

IgA is a 7S globulin of molecular weight 160 000 daltons but it may polymerize giving 9S and 11S fractions and molecular weights of up to about 360 000 daltons. Each molecule has two or more combining sites (Fig. 22D). IgA has a serum concentration of 1.4–4.2 g/litre. It is actively secreted into colostrum, milk, saliva, respiratory secretions and intestinal juice and may reach higher concentrations than IgG in these fluids. The secreted form of IgA consists of two immunoglobulin units and an additional poly-peptide chain, the secretory component, synthesized by the local epithelial cells. IgA plays a protective role on mucous surfaces, particularly against viruses.

IgM is a 19S macroglobulin with a molecular weight of 900 000 daltons. The molecule consists of five of the basic immunoglobulin units and has ten identical combining sites (Fig. 22C). IgM is predominantly intravascular and has a serum concentration of 0.5–2.0 g/litre. IgM is the main immunoglobulin produced in the very early response to an antigen encountered for the first time

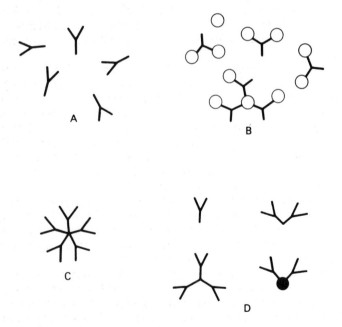

Fig. 22 Classes of immunoglobulins. A, IgG, consisting of single units. B, IgG plus antigen, showing the two combining sites of IgG. C, IgM, consisting of five units. D, IgA, consisting of one, two or three units, and its secreted form of two units plus the secretory component.

(primary response). Because of its multiple combining sites, IgM is adapted to dealing with large particulate antigens such as the surface of cells which have large numbers of identical antigenic sites. It is particularly effective in promoting agglutination, opsonization and, in the presence of complement , lysis of bacteria.

IgE is normally present in the serum in extremely small amounts (about 40 μg/litre). It is the homocytotrophic antibody (reagin) responsible for the anaphylactic type of hypersensitivity. High levels of IgE occur in infections with intestinal worms. It may play a role in the defence against such parasites.

IgD has no readily detectable antibody function. It has been suggested that it acts as an antigen receptor on the surface of lymphocytes.

Specificity

The most striking property of an antibody is that it is specific in its action, e.g. an antibody produced against tetanus toxin has no action against diphtheria toxin and *vice versa*. However, specificity is not an absolute term. It implies that an antibody reacts most strongly with the antigen that stimulated its production. The antibody usually has weaker activity against closely related antigens.

If human serum is injected into a rabbit, antibodies are produced which react strongly with human serum but not at all with the serum of horses, cows, cats, dogs, rats, mice or chickens. They may, however, give quite a strong reaction with the serum of chimpanzees and other apes and may give a weak reaction with the serum of some monkeys. Similarly, antibodies against artificial antigens react strongly with the conjugated protein or haptenic group used for immunization, but give lesser reactions with haptens of similar chemical structure.

Specific antibody activity must depend on the chemical structure of the individual immunoglobulins. The light and heavy chains of immunoglobulins are peculiar in having *variable* and *constant* regions of amino acid composition. Specificity is mediated by particular amino acid sequences in the variable regions of the light and heavy chains. These are situated in a part of the molecule known as the antigen-binding fragment or Fab fragment (Fig. 21, p. 99). The basic immunoglobulin unit has two Fab fragments, each with a single combining site. The remainder of the immuno-globulin molecule, a single fragment known as the Fc fragment, has other functions. Thus the 'complement cascade' is triggered by a conformational change in the Fc fragment brought about by the specific combination of the Fab fragments with antigen.

Immunoglobulin molecules themselves bear antigenic determinants, some of which are unique or idiotypic. When an antibody (Ab-1) is used as an antigen the resulting antibodies (Ab-2) may be: *anti-isotypes* which bind to the Ab-1 that induced them as well as to other antibodies of the same class; *anti-allotypes* which react with all antibodies from the individual which produced Ab-1; or *anti-idiotypes* which react only to the antibody elicited by a single antigen. Anti-idiotypes themselves bear idiotypes and can in turn stimulate production of anti-anti-idiotypes (Ab-3), and so on. Because anti-idiotypes recognize the molecular individuality of the primary antibody and carry an 'internal image' of the original antigen it is likely that in the future anti-idiotypes will be used as vaccines against infectious agents.

Antibodies are sometimes encountered which have an unexpectedly wide range of reactivity. They are not an exception to the rule that antibodies are specific, but reflect the fact that some antigens (heterophile antigens) are shared by completely different types of living organisms.

'C-reactive protein', so called because it precipitates pneumococcal C substance, appears in increased amounts in the blood of patients with a wide variety of diseases. It owes its reactivity to chance chemical structure. It is *not* an antibody. Like a raised erythrocyte sedimentation rate (ESR) it is a non-specific indicator of inflammation and tissue damage.

Site of formation

Antibodies are formed by cells of the lymphoid tissues, particularly in the spleen, lymph nodes and bone marrow. When an animal has been sufficiently stimulated with antigens a high concentration of antibodies can be detected in the spleen and lymph nodes and these organs continue to produce antibodies if grown in tissue culture or transplanted into other animals.

Antibody formation is to some extent a local process. The most active cells are those which are most exposed to the antigen. Thus following injection of antigen into the foot-pad or ear of a rabbit antibodies are detected first and in highest concentration in the local lymph nodes and their efferent lymphatics. The spleen is the most important single source of antibodies when antigens gain access to the blood.

By using fluorescent antibody techniques to stain antigens and antibodies in tissue sections it has been shown that macrophages are mainly responsible for taking up antigens and that plasma cells are responsible for forming antibodies. Following immunization there is a great increase in the number of plasma cells in the red pulp of the spleen and the medulla of lymph nodes, and special staining shows that antibody is almost entirely confined to these cells. Single plasma cells suspended in fluid have been shown to produce antibody. Indirect evidence for this special role of plasma cells is given by the almost complete absence of plasma cells and antibodies in germ-free animals and individuals with agammaglobulinaemia and the association of large numbers of plasma cells and hyperglobulinaemia in myelomatosis.

By using fluorescent antibodies specific for the heavy and light chains of immunoglobulins it can be shown that individual plasma cells are restricted in the immunoglobulins they can produce, e.g. a particular plasma cell might produce IgG but not IgA or IgM; further, the molecules of IgG in that cell will have κ and λ chains but not both. However, in certain circumstances a plasma cell can switch production from one class of immunoglobulin to another, e.g. from IgM to IgG. The full range of immunoglobulins found in an individual depends on a mixed population of plasma cells, with individual cells manufacturing a particular immunoglobulin.

This specialization of immunoglobulin producing cells is reflected in the immunoglobulins synthesized in the diseases myelomatosis and macroglobulinaemia. In virtually every case the immunoglobulins are remarkably homogeneous in class, type and minor antigenic features, e.g. in myelomatosis the Bence Jones protein in the urine consists of light chains of one or other type corresponding to the type of the abnormal protein in the plasma. In certain syndromes associated with deficiency of antibody production a selective depression of immunoglobulin synthesis occurs and one or two of the main classes or subclasses of immunoglobulins fail to appear.

Mechanism of formation

The way in which an antigen directs globulin synthesis to the production of molecules specifically orientated towards itself is still obscure, but experimental findings are consistent with the *clonal selection theory*. It is assumed that the antibody-forming tissues consist of a mixed population of genetically distinct cells which collectively can synthesize globulins with a vast number of different configurations capable of reacting with all possible antigens but which individually can only synthesize globulins capable of reacting with a single antigen or a small range of antigens. When an antigen is introduced into the body it combines with the small number of pre-existing cells which produce globulins with the appropriate configuration and by some selective process preferentially stimulates multiplication of this type of cell. The result is a family or *clone* of cells all producing globulin (antibody) of the same sort. Because an antibody normally represents the combined products of many different clones it is described as *polyclonal*. The great diversity of antibodies is largely explained by the fact that they are encoded by several hundred scattered gene fragments which can combine in millions of different ways.

Monoclonal antibodies

Large quantities of highly specific antibodies can be obtained by cell-fusion techniques. Plasma cells are short-lived and produce only minute quantities of antibodies in tissue culture. However, by taking plasma cells from the spleen of a mouse immunized against a particular antigen and fusing them with suitable malignant cells such as mouse myeloma cells it is possible to obtain antibody-producing hybrid cells or *hybridomas* which will replicate themselves indefinitely. By selection it is possible to obtain a clone which manufactures a single antibody of the required specificity. The clone can be frozen for long-term storage. Cells can subsequently be grown in tissue culture or they can be injected into a mouse where they induce myelomas which produce the antibody. Monoclonal antibodies are important tools used to identify antigens of bacteria and viruses, to purify substances such as interferon and antigens used for bacterial and viral vaccines, and for blood and tissue typing and the immunohistological classification of lymphomas and other malignant tumours. It is also possible to create human hybridomas, e.g. a human monoclonal antibody against *E. coli* endotoxin has been used to treat gram-negative bacteraemia. If malignant cells are found to possess specific surface antigens monoclonal antibodies could form the basis for new therapeutic agents which attack cancer cells but spare normal ones, e.g. monoclonal antibodies linked to the poison ricin.

Factors influencing antibody formation

Number and spacing of doses of antigen

The immune response when an animal encounters an antigen for the first time is different from the response when it encounters the same antigen on subsequent occasions. This applies in humoral immunity and in cellular immunity, and is best illustrated in terms of antibody production (Fig. 23).

Primary response. Following a first injection of a soluble antigen there is a *latent period* (commonly a week or more) before antibodies (mainly IgM) can be detected. There is then a *slow rise* to reach a *low maximum level*. This is followed by a slow decline in

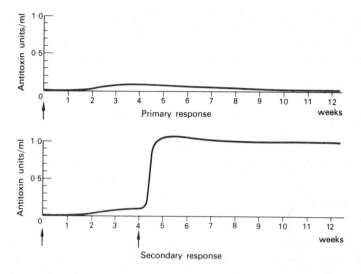

Fig. 23 Primary and secondary responses. Antibody titres (units of tetanus antitoxin/ml) in a patient's serum after subcutaneous injection of an antigen (tetanus toxoid) at the times indicated by the arrows.

which antibody may be detected in very small amounts for some months.

Secondary response. If a second injection is given at this stage antibodies (mainly IgG) are produced with *little delay* (usually a day or so). There is a *rapid rise* to reach a *high maximum level.* The level then falls, rapidly at first, but *persists* for a longer period and at a higher level than in the primary response.

The response to further injections resembles the secondary response. The level of antibodies becomes greater and more sustained until it reaches a maximum for the individual.

The importance of the primary response is not the production of antibodies, which may be negligible, but the conditioning or education of the antibody-forming tissues to respond promptly and powerfully on subsequent occasions. Full development of this *immunological memory* takes several weeks. A second injection given the day after the first injection will excite no additional antibody response and for the next few days the additional response to a further injection is usually trivial. In the immunization of human beings there is nothing to be gained by injecting an antigen at intervals of less than 7−10 days and the ultimate response is invariably greater if the interval is four weeks or longer. Once immunological memory has been established it lasts for life. Even when circulating antibodies are no longer detectable the specific reactivity remains and the antigen may excite a typical secondary response.

Physical state of antigen

Particulate antigens such as intact bacterial cells usually give a better immune response than soluble antigens. This is probably because particulate antigens are eliminated more slowly. The antigenicity of soluble antigens is enhanced if they are adsorbed to *adjuvants*, e.g. aluminium compounds increase the antigenicity of diphtheria and tetanus toxoids for human use. Antigens become fixed in the area of inflammation produced by the adjuvant.

Route of administration of antigen

Antigens reach the tissues spontaneously in the course of overt infections and in the repeated minor intrusions into the body by organisms of the normal flora. Soluble antigens may sometimes gain access through the intestinal tract, but most are either digested or very poorly absorbed. Some antigens can enter in small amounts through the respiratory tract. Hypersensitivity to pollens and dusts is probably acquired by this route. Antigens are deliberately introduced into the tissues in the course of immunization. The route of injection is not normally critical although some antigens are more effective if introduced by one route rather than by another.

Dose of antigen

No antibodies appear if the dose is below a threshold value, but a minute dose is often enough to condition the antibody-forming tissues. The response increases with size of dose, but once a well-defined response is obtained a large increase in dose results in a relatively small increase in response. A given amount of antigen is more effective if given in several spaced doses.

Mixtures of antigens

The body can respond to several distinct antigens given simultaneously. Rabbits given a mixture of 35 distinct antigens produced separate antibodies to 34 of them. A combined vaccine of tetanus toxoid, diphtheria toxoid and *Bordetella pertussis* gives excellent results in children. The body responds preferentially to an antigen present in excessive amount, but if antigens are present in ideal proportions the response to each may be as great as if it were administered alone.

Age of animal

Immunoglobulin formation begins in fetal life but only minute amounts are produced before birth. Newborn infants have few plasma cells in their tissues and the small amount of immunoglobulin in their blood is mainly of maternal origin. Ability to produce immunoglobulins develops slowly and is not efficient for several months.

Individual variation

The response to a standard dose of antigen varies enormously. Some individuals are incapable of producing antibodies (agammaglobulinaemia, see below). Selective breeding in animals has shown that variations in antibody response depend on genetic factors.

Agammaglobulinaemia

In its most severe form this is a rare congenital disease affecting males, characterized by repeated bacterial infections beginning in infancy or early childhood. No antibodies are produced as a result of natural infections or injected antigens and normal blood group antibodies fail to appear. The serum contains no gamma-globulins (immunoglobulins) or only traces and the tissues contain few or no plasma cells. The disease represents a deficiency of B-cell function. Study of these cases has confirmed that mechanisms other than those involving circulating antibodies are important in human immunity. Common viral infections such as measles, chickenpox and mumps may run a normal course and, although exceptions have been reported, be followed by clinical immunity. The patients also develop the delayed type of hypersensitivity, e.g. to tuberculin following vaccination with BCG. These processes depend on cell-mediated immunity which is a T-cell function. Similar though less severe forms of the disease may occur in either sex as a transient state in early infancy or as an acquired disease at any time in life. Patients with agammaglobulinaemia or hypogammaglobulinaemia can usually be maintained in good health by means of antibiotics and injections of immunoglobulin. In severe combined immunodeficiency (SCID) agammaglobulinaemia is associated with defective cellular immunity and the outlook is bleak.

Presence of preformed antibody

Preformed antibody diminishes the response to the antigen by combining with it and hastening its elimination. A fall of antibody level, or *negative phase*, is often seen in the first stages of a secondary response, particularly when the antigen is introduced directly into the circulation. Because of the effects of preformed antibody it is usually advisable to postpone the immunization of infants against measles until they are at least nine months old and have had time to eliminate any antibodies they may have acquired from the mother. Antigens and antibodies never entirely neutralize each other in the body. If essential, it is possible to give a non-immune person both immediate and future protection against diphtheria or tetanus by injecting a small dose of preformed antibody (antitoxin) in one site and antigen (toxoid) in another.

Anamnestic reaction

In an individual who has been well immunized with a particular antigen a rise in the level of specific antibody may be brought about by *non-specific* stimuli such as injection of unrelated antigens, intercurrent infections and fever. The mechanisms are obscure.

Immunological tolerance and autoimmunity

An animal can readily produce an immune response (humoral and cell-mediated) against 'foreign' antigens but does not normally react against the innumerable antigens present in its own tissues. This aversion to self-destruction was called by Ehrlich *horror autotoxicus*. The immunological mechanisms must somehow be able to distinguish 'self' and 'non-self'. In fact this distinction is not absolute. In certain circumstances the body fails to react against foreign antigens (*immunological tolerance*) and in other circumstances it produces an immune response against its own antigens (*autoimmunization*).

Immunological tolerance

If a foreign antigen is repeatedly encountered at an early stage of development the antigen becomes accepted as 'self' and ability to produce an immune response against it is delayed and sometimes suppressed indefinitely. This is a naturally occurring state of affairs in a *chimera*, an animal in which living cells of another individual coexist with its own. Thus in dizygotic (binovular) cattle twins the blood of each individual not infrequently contains a mixture of two antigenically distinct types of red cells, one derived from each twin. Haemopoietic tissue has evidently been exchanged across the shared fetal membranes *in utero* and the 'foreign' cells from the other twin have been permanently accepted as 'self'. A similar condition occurs very rarely in human dizygotic twins.

Immune tolerance can be analysed more thoroughly in artifical chimeras. *Allografts*, i.e. grafts between dissimilar strains of the same species, fail to take because the grafts are destroyed by cell-mediated processes (allograft reaction). If, however, a fetal mouse is inoculated while still *in utero* with living donor cells of a dissimilar strain the normal immunological response is suppressed and skin grafts from that donor will be accepted in later life. The tolerance acquired is specific and there is no impairment of ability to reject grafts from a third unrelated strain. Tolerance is abolished if the tolerant recipient bearing a foreign skin graft is injected with lymph node or spleen cells from a mouse of the same strain that has previously been immunized against donor-strain skin: there is rapid rejection of the hitherto tolerated graft.

Persistence of the antigenic stimulus is necessary to maintain immunological tolerance. The lifelong tolerance of allografts is probably due to the continued presence of descendants of the cells originally injected. Non-living antigens such as red cells, simple proteins and bacterial and viral antigens can produce varying degrees of tolerance, but tolerance will often change to active immunity if the animal is not repeatedly exposed to the particular antigen.

Autoimmunization

A limited number of body constituents which are normally se-gregated from the antibody-forming tissues and which are there-fore unable to establish or maintain immunological tolerance behave as foreign antigens and stimulate the production of anti-bodies (*autoantibodies*) if they are injected into the same animal from which they were obtained. Thus a rabbit can be immunized against its own spermatozoa or the lens protein from its own eyes. In general, however, injection of unmodified tissue extracts does not stimulate autoantibody production, although this will often occur if the extracts are injected with a powerful adjuvant. The appearance of autoantibodies is often associated with pathological lesions in the organ from which the antigen was obtained, e.g. injection of brain tissue produces demyelinating encephalomyelitis; injection of thyroglobulin produces thyroiditis.

The spontaneous appearance of circulating autoantibodies and the development of delayed hypersensitivity to tissue antigens indicate that many human diseases depend at least in part on autoimmunization. Sensitive immunofluorescent techniques for detecting autoantibodies have been particularly valuable in drawing attention to the frequency and diversity of such diseases. They range from those which are organ-specific to those which affect many organs. They include Hashimoto's thyroiditis (inflammation of the thyroid; antibodies react with thyroglobulin and other thyroid antigens), thyrotoxicosis (hyperthyroidism; antibodies react with surface antigens of thyroid cells and cause cell stimulation), pernicious anaemia (macrocytic anaemia; antibodies react with intrinsic factor and parietal cells of the stomach and interfere with absorption of vitamin B12), autoimmune haemolytic anaemia (haemolysis; antibodies react with red cells), sympathetic ophthalmia (damage to one eye results in uveitis and loss of sight in the other eye; antibodies react with the iris, ciliary body, etc.), rheumatoid arthritis (widespread lesions; 'rheumatoid factors' react with altered IgG), and systemic lupus erythematosus (lesions throughout the body; 'antinuclear factors' react with DNA, cell nuclei and many other antigens). In other autoimmune diseases the brunt of the damage falls on the central nervous system (certain demyelinating diseases), adrenals (Addison's disease), spermatozoa (some cases of male infertility), skin (pemphigus vulgaris), platelets (idiopathic thrombocytopenic purpura), salivary and lacrimal glands (Sjögren's syndrome), liver (some types of hepatitis and cirrhosis), kidney (some types of nephritis), pancreas (juvenile diabetes), colon (ulcerative colitis) and various tissues (dermatomyositis). Some autoimmune diseases are due to the action of antibodies against hormone and transmitter receptors on cell surfaces, e.g. acetylcholine receptors of muscle in myasthenia gravis; insulin receptors in one type of diabetes.

Overlap of autoimmune diseases. This is common, e.g. about 10% of patients with autoimmune thyroiditis develop pernicious anaemia and 30% of them have parietal cell antibodies in their serum.

Genetic factors. Autoimmune diseases tend to be familial, e.g. blood relations of patients with autoimmune thyroiditis show a high incidence of thyroid autoantibodies and thyroiditis.

Age and sex. Most autoimmune diseases are more common in women than men. The incidence increases steadily with age and low titres of autoantibodies and minor histological evidence of autoimmune disease can be detected in nearly a quarter of all people over 70.

9

Antigen-Antibody Reactions

> By the action of dilute sera of highly immunized ani-
> mals microbes are caused to aggregate together in
> 'clumps'.
>
> H. E. Durham, 1896

Antigen-antibody reactions are the methods by which antigens
and antibodies are measured. Since the source of antibody is
usually serum the subject is known as *serology*, although other
antibody-containing fluids, e.g. saliva, can be used if necessary.
The observable reactions between antigen and antibody may take
various forms (precipitation, agglutination, etc.) which depend
on the way the antigen is presented to the antibody. Most antibodies can be detected in many different ways.

Heterogeneity of antibodies

An antibody produced in response to a single antigen consists of
large numbers of different immunoglobulin molecules. These will
usually include representatives from the three main classes, IgG,
IgA and IgM, which differ greatly in their effectiveness in bringing
about different types of antigen-antibody reactions. Different
immunoglobulin molecules also vary in the firmness with which
they combine with the antigen. Moreover, some of them may be
specific for one determinant group (combining site or *epitope*) of
the antigen while others are specific for another part of the
antigen molecule.

When one refers to antibodies one normally implies *classical
antibodies* which are detectable by tests such as precipitation and
agglutination. However, some antibodies combine with the antigen
but cannot be detected by the ordinary tests. These non-precipitating
and non-agglutinating *incomplete antibodies* can be detected only
in special ways, e.g. the antiglobulin test. Sometimes they block
the action of classical antibodies and are known as *blocking antibodies*. Most of the phenomena attributed to incomplete antibodies
can be explained by differences in the behaviour of the three
main classes of immunoglobulins or by structural peculiarities of
particular antigens.

Method of measurement

Serological tests can be used in two ways: a known antibody can be used to detect and measure an unknown antigen, or a known antigen can be used to detect and measure an unknown antibody. Quantitative results are normally expressed in terms of the *titre* of the serum, the highest dilution of the serum at which a particular effect can be demonstrated. For example, a titre of 160 means that in the reaction being studied the serum shows the effect when it is diluted 1 in 160. The titre is thus a measure of the amount of antibody in a unit volume of the original serum.

When antibodies are being sought in a patient's serum to confirm a clinical diagnosis, a single observation may be of no value: antibodies may not have had time to appear or the patient may already possess antibodies from previous infection, subclinical infection or immunization. It is always preferable to repeat the observation after a week or so and look for evidence of a *rising titre*. Antibodies will retain their activity if the serum is kept in the deep-freeze.

Serological and other tests used in medicine vary greatly in their ability to provide a correct diagnosis. In evaluating a test it is important to distinguish:

Sensitivity: the percentage of patients with the disease in which the test is positive.
Specificity: the percentage of patients free of the disease in which the test is negative.

Thus a test with a sensitivity of 95% will detect 95 out of 100 patients with the disease, but 5 patients will have false negative results. Similarly, a test with specificity of 98% has the drawback that 2 out of every 100 healthy people will have false positive results. No serological test is 100% sensitive or 100% specific.

Combination of antigen and antibody

The relationship between antigen and antibody has been likened to that between lock and key. Their combining sites are complementary in shape and chemical reactivity. The combining forces between the two molecules depend on hydrogen bonding, attraction between oppositely charged groups, hydrophobic bonding and van der Waals forces. The number of combining sites, or valency, of antibodies is two in IgG, two or more in IgA and ten in IgM (Fig. 22, p. 100). Incomplete antibodies behave as though they are univalent. Antigens are multivalent: the larger the antigen the higher the valency, i.e. the more combining sites (epitopes) it contains. Antigen and antibody combine in varying proportions depending on their relative concentrations. To begin with the molecules combine to form a network or lattice. As the complex increases in size the hydrophilic groups of the antigen become masked and the complex as a whole becomes susceptible to precipitation and agglutination by the non-specific influence of electrolytes which are essential for the final stages of the reaction.

Various puzzling phenomena depend on the fact that antigen and antibody combine in varying proportions. If one reagent in a precipitation reaction is present in excess the expected reaction may not take place, i.e. the combining sites on the reagent present in smaller amounts are used up before the complexes are large enough to be precipitated. If a certain dose of toxin is added to a given quantity of antitoxin it is exactly neutralized; but if the same dose is divided into two parts and these are added separately with a short interval in between, the mixture remains toxic (Danysz phenomenon), i.e. when the toxin is added in two fractions the first forms complexes containing a relatively high proportion of antitoxin and insufficient antitoxin is left over to neutralize the second.

Precipitation

When an antibody combines with an antigen in solution a precipitate is formed, i.e. the antigen-antibody complex is thrown out of solution. The reaction may be carried out in various ways:

1 *Simple mixture.* A solution of the antigen is mixed with antibody in a tube and observed for precipitation. The reaction is quickest and the precipate most heavy when antigen and antibody are present in *optimal proportions*. Excess of antigen or antibody may inhibit the formation of the precipitate (prozone phenomenon).

2 *Ring test.* A solution of antigen is layered on the surface of the antibody in a small tube. A narrow ring of precipitate occurs near the junction of the two fluids.

3 *Gel-diffusion (double diffusion) precipitation.* Antigen and antibody are allowed to diffuse towards each other in an agar medium, e.g. from separate wells cut in an agar plate, or an organism may be streaked at right angles to a strip of filter paper containing the serum. Where antigen and antibody meet in optimal proportions they produce a thin line of precipitate. Usually there are several lines because the serum

contains several distinct antibodies and the antigen is a mixture of antigens. By using known controls particular antigens and antibodies can be identified. If the lines emerge at the same angle and fuse they have been produced by the same antigen-antibody reaction. If they emerge at different angles and cross each other the reactions are not the same (Fig. 24).

4 *Single radial immunodiffusion.* The antigen is placed in a well cut in an agar gel containing suitably diluted antibody. A ring of precipitate forms where the reactants meet in optimal proportions. The higher the concentration of antigen, the greater is the diameter of the ring.

5 *Immunoelectrophoresis.* This consists of electrophoresis followed by gel-diffusion precipitation. An electric current is used to separate the components of an antigen mixture on an agar-coated slide. A trough is cut in the agar parallel to the axis of electrophoresis and filled with antibody. Diffusion is then allowed to take place.

6 *Countercurrent immunoelectrophoresis (CIE).* This is a rapid and more sensitive variant of the double diffusion method in which an electric current is used to drive the antigen towards the antibody.

Uses

The precipitin reaction is mainly used for detection of antigens, e.g. in the grouping of streptococci according to Lancefield's scheme polysaccharide haptens extracted from the organisms are identified by using known sera in the ring test. Gel-diffusion has been used for recognizing toxin production by *Corynebacterium diphtheriae* and for identifying some viral antigens, e.g. herpes

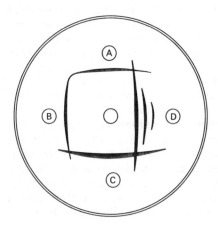

Fig. 24 Gel-diffusion technique. The centre well contains antiserum; the peripheral wells contain antigen solutions. Antigens A and B are identical (fusion of lines), but differ from antigen C (crossing of lines). Antigen D contains three different antigenic components.

virus in vesicle fluid. Immunoelectrophoresis is a delicate technique for analysing complicated mixtures of antigens and antibodies. It is of great value in identifying immunoglobulins, other
serum proteins (including the components of complement) and
microbial antigens. CIE has been used for the rapid detection of
bacterial antigens in clinical specimens such as cerebrospinal
fluid (CSF) and sputum. The precipitin reaction has an important
medico-legal use in identifying proteins (e.g. blood stains) of
human and animal origin. The VDRL test and other 'flocculation'
tests for syphilis are important applications of the precipitin test
for detecting antibodies.

Agglutination

When an antibody combines with an antigen which forms part of
a cell the cells agglutinate, i.e. form clumps. The reaction may be
carried out in two ways:

Slide test. This is usually a provisional or qualitative procedure.
The cells (living or dead bacteria, red blood cells, etc.) are suspended in a drop of saline on a slide and a small drop of antiserum
is added. The slide is gently rocked for a minute or two and the
presence or absence of clumping is noted. A control suspension
in saline excludes the possibility of spontaneous agglutination.

Tube test. This is usually a confirmatory and quantitative procedure. A standard amount of the cell suspension is dispensed
into tubes and serial dilutions of the antiserum are added. The
tubes are incubated and the highest dilution of the antiserum at
which agglutination occurs is recorded as the titre. High concentrations of antibody may inhibit agglutination: such *prozones* (Fig.
25, p. 116) are often encountered in the agglutination of suspensions
of *Brucella abortus.* Agglutination tests are complicated by the anti
genic complexity of bacteria. Thus an unknown serum may have
to be tested separately against the flagellar (H) and somatic (O)
antigens of various bacteria. Conversely the identification of an
unknown organism may require a series of antisera each of
which is capable of reacting with a single known antigen.

Bacterial suspensions

H suspensions. If motile organisms are treated with formalin the
H antigens are preserved and the activity of the O antigens is
annulled. H agglutination is best observed in conical tubes incubated at 50°C for 2 hours and read immediately. The bacteria
adhere by their flagella in the form of a network and produce a
loose, flocculent deposit. H agglutination is usually obvious.

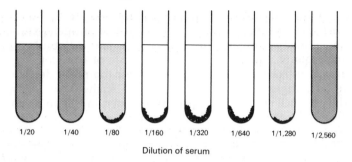

Dilution of serum

Fig. 25   Agglutination reaction showing the prozone phenomenon. Each tube contains a standard amount of bacterial suspension. The dilution of serum ranges from 1 in 20 to 1 in 2560. There is inhibition of agglutination at high concentrations of antibody (1 in 20 to 1 in 80).

O suspensions. If motile organisms are treated with heat or ethanol the O antigens are preserved and the activity of the H antigens is annulled. Non-motile organisms can only produce O suspensions whatever method is used to kill them. O agglutination is best observed in round-bottomed tubes incubated at 37°C for 2 hours and read after storage overnight at 4°C. The bodies of the bacteria adhere closely to one another and produce a *compact, granular deposit.* O agglutination is less obvious than H agglutination and it is important to check that there has been clearing of the supernatant fluid and that the deposit does not break up when the tube is lightly tapped.

Diagnostic sera

Bacteria invariably contain several antigens, some of which are specific and others of which are shared with other species. When intact organisms are injected into an animal the usual result is a mixture of antibodies some of which cross-react with other organisms. Occasionally only one antibody is produced or the level of unwanted antibodies is so low that they can be disregarded. At other times the effects of certain antigens can be annulled before the organisms are injected. When necessary a specific antibody can be obtained from a mixture by *absorption of agglutinins.* This depends on the fact that an antigen only combines with its specific antibody and leaves other antibodies unaffected. The principle is as follows:

If an organism with antigens A, B and C is injected into a rabbit three separate antibodies *a*, *b* and *c* will be produced. If a sufficient mass of another organism containing antigens B, C and D is mixed with serum, B combines with *b*, C combines with *c*, D has nothing to combine with and *a* is left free. If the mixture is centrifuged to remove the bacteria the supernatant fluid is found to contain antibody *a*, i.e. it will now agglutinate only bacteria containing antigen A.

Uses

Specific diagnostic sera are widely used for identifying species of *Salmonella* and *Shigella* and serological types of *Escherichia coli, Haemophilus influenzae, Neisseria meningitidis* and *Streptococcus pyogenes*. Standard suspensions of organisms are used for detecting antibodies in salmonella infections (Widal reaction), brucellosis, leptospirosis and rickettsial diseases.

Other types of agglutination test

Antiglobulin (Coombs) test. So-called 'incomplete' antibodies may combine with the surface antigens of a cell but fail to cause agglutination. If cells coated with incomplete antibodies are washed and resuspended in saline they can be agglutinated by a specific antiglobulin serum. In haematology an anti-human globulin serum prepared in rabbits is used to detect red cells coated with antibodies, e.g. rhesus antibodies (human globulins) formed as a result of immunization with rhesus red cell antigens. Incomplete antibodies against bacterial antigens are often encountered if specifically looked for. In infections caused by salmonellae and brucellae the antiglobulin test may be positive when ordinary agglutination tests are negative.

Indirect haemagglutination. Bacterial polysaccharide antigens and haptens will spontaneously adsorb to red cells. Protein antigens and some viruses will adsorb if the red cells are first treated with tannic acid. Such cells are readily agglutinable by sera against the particular antigens. The method is more sensitive than ordinary precipitin reactions and can be applied to tissue antigens, viruses, etc., which are difficult to study by other means.

Latex particle test. This resembles indirect haemagglutination, but instead of using red cells the antigen (or antibody) is adsorbed on polystyrene latex particles. Many latex tests are available commercially, e.g. for grouping streptococci, detecting bacterial antigens in CSF and detecting and measuring hepatitis B surface antigen (HBsAg), 'rheumatoid factors' and aminoglycoside antibiotics in blood.

Empirical tests. These include the agglutination of sheep red cells in glandular fever (Paul-Bunnell test), agglutination of human group O red cells at low temperatures ('cold agglutinins') in mycoplasmal pneumonia and agglutination of strains of *Proteus* in rickettsial infections (Weil-Felix reaction).

Lysis and bactericidal action

When an antibody combines with an antigen which forms part of the surface of *certain* cells (e.g. a few species of gram-negative bacilli and red blood cells) and provided complement is also present the cells are *lysed*, i.e. dissolved. The cells may also be agglutinated, but this is an incidental feature. Sometimes bacteria are killed without lysis occurring.

Bacterilysis

Pfeiffer and Bordet showed that lysis of *Vibrio cholerae* by serum depends on two factors: a specific heat-stable factor, or antibody, and a non-specific heat-labile factor, or complement, which is normally present in serum. Bacterilysis and bactericidal action are important defence reactions but are of little practical use in the laboratory.

Haemolysis

Lysis of red cells by antibody depends on the same mechanisms, and provides a simple method for detecting complement.

Haemolytic system. By injecting sheep red cells into a rabbit a serum can be obtained which will cause lysis of sheep red cells. If the serum is heated (55°C for 30 minutes) it will no longer cause lysis because complement is destroyed. If complement, e.g. fresh normal serum, is added the ability to cause lysis is restored. In summary:

Cells + unheated serum (contains complement)→lysis
Cells + heated serum (complement destroyed)→no lysis
Cells + heated serum + added complement→lysis

This system of red cells and heated specific anti-red cell serum can therefore be used as a test for complement.

Single radial haemolysis

Haemolysis by antibody can also take place in solid media. Thus a useful screening test for rubella antibodies is provided by measuring the zone of haemolysis produced when the patient's serum is placed in a well in an agar gel containing complement and sheep red cells coated with rubella antigen.

Complement fixation

When an antibody combines with an antigen, regardless of the type of reaction which takes place and even when no readily observable reaction takes place, complement if present is usually *fixed*, i.e. rendered undetectable.

Complement may be defined as a non-specific, heat-labile complex present in the serum of normal animals, fixed in antigen-antibody reactions and essential for the production of lysis by antibody. These properties may be amplified:

1 *Non-specific*: it is always the same substance and is not increased by immunization.
2 *Heat-labile*: it is destroyed when heated to 55°C for 30 minutes unlike antibodies which survive this treatment.
3 *Complex*: it consists of a highly complex group of serum proteins with nine main components (C1 to C9) and many subcomponents, but for most practical purposes can be considered as a single substance.
4 *Present in serum*: the components vary slightly in different animals; guinea-pig serum is most satisfactory for routine work.
5 *Fixed*: the interaction between an antigen and its antibody (IgM or IgG) can induce a structural change in the Fc portion of the immunoglobulin molecule which activates the first step in the 'complement cascade'. This is a sequence of reactions involving the complement complex in which a number of short-lived intermediates are formed. The net result is the very localized activity of an end-product which damages cell membranes and causes cell lysis. As a result of the cascade the individual components of the complement complex are used up or fixed. If there is a limited amount of complement present initially its disappearance can be demonstrated by the complement fixation test.

Activition of the complement system can take place not only by the *classical pathway* initiated by an antigen-antibody reaction but also by an *alternative (properdin) pathway* acting independently of antibody and initiated by such agents as bacteria, their endotoxins and other products. This alternative pathway is an important mechanism of innate (non-specific) immunity.

Complement fixation test

The complement fixation test involves two stages: a test system in which antigen and antibody are allowed to react in the presence of a limited amount of complement and a haemolytic system in which it is determined whether or not complement has been fixed. Since human sera contain a variable and unknown quantity of complement all sera used in the test are heated (55°C for 30 minutes) and a known amount of complement is provided in the form of fresh or specially preserved guinea-pig serum.

1 *Test system.* Antigen, antibody and complement are mixed, incubated and allowed to react. If the antigen encounters its specific antibody they combine and complement is fixed. If the antigen does not encounter its specific antibody no reaction takes place and the complement remains. When the reaction has had time to go to completion the presence or absence of complement in the test mixture is determined in a separate experiment by using the haemolytic system.

2 *Haemolytic system.* This consists of a suspension of sheep red cells sensitized with anti-sheep red cell serum (p. 118). The suspension is mixed with the test mixture and incubated. If antigen has combined with specific antibody, complement is fixed and is not available for haemolysis: the red cells remain intact and the result is positive. If antigen has not combined with specific antibody, complement is still present and haemolysis can take place: the red cell suspension clears with release of haemoglobin into solution and the result is negative. In summary:

Positive test
Antigen + specific antibody + complement→complement fixed
        (heated 55°C   (guinea-pig
        for 30 min)   serum)
                                    Result: no haemolysis

Negative (control) test
Antigen + normal serum + complement→complement remains
        (heated 55°C   (guinea-pig
        for 30 min)   serum)
                                    Result: haemolysis

The test is performed quantitatively by using serial dilutions of the antibody or semi-quantitatively by varying the amount of complement. Preliminary titration of complement and anti-red cell serum is necessary to find out how much to use in the test. It is also essential to have known positive and negative controls as well as controls to exclude the possibility of non-specific complement fixation (anticomplementary effect) by antigen or antibody.

Complement fixation tests offer obvious advantages when it is difficult or impossible to obtain sufficiently concentrated solutions of antigens or suspensions of cells for precipitation or agglutination reactions. Complement fixation is widely used for detecting antibodies in diseases caused by rickettsiae (including *Coxiella burneti*), chlamydiae, mycoplasmas, viruses, protozoa and helminths.

Opsonization

When an antibody combines with an antigen which is part of the surface of a bacterial cell and phagocytes are present the bacteria are opsonized, i.e. rendered enormously more susceptible to phagocytosis. Intermediates formed as a result of complement activation enhance phagocytosis and when antibody is present in low concentration complement may be essential.

Opsonic tests are not used for routine purposes since the same antibodies can be measured more accurately by the much simpler agglutination test.

Toxin neutralization

When an antibody combines with a toxin, the toxic effects of the toxin are neutralized, i.e. it is rendered harmless. Since the toxin is an antigen in solution it is also precipitated.

Toxins and antitoxins can be measured by lethal tests in animals, intradermal tests in animals and man (e.g. Schick test), neutralization tests on cells in tissue culture and by ordinary serological tests, e.g. precipitation or enzyme-linked immunosorbent assay (ELISA). Antitoxins will also neutralize any *in vitro* effects shown by a toxin, e.g. the lecithinase of *Clostridium perfringens* is inhibited by *Cl. perfringens* antitoxin (Nagler reaction); the haemolytic activity of streptolysin O is neutralized by antistreptolysin O which appears in the serum of patients infected with most strains of haemolytic streptococci of groups A, C and G.

Neutralization is not invariable. Endotoxins of gram-negative bacteria may combine with their specific antibodies but still be toxic. Some enzymes may be precipitated by antibodies but still retain their specific catalytic activity.

Capsule swelling

When an antibody combines with an antigen which forms the capsule of an organism the capsule appears to swell.

The phenomenon is also referred to as the Neufeld *Quellung* (swelling) reaction or the specific capsular reaction. It can be used for serological typing of capsulated organisms such as pneumococci, klebsiellae and *H. influenzae*.

Virus neutralization

When an antibody combines with a surface antigen of a virus the virus is neutralized, i.e. rendered non-infective.

Suitable mixtures of virus and antibody are introduced into a living host system which will serve as an indicator of the presence or absence of active virus, e.g. animals (especially the mouse), the embryonated hen's egg, tissue cultures and, in the case of phage, cultures of bacteria. The neutralization test is widely used in virology to estimate antibodies and to identify viruses. The antibodies it measures are not always the same as the antibodies detected by complement fixation and other methods.

Haemagglutination-inhibition

Many viruses agglutinate red cells. Since the process is specifically inhibited by antibodies against the virus, haemagglutination-inhibition can be used as an *in vitro* test for identifying viruses and measuring antibodies (Fig. 26). In practice it is necessary to exclude non-specific inhibitors from the test systems.

Immune electron microscopy

When viruses in suspension are exposed to specific antibody they form clumps and become much more readily detectable when viewed in the electron microscope. In this way it is possible to demonstrate viruses which are not detectable by ordinary methods, e.g. hepatitis A virus can be identified in faeces by using convalescent serum to aggregate the particles. The technique is of value in identifying new viruses and investigating their role in disease.

Radioimmunoassay (RIA)

When an antibody reacts with a mixture of an antigen and the same antigen labelled with a radioactive marker the unlabelled and labelled antigens compete for the binding groups of the antibody. When the reaction is complete, free antigen and antibody-

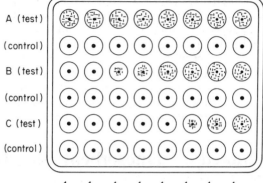

A (test)
(control)
B (test)
(control)
C (test)
(control)

$\frac{1}{10}$ $\frac{1}{20}$ $\frac{1}{40}$ $\frac{1}{80}$ $\frac{1}{160}$ $\frac{1}{320}$ $\frac{1}{640}$ $\frac{1}{1280}$

Fig. 26 Haemagglutination-inhibition. Measurement of rubella antibody is depicted. A standard volume of patient's serum varying in dilution from 1 in 10 to 1 in 1280 and a standard amount of rubella antigen (haemagglutinin) are placed in wells in a plastic tray. Chick red cells are added. Test A is negative (antibodies not detected): there is agglutination of red cells at all dilutions. Test B is weakly positive: there is inhibition of agglutination at a titre of 20. Test C is strongly positive: there is inhibition at a titre of 160. Controls without rubella antigen check that the patient's serum does not agglutinate chick red cells.

bound antigen can be separated and the radioactivity of each fraction determined. By comparison with suitable standards, unlabelled antigen can be measured by the extent to which it prevents the binding of labelled antigen. RIA is a highly sensitive technique and can be used to measure protein hormones, enzymes, complement components, immunoglobulins, viral antigens and, by using antisera produced against haptens, small molecules such as antibiotics (especially aminoglycosides), steroids, thyroxine, digoxin and morphine.

Other radioactive binding techniques

Solid-phase immunoradiometric assay. Unlabelled antibody is first firmly attached to a solid phase such as the surface of a well in a plastic tray. The test sample containing antigen is allowed to react with this antibody-coated surface. The amount of antigen bound to the surface is then measured by means of a labelled antibody. The technique can be used to detect hepatitis A virus and measure its antibody.

Radioallergosorbent test (RAST). This technique is used to measure IgE antibodies to specific antigens ('allergens') in patients with atopic hypersensitivity. The allergen obtained from pollens, mites, etc., is bound to a solid phase support such as a paper disc and is allowed to react with the patient's serum. IgE binds to the allergen. After washing, the disc is allowed to react with a radio-labelled anti-human IgE antibody which binds to the allergen-IgE complexes. After further washing, the residual radioactivity gives a measure of the amount of IgE in the patient's serum.

Enzyme-linked immunosorbent assay (ELISA)

Antibodies can be labelled by linking them to a readily detectable enzyme. In the commonly used indirect ELISA technique for measuring antibodies the antigen is first firmly attached to the surface of a well in a plastic tray and is then allowed to react with the test serum. Excess serum is removed by washing and an antiglobulin serum conjugated with a suitable enzyme is added. The conjugate becomes attached to the antibody bound to the original antigen. After further washing the amount of conjugate retained is measured by adding enzyme substrate and determining enzymic activity by means of a colour change. The ELISA technique is sensitive and suitable for routine work. It avoids the risk of radioactivity and the need for the specialized equipment used in radioimmunoassay.

IgM-capture ('μ-capture') ELISA. Anti-human IgM is attached to the solid phase and allowed to react with the patient's serum. All the IgM in the patient's serum is captured. The presence of IgM against a particular antigen is detected by adding the antigen, followed by an enzyme-labelled antibody against it and finally an appropriate substrate. IgM-capture ELISA is more sensitive and more specific than indirect ELISA.

Competitive enzyme immunoassay. Competition for binding to immobilized antigen of human immunodeficiency virus (HIV) between the test serum and an anti-HIV serum conjugated to an enzyme (horseradish peroxidase) is the basis of a valuable screening test for antibodies to HIV.

Immunoblot techniques (western blot)

The antigenic material is separated into its individual components by electrophoresis on a slab of polyacrylamide gel. The separated components are then electrophoretically transferred to a sheet of nitrocellulose. The sheet is cut into strips and individual strips are incubated with the unknown serum. The strip is allowed to react with an enzyme-linked antiglobulin serum and finally with a chromogenic substrate. Western blot analysis is a specific and highly sensitive method for detecting antigens and antibodies, e.g. it is probably the most sensitive method for detecting antibodies against HIV.

Fluorescent antibody techniques

Antigens (bacteria, viruses, etc.) can be detected in smears and frozen tissue sections by staining with a specific antibody which has been coupled to a fluorescent compound such as fluorescein isothiocyanate. The slides are examined under ultraviolet light and the sites where antigen and antibody have combined can be detected by their fluorescence (Fig. 27A).

Antigens can often be detected more readily by an indirect or double layer method. The material under investigation is allowed to react with an unlabelled specific antibody (globulin) of a particular species. The localization of this antibody is subsequently detected by means of a fluorescein-labelled antiglobulin serum prepared against that species, e.g. a labelled anti-human globulin serum prepared in rabbits can be used to detect human antibodies (Fig. 27B).

Antibodies can be detected by the 'sandwich' method. The material is treated with a solution of antigen and, after washing, is exposed to fluorescent antibody (Fig. 27C).

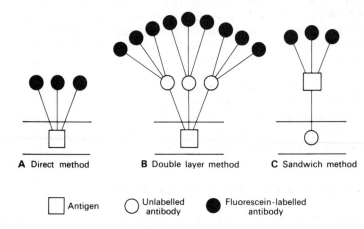

A Direct method   **B** Double layer method   **C** Sandwich method

☐ Antigen   ○ Unlabelled antibody   ● Fluorescein-labelled antibody

Fig. 27 Fluorescent antibody techniques.

Immunofluorescent techniques are of general applicability in all branches of microbiology and are used in research and in diagnostic tests. Because they combine the sensitivity and specificity of immunology with the precise visual localization inherent in microscopy they have yielded information that could not have been readily obtained in other ways. Thus they have been of value in studying the distribution of bacteria, viruses, antigens and antibodies in tissues and cells, the site and mechanisms of antibody formation and the processes involved in autoimmunity. Routine tests for viral antibodies can be carried out using stock sets of virus-infected tissue culture cells dried on slides. The cells are allowed to react with the patient's serum and are then stained with a fluorescent anti-human globulin serum. By using conjugated anti-human IgM and anti-human IgG sera it is possible to distinguish IgM and IgG antibodies. Many routine tests for human autoimmune diseases are based on fluorescent antibody techniques, e.g. the antibody ('antinuclear factor') which appears in the serum of patients with systemic lupus erythematosus can be detected by allowing the serum to react with a frozen section of normal tissue rich in cell nuclei and subsequently staining with a fluorescent anti-human globulin serum. Immunofluorescent tests are of value in detecting antibodies in protozoal and helminth infections. The fluorescent treponemal antibody test is an important test for antibodies in syphilis.

Immunofluorescent techniques possess the advantage of speed and can be used for rapid identification of organisms in clinical specimens, e.g. poxviruses and herpesviruses in vesicle fluid; *Legionella pneumophila*, influenza and parainfluenza viruses, respiratory syncytial virus, adenoviruses and measles virus in sputum and nasopharyngeal secretions; viruses in cells of the CSF from patients with viral meningitis; *Shigella sonnei* and enteropathogenic *Escherichia coli* in smears of faeces. The techniques are of value for identifying viruses in post-mortem specimens, e.g. in investigation of 'cot death' in infants. They can also be used to examine material which has been dried and fixed on slides and sent by post from areas which lack facilities for studying viruses. In many viral infections immunofluorescent techniques can establish a precise diagnosis within a few hours and so replace conventional isolation procedures. Staining by fluorescent antibody is also of value in speeding up the identification of organisms growing in culture, e.g. to distinguish *N. gonorrhoeae* and *N. meningitidis* from other neisseriae, and to identify viruses in tissue culture.

Acquired Immunity and Immunization

...I selected a healthy boy, about eight years old, for the purpose of inoculation for the Cow Pox. The matter was taken from a sore on the hand of a dairymaid, who was infected by her master's cows...

Edward Jenner, 1798

Immunity may be defined as the resistance the body possesses to infectious disease. By extension the term immunology has come to mean the study of the reactions of the body to 'non-self' materials such as microbial products, foreign proteins, tissue transplants and other antigens.

Acquired immunity develops as a result of contact with organisms and their products. It is specific and is of two types: antibody-mediated ('humoral') and cell-mediated. Usually both types of immunity develop in parallel, but their relative importance varies in different conditions. Thus the response to a soluble antigen such as diphtheria toxin is almost entirely due to the production of antibody whereas cell-mediated immunity plays a large part in immunity to viruses and predominantly intracellular bacteria such as *Mycobacterium tuberculosis*. Some types of specific acquired response such as delayed hypersensitivity and the rejection of allografts appear to depend exclusively on cell-mediated mechanisms.

For day-to-day clinical purposes acquired immunity to infectious diseases can be considered in terms of antibodies. Acquired humoral immunity may be active or passive.

1 *Active immunity*. The individual makes his own antibodies in response to the stimulus of an antigen. Immunity develops slowly, persists for a long time (often years) and is associated with long-lasting specific reactivity of the antibody-forming tissues (immunological memory).

2 *Passive immunity*. The individual acquires ready-made antibodies from another animal. Immunity is rapidly established, is of short duration, at most a few months, and disappears completely when the foreign antibodies have been eliminated.

There is no education of the antibody-forming tissues and therefore no immunological memory.

Naturally acquired active immunity

Infectious diseases are followed by variable degrees of immunity. Measles and diphtheria are followed by a high degree of immunity and second attacks are rare. On the other hand, boils and gonorrhoea produce weak and short-lived immunity and repeated attacks are common. In some diseases lack of immunity is more apparent than real. Thus an individual may have several attacks of sore throat due to *Streptococcus pyogenes*, but the serological type is usually different in each attack. Similarly, a large number of different viruses can cause a common cold.

Subclinical infections may provide an important source of immunity when a disease is endemic in a community. Thus in some tropical countries paralytic poliomyelitis is rare, but nearly every child acquires antibodies against all three types of the virus before the age of four. Inapparent infections caused by herpesviruses, adenoviruses, coxsackieviruses, echoviruses, hepatitis viruses, mycoplasmas and chlamydiae are extremely common. Diphtheria, enteric fever, dysentery, tuberculosis and yellow fever produce inapparent infections in parts of the world where they are endemic. Subclinical infections do not occur in syphilis, chickenpox or measles and were never found in smallpox.

Organisms of the normal flora and *non-microbial antigens* acquired by ingestion or inhalation contribute to the production of immunity.

Artifically acquired active immunity

Living vaccines

Smallpox

Prevention of smallpox by case-to-case inoculation of pus from the lesions of a mild case was established in India and China over 2000 years ago. The well-founded popular belief that milk-maids who acquired cowpox were immune to smallpox led to the introduction by Jenner (1796) of the safer method of vaccination using material from lesions of cowpox.

The modern vaccine consists of vaccinia virus. Its precise lineage is obscure but it is probably either a hybrid produced by genetic recombination of smallpox and cowpox viruses or a strain of smallpox virus that has been *attenuated,* i.e. rendered less virulent, by passage through calves. It is available in the form of a freeze-dried vaccine with a long shelf-life. The virus is introduced into the skin by multiple pressure or scratch techniques.

Now that smallpox has been eradicated there are no medical indications for vaccination except for the compulsory vaccination and regular revaccination of workers in laboratories that still hold smallpox virus and staff in designated smallpox hospitals. Vaccination should also be offered to the families of those vaccinated and people engaged in the manufacture of the vaccine or who perform vaccination. Details of the technique, reactions and complications of vaccination can be found in larger text-books and in *Memorandum on Vaccination against Smallpox* (HMSO, London) which should be consulted before undertaking this potentially dangerous procedure.

Tuberculosis

BCG (*Bacille Calmette-Guérin*) is a strain of *Mycobacterium bovis* attenuated by growth for many years on a medium containing bile. The vaccine is usually introduced by *intradermal injection.* A nodule appears after a few weeks and often breaks down to form a small discharging ulcer. The lesion heals in 2–3 months and leaves a small scar.

BCG should be offered to all tuberculin-negative children at the age of 10–13 years and to tuberculin-negative individuals who have been in contact with known cases or whose work exposes them to special risk, e.g. doctors, nurses and students. More widespread inoculation of the population is desirable, particularly among immigrant communities. In a trial in the UK involving over 50 000 healthy adolescents who were followed up for 15 years, vaccination with BCG reduced the incidence of tuberculosis by nearly 80% and greatly reduced serious complications in those who did acquire the disease. For unknown reasons BCG provides little or no protection in some developing countries, e.g. Puerto Rico and India.

Complications. A small abscess may occur at the site of inoculation, particularly if the vaccine is injected too deeply. Slight enlargement and tenderness of the regional lymph nodes is normal but abscess formation is rare. Localized invasion of the skin, lupus, is very rare. Generalized tuberculosis is almost unknown.

Poliomyelitis

Sabin oral vaccine consists of living viruses of types 1, 2 and 3 attenuated by growth in tissue culture. It is given by mouth on a lump of sugar or in syrup. Because there is a possibility that one type of the virus will interfere with the growth of the other types the vaccine is given in *three* doses, usually at intervals of 4–8 weeks. This ensures that each type is given an opportunity of establishing immunity. The vaccine is safe and very effective. Paralytic poliomyelitis is an extremely rare complication among vaccine recipients and their contacts.

Measles

The vaccine consists of living measles virus attenuated by growth in chick embryo cells. A single injection reduces the attack rate by 95%. A non-communicable, measles-like illness often occurs 6–12 days after injection, but serious complications are rare. Children with a personal or family history of fits should be given a simultaneous injection of specially diluted human normal immunoglobulin. A combined measles-mumps-rubella vaccine is normally given at the age of 15 months.

Mumps

An effective live attenuated mumps vaccine is available (see above).

Rubella

The vaccine consists of living attenuated rubella virus grown in tissue culture. It is usually given in combination with live measles and mumps vaccine at the age of 15 months. The aim of immunization is to prevent the occurrence of rubella in pregnancy because of the serious effects that the virus can have on the developing fetus. As far as possible all girls should be immunized before they reach child-bearing age. Because there is a possibility that the vaccine virus could itself infect and damage the fetus, pregnant women must not be immunized. Women of child-bearing age should first be tested for rubella antibodies. If they possess antibodies there is no need for immunization; if the results are negative they should be immunized and advised to take contraceptive precautions for the next three months. Staff, both male and female, working in antenatal clinics should be immunized if they are seronegative. A single injection of rubella vaccine stimulates production of antibodies in 95–100% of patients. Side effects are uncommon but some patients develop transient arthritis, enlarged glands, a rash and malaise about the ninth day after injection. Rarely, patients may develop chronic arthritis. Person-to-person transmission of the vaccine virus does not seem to occur.

Yellow fever

The vaccine consists of a strain of yellow fever virus attenuated by repeated growth in tissue culture and prepared in chick embryos. It is a highly effective vaccine. There is a slight risk of encephalitis particularly in infants under nine months of age. International certificates are valid for ten years.

Rabies

Pasteur's vaccine prepared from the spinal cords of infected rabbits is now obsolete. The vaccine contains central nervous system tissue (myelin) and some patients develop a severe demyelinating encephalomyelitis.

A vaccine consisting of virus attenuated by repeated passage in chick embryos largely avoids the risk of neurological complications, but most authorities prefer a killed vaccine.

Other diseases

A live oral typhoid vaccine (Ty21a) in enteric-coated capsules is less effective than killed vaccines but does not cause adverse reactions. A live vaccine has been used against plague. BCG gives considerable protection against tuberculoid leprosy.

Killed vaccines

Killed vaccines do not provide such a prolonged antigenic stimulus as living vaccines and two, three or more subcutaneous or intramuscular injections are usually required. Vaccines can be given in smaller doses by the intradermal route to reduce side effects, e.g. typhoid vaccine, or expense, e.g. rabies vaccine. Vaccines containing adjuvants must *never* be given intradermally as they may produce granulomatous or necrotic lesions. In preparing the vaccines fully virulent organisms are killed by the mildest possible treatment so as to leave their antigens intact.

Typhoid fever

Typhoid vaccine consists of a suspension of killed *Salmonella typhi*. Fever, rigors and headache are common complications. The immunity produced is only moderate and reinoculation every two or three years is desirable for those at special risk. TAB vaccine which contains *S. typhi* and *S. paratyphi* A and B is ineffective against the paratyphoid fevers and is no longer recommended.

Whooping cough

A vaccine containing killed virulent (smooth-phase) *Bordetella pertussis* gives substantial protection. Severe encephalopathy is an extremely rare complication. It is difficult to assess the risks accurately because convulsions due to other causes are common in very young children. Although a tiny proportion of children given whooping cough vaccine develop convulsions within seven days, and some of them die or are left with permanent brain damage, most of these cases are probably coincidental. Nevertheless the vaccine inevitably gets the blame. On balance the advantages of the vaccine outweigh the risks. It is inadvisable to give it to children with a history of brain damage or convulsions.

Poliomyelitis

Salk vaccine contains the three types of poliovirus grown in monkey kidney tissue culture and killed by low concentrations of formalin. It contains a small amount of penicillin (and streptomycin), but hypersensitivity reactions are only rarely produced. The vaccine provides substantial protection and has been just as effective in eliminating poliomyelitis in Scandinavia as has the oral vaccine elsewhere.

Rabies

Human diploid cell vaccine is the safest and most reliable rabies vaccine. It consists of rabies virus grown in cultures of human diploid cells and inactivated with β-propiolactone. It is suitable for prophylactic immunization of people at special risk and, in conjunction with human antirabies immunoglobulin, for treatment of patients who have been bitten by rabid animals. High antibody levels are obtained and side effects are clinically unimportant

Killed vaccine prepared from virus grown in duck embryos is still used. It is safe but its antigenicity is poor.

Influenza

Vaccines are prepared from virus grown on chick embryos. The most satisfactory vaccines ('subunit vaccines') contain highly purified haemagglutinin and neuraminidase antigens adsorbed on aluminium hydroxide. Side effects are usually trivial, but patients sensitive to egg may show severe reactions. Guillain-Barré syndrome is a rare but serious complication, probably associated with the myelin content of particular batches of vaccine. Influenza vaccines are of most value for those at special risk, e.g. patients with chronic chest disease and the elderly living in residential homes, and for people such as doctors, nurses and ambulance men. Antigenic variants of influenza virus encountered in different epidemics limit the effectiveness of the vaccines although some success has been achieved by using vaccines prepared from recombinant strains of virus.

Hepatitis B

A recombinant vaccine consisting of hepatitis B surface antigen produced by a yeast is available for individuals at special risk, e.g. health care workers, patient contacts, police and prison staff, homosexuals, drug abusers and travellers to countries where the incidence of hepatitis B is high. Protection lasts 3–5 years.

Other diseases

Killed suspensions of *Vibrio cholerae* and *Yersinia pestis* are of vaccine containing the alum-precipitated protein antigen of *Bacillus anthracis* is available for workers at special risk. Yolk-sac suspensions *thracis* is available for workers at special risk. Yolk-sac suspensions of rickettsiae are used in vaccines against epidemic typhus, murine typhus and Rocky Mountain spotted fever. A yolk-sac vaccine of *Coxiella burneti* has been used in Australia to prevent Q fever among workers in abattoirs. Mouse-brain and hamster-kidney vaccines are effective against Japanese encephalitis. A pneumococcal vaccine containing purified polysaccharide capsular antigens from the 23 commonest serological types of *Streptococcus pneumoniae* provides useful protection against pneumococcal pneumonia, particularly in the elderly and in patients who have had splenectomy. The vaccine should be given once only as reinoculation does not lead to a booster effect and produces local and systemic reactions in about half the recipients. Penicillin-resistant pneumococci have emerged in a few parts of the world and the vaccine could prove of special value if antibiotic resistance becomes common. A vaccine containing the capsular polysaccharide of *Haemophilus influenzae* type b protects against haemophilus meningitis and epiglottitis. It is given as a single dose to children aged two. It is not immunogenic in younger children. A vaccine containing the capsular polysaccharides of *Neisseria meningitidis* groups A and C is available for travellers to countries where meningococcal infections are epidemic. Group B polysaccharides are poorly immunogenic and there is no effective vaccine. A vaccine prepared from *M. leprae* grown in armadillos provides protection against leprosy. A leprosy vaccine made by genetic engineering is being developed.

Products of organisms (toxoids)

Immunity to diphtheria and tetanus depends on the possession of antitoxins. Toxins themselves are too dangerous to use as immunizing agents, but they can be converted into harmless toxoids by treatment with formalin.

Diphtheria

Diphtheria formol toxoid is suitable for immunization at all ages, but is less effective than preparations which contain an adjuvant. It can be used in combination with other immunizing agents, e.g. 'adsorbed triple vaccine' contains diphtheria toxoid, tetanus toxoid and whooping cough bacilli, together with an adjuvant.

Adsorbed diphtheria vaccines prepared from toxoid and a mineral carrier such as aluminium hydroxide or phosphate give a prolonged antigenic stimulus (adjuvant effect). They are used mainly for young children as they tend to cause reactions in older patients. They may provoke paralysis in the injected limb in patients incubating poliomyelitis (*provocation paralysis*). This hazard has been virtually eliminated by the extensive use of poliomyelitis vaccine.

Diphtheria vaccine for adults (adsorbed) contains a reduced amount of toxoid. It seldom causes reactions and can be used to immunize persons over 10 years of age without prior Schick testing (see below).

Complications. Immunization may cause inflammation at the site of injection and a febrile illness. Reactions are not common in very young children but become more common and more severe with increasing age. Individuals who are already immune because of subclinical infection or previous immunization may react severely and in any case do not require further immunization. Such individuals can be detected by laboratory estimation of diphtheria antitoxin or by the Schick test.

Schick test. This test is now rarely used. A standard skin test dose of diphtheria toxin (*not toxoid*) is injected intradermally into the left forearm ('test') and heat-inactivated toxin into the right ('control'). The results are read at 48 hours and again at 1 week.

Positive: the test arm shows a red area (1—5 cm diameter) at 48 hours which persists for 1—2 weeks. The control shows no reaction. The patient has insufficient antitoxin to neutralize the toxin and is considered 'susceptible'.

Negative: there is no reaction on either arm. The patient has sufficient antitoxin to neutralize the toxin and is considered 'immune'.

Pseudo-reactions: reactions occur on both arms. This indicates a non-specific reaction to some component other than the toxin. Pseudo-reactions are difficult to interpret. Occasionally they are well marked and persistent. Such patients usually possess a large amount of antitoxin and are liable to react very severely to immunization.

Newborn infants may be Schick-negative because of antitoxin acquired from the mother. They possess temporary immunity and respond poorly to immunization. In a few months the antitoxin disappears and they become Schick-positive.

Children up to the age of 10 years are assumed to be Schick-positive and are immunized without testing. Older children and adults should either be immunized with *diphtheria vaccine for adults* or they should be tested and those shown to be Schick-positive can then be immunized with conventional diphtheria vaccines.

Tetanus

Normal unimmunized individuals possess extremely small amounts of tetanus antitoxin (presumably the result of growth of *Clostridium tetani* in the bowel) and with rare exceptions are susceptible to the disease. Tetanus toxin does not produce skin reactions analogous to those used in the Schick test.

Tetanus formol toxoid is safe and effective but has been superseded by *adsorbed tetanus toxoid*. This consists of toxoid and a mineral carrier and is a much better antigen than the soluble toxoid. Local reactions are uncommon and seldom severe. A patient who gets a severe local reaction can be immunized by giving a small dose of formol toxoid (*not adsorbed toxoid*) intradermally. When combined active and passive immunization is required, adsorbed toxoid should always be used as tetanus antitoxin severely depresses the antigenicity of ordinary tetanus toxoid.

Naturally acquired passive immunity

The fetus acquires maternal IgG antibodies via the placenta and the infant is born with some degree of temporary immunity to various infectious diseases, e.g. measles and chickenpox are almost unknown in the first few months of life. Undesirable antibodies such as those responsible for rhesus disorders may also reach the fetus.

In the first few days of life the mucous membranes of the intestinal tract are relatively permeable to unaltered proteins, and antibodies in small amounts may be acquired from colostrum. The secreted form of IgA is resistant to digestion and in breast-fed infants the IgA of breast milk protects the gut against attack by organisms causing gastroenteritis.

Artificially acquired passive immunity

The patient acquires temporary immunity following injection of antibodies of human or animal origin.

Human normal immunoglobulin (gammaglobulin) prepared from pooled normal plasma is used to protect susceptible contacts of certain viral diseases, e.g. prevention of hepatitis A (infective hepatitis) in institutional outbreaks and in travellers to countries where the disease is endemic; and prevention or attenuation of measles in children under three or suffering from intercurrent illness. It is also used for treatment of patients with hypogamma-globulinaemia.

Human specific immunoglobulins are rich in particular antibodies. Antitetanus immunoglobulin from individuals vaccinated against tetanus is used for passive immunization against this disease. Antirabies immunoglobulin from individuals vaccinated against rabies is used in conjunction with active immunization to treat non-immune patients who have been exposed to the disease. Antihepatitis B surface antigen (anti-HBsAg) immunoglobulin from blood donors found to have the antibody on routine screening is used to protect patients who have been accidentally inoculated with material containing hepatitis B virus, including newborn infants of women who are chronic carriers. Antivaricella-zoster immunoglobulin (often called ZIG or zoster immune globulin) and antimumps immunoglobulin are used for patients at special risk, e.g. during immunosuppressive therapy. Anti-D immuno-globulin is used to prevent haemolytic disease of the newborn (p. 145).

Human immunoglobulin should be given by intramuscular injection. It produces no reactions. If intravenous injection is essential the solution should be diluted and given slowly or mild reactions may occur. Immunoglobulin is prepared by a method which kills the viruses causing hepatitis B and AIDS. Concentrated IgG preparations suitable for intravenous infusion are used for treating hypogammaglobulinaemia and infections caused by particular organisms, e.g. *Pseudomonas aeruginosa*.

Antiviral sera (other than human immunoglobulin) are rarely used. Antirabies serum prepared in horses is still in use, but hypersensitivity reactions are common and human antirabies immunoglobulin (see above) is preferred.

Antibacterial sera prepared in animals were at one time used for treating bacterial infections, e.g. pneumococcal pneumonia, but chemotherapy has rendered such treatment obsolete.

Antitoxic sera prepared in animals, usually the horse, are still occasionally used to give non-immune individuals temporary protection against diphtheria. Antitetanus serum is now obsolete. Antitoxic sera are dangerous substances because the patient may be sensitive to horse protein and develop anaphylactic shock. A test dose should precede the main dose and a syringe loaded with 1 in 1000 adrenaline should be at hand. Foreign serum is eliminated more rapidly than human immunoglobulin and to ensure protection further doses of antitoxin may be required after a few days.

Antitoxins are also occasionally used in treatment. They are given in large doses at the earliest possible moment. Diphtheria antitoxin is of great value in the treatment of diphtheria. Polyvalent (*Clostridium perfringens, Cl. novyi* and *Cl. septicum*) gas gangrene antitoxin and polyvalent (types A, B and E) *Cl. botulinum* antitoxin are of less value. Specific antivenoms may be life-saving following snake-bite in some countries, but in Great Britain an injection of antivenom is more dangerous than the bite of the only poisonous British snake, the adder or viper.

Fab fragments (antigen-binding fragments) prepared from IgG from sheep immunized against digoxin are of value in treating severe digoxin poisoning in man.

Future vaccines

Vaccines have been produced against virtually all infectious diseases, including syphilis, gonorrhoea, herpesvirus infections and malaria. Use of such vaccines has been limited because of their doubtful effectiveness or concern about their long-term effects. Genetic manipulation of viruses provides mutants suitable for live attenuated vaccines. New techniques are being developed to obtain increased amounts of desired antigens and eliminate unwanted materials. Subunit vaccines, which have proved to be effective against influenza virus, are likely to be developed against other organisms. Of the many antigenic sites in a protein only a few give a strong antibody response and synthetic peptides corresponding to these sites can sometimes be used as the basis of vaccines. Recombinant DNA techniques may prove ideal for preparing purified viral antigens. A large virus such as vaccinia whose DNA can accommodate large numbers of foreign genes could form the basis of polyvalent vaccines providing simultaneous immunization against many different infective agents. Vaccines prepared from anti-idiotype antibodies could prove to be more useful than vaccines prepared from organisms and their antigens. New methods of vaccine administration are being investigated, e.g. use of intranasal aerosols against respiratory disease viruses.

Routine immunization in childhood

An ideal scheme provides maximum protection with the least risk of complications and the smallest number of injections. In practice it is necessary to accept a compromise. The following is a workable schedule:

Age	Vaccine	Interval
3—6 months	Diphtheria-Tetanus-Pertussis Poliomyelitis (oral)	6—8 weeks
	Diphtheria-Tetanus-Pertussis Poliomyelitis (oral)	4—6 months
	Diphtheria-Tetanus-Pertussis Poliomyelitis (oral)	
15 months	Measles-Mumps-Rubella	*
5 years	Diphtheria-Tetanus Poliomyelitis (oral)	*
10—13 years	BCG	*
15—19 years	Tetanus Poliomyelitis (oral)	*

*An interval of 3 weeks should normally be allowed between the administration of any two live vaccines.

The following points have been considered:

1 The mother is more likely to accept advice if immunization is started early in life.
2 In the first 6—9 months of life antibody response is poor and antibodies acquired from the mother may inhibit active immunity. However, two-thirds of the deaths from whooping cough occur under the age of one year. There are therefore advantages in giving whooping cough vaccine as early as possible. Diphtheria and tetanus are rare in the first year of life, but immunity can be given at the same time ('triple vaccine'), even though the response may not be maximal. Oral poliomyelitis vaccine can be given concurrently. Immunization is best commenced at the age of three months.
3 Measles vaccine should not be given to children below the age of 9 months because of the inhibitory effect of maternal antibodies.
4 BCG can be given in infancy. This is recommended in conditions of special risk.

Other immunizing procedures

Individuals going to tropical countries may require immunization against a large number of infectious diseases. As far as possible injection of a live vaccine should be separated from other inoculations by an interval of three weeks. All inoculations should be properly spaced and the information which comes with the vaccines should not be ignored. In an emergency it is possible to immunize against several diseases simultaneously, e.g. one arm is used for yellow fever vaccine, the other for various killed vaccines or toxoids.

Herd infection and herd immunity

When an infectious disease is always present in a community and produces a steady rain of infection which varies little in intensity from year to year it is said to be *endemic*. Occasionally, a disease may spread rapidly over an area and infect an unusually large number of individuals. The disease is then said to be *epidemic*, or if it spreads over most of the world, it is *pandemic*.

The factors which determine the behaviour of an infectious disease in the community are complex. They include: (*a*) peculiarities of the particular host-parasite relationship, e.g. how the parasite enters and leaves the host, incubation period, period of infectivity; (*b*) environmental factors which influence contact between individuals and the transmission of infection, e.g. population density, movement of populations, personal hygiene, sanitation, climate, prevalence of insect vectors; (*c*) herd immunity, i.e. immunity possessed by the population as a whole and which, if it is high, hinders the spread of disease and the development of an epidemic. In a few diseases such as diphtheria and poliomyelitis a high degree of herd immunity can be achieved by immunization, but usually the main source of herd immunity is naturally occurring infectious disease.

An epidemic represents a temporary spread of a micro-organism in a susceptible herd. Epidemics of many of the common infectious diseases occur at fairly regular intervals. Infection dies down when the supply of susceptibles is exhausted and reappears when the number rises above a critical level. In other diseases epidemics may be due to such factors as breakdown of sanitary control, importation of an organism from abroad, transportation of troops to foreign countries, and, rarely, production by an organism of mutants with new antigenic properties.

Isolated communities such as Eskimo settlements, inhabitants of remote islands, and inaccessible native tribes seldom suffer from the common infectious diseases, but on rare occasions when such a disease is introduced from the outside world it is likely to spread through the entire community. Sometimes the disease spreads with devastating severity, e.g. in 1875 an epidemic of measles in the Fiji Islands affected all age groups and killed a quarter of the population. Such an event is liable to occur when a population encounters a parasite for the first time in history. In the rest of the world the more susceptible individuals have been eliminated by natural selection over the centuries and the basic immunity of the inhabitants is much greater.

Hypersensitivity

> What is food to some men may be fierce poison to
> others.
>
> Lucretius (*c*. 98–55 B.C.)

Hypersensitivity may be defined as a specific, acquired deleterious
reactivity of the body to a substance which in similar amounts
does not provoke such a reaction in previously unexposed
members of the same species. The term *allergy*, implying an
'altered reactivity', is used more or less synonymously. Hypersensitivity may express itself in a variety of ways, but the underlying mechanisms have certain features in common:

1 The substances which induce the hypersensitive state (*allergens*)
   are either antigens or haptens.
2 Hypersensitivity takes time to develop: the induction period
   is commonly 7–10 days as with other immunological responses.
3 The reactions are specific: only the specific antigen or hapten
   will excite the reaction.
4 Antibodies or specifically sensitized lymphocytes can be
   demonstrated in sensitized individuals.
5 The antigen combines with antibodies or the receptors of
   sensitized lymphocytes in the tissues.
6 Tissue cells are damaged as a result of this combination.

Hypersensitivity reactions fall into two groups:

Antibody-mediated reactions depend on the activity of antibodies
(immunoglobulins) and hypersensitivity can be transferred to a
normal individual by injection of serum. Three types of reaction
are recognized: type I or *anaphylactic* type; type II or *cytotoxic*
type; type III or *complex-mediated* type. The reaction to the allergen,
especially in type I hypersensitivity, often develops within a few
seconds or minutes and the term *immediate hypersensitivity* is
sometimes given to antibody-mediated reactions.

Cell-mediated reactions depend on the activity of lymphocytes
bearing specific antigen-binding receptors on their surface.
Antibodies play no part in the reaction and hypersensitivity
cannot be transferred to another individual by means of serum. It

can, however, be transferred by lymphocytes. Cell-mediated reactions can be assigned to a single type: type IV or *delayed* type. The reaction develops slowly and does not appear until 24 hours or more after contact with the allergen.

Type I. Anaphylactic type of hypersensitivity

Antigen reacts with tissue mast cells (basophils) previously sensitized with a coating of antibody (mainly IgE). Damage is caused by liberation of histamine and other pharmacologically active substances.

Anaphylaxis

If a laboratory animal is injected with a very small dose of a harmless antigen such as horse serum, i.e. a *sensitizing dose,* and after an interval of not less than ten days is given a much larger dose of the same antigen by the intravenous route, the *shocking dose,* the animal rapidly develops severe symptoms known as anaphylactic shock and it usually dies. The main symptoms can be accounted for by damage to capillary endothelium and contraction of smooth muscle. The tissues mainly affected vary in different species. In man there is usually acute respiratory embarrassment, circulatory collapse and widespread urticaria and oedema. Other changes include decreased coagulability of the blood, leucopenia, thrombocytopenia and depletion or disappearance of complement. The average human being is not highly susceptible to anaphylaxis. Individuals with atopy are more sensitive than most. Anaphylaxis is a potential hazard following injection of foreign serum, particularly antitoxins prepared in horses; vaccines, particularly viral and rickettsial vaccines grown in eggs; drugs, of which penicillin is the worst offender; and specific allergens, e.g. pollens, etc., used in desensitization of atopy. It may rarely follow bee or wasp stings or the rupture of a hydatid cyst following injury or during surgery.

Role of histamine

The main symptoms resemble those of acute histamine shock: the effects on capillaries and smooth muscle are similar; the different reactions in different species closely parallel differences in their response to histamine; the symptoms can be prevented or treated with antihistamine drugs and adrenaline. The antigen-antibody reaction results in degranulation of mast cells and release of histamine. Other substances such as serotonin, prostaglandins and certain leukotrienes ('slow reacting substances') are liberated in shock and also play a part. Eosinophils are attracted to the site of mast cell degranulation and neutralize the effects of histamine and other mediators.

Skin reaction

Injection of a minute amount of antigen into the skin of a sensitized person produces a 'triple response'.

Passive transfer

Sensitivity can be transferred to a normal animal by injecting it with a small amount of serum from a sensitized animal. This provides conclusive evidence that antibodies are involved in anaphylaxis. IgE antibodies are mainly responsible. They are non-precipitating antibodies known as *homocytotrophic antibodies* or *reagins*. Their most characteristic property is their ability, independently of any antigen-antibody reaction, to attach themselves firmly to skin and tissue cells, particularly mast cells and circulating basophils.

Desensitization

Animals which recover from shock are temporarily refractory to further shock. Apparent desensitization can be produced without causing shock by injecting very small and gradually increasing doses of antigen over a period of several hours. This technique can be used as an emergency measure when serum or some drug has to be injected into a hypersensitive patient. It is assumed that the antigen gradually neutralizes the antibodies fixed to the tissue cells or exhausts some other link in the mechanism of anaphylaxis. Sensitivity returns in a few days. True desensitization, a process which takes several weeks, is used for patients who develop life-threatening anaphylactic reactions following bee and wasp stings.

Atopic hypersensitivity (atopy or idiosyncrasy)

Many human diseases are due to an immediate-type hypersensitivity to substances the individual encounters in everyday life. Some of the allergens are protein and therefore antigens; others have smaller molecules and presumably couple to body proteins and function as haptens.

Contact with the allergen occurs through the respiratory or intestinal tracts. Inhalation of pollens (particularly timothy grass in the UK and ragweed in the USA), moulds, and vegetable and animal dusts may produce hay fever or asthma. Domestic dust containing the house dust mite (*Dermatophagoides* spp.) accounts for many cases. Ingestion of egg, milk, fish, shellfish and some drugs may produce asthma but is more likely to produce urticarial rashes and gastrointestinal upsets.

The tendency to develop atopic hypersensitivity has a strong hereditary basis, but the particular allergen to which the individual becomes sensitive is largely a matter of chance. Infantile eczema is frequently associated with asthma and hay fever and the underlying mechanisms are probably similar.

Skin reaction

If the allergen is injected or pricked into the skin the result is an immediate weal-and-flare reaction, i.e. a histamine-like 'triple response' of capillary dilatation, local oedema and a peripheral zone of arteriolar dilatation. Skin tests are used to identify the allergens responsible for symptoms.

Passive transfer

If serum from a sensitized individual is injected into the skin of a normal individual a weal-and-flare reaction develops when the allergen is injected into the same area (Prausnitz-Küstner reaction). The antibodies responsible for atopic hypersensitivity are mainly IgE. They can be measured by the radioallergosorbent test.

Desensitization

Relief of symptoms, particularly in hay fever, can sometimes be achieved by a course of injections of the antigen. It is thought that production of conventional antibody blocks the access of the allergen to the tissue-fixed IgE. If desensitization is attempted, facilities for cardio-respiratory resuscitation must be at hand. The drug sodium cromoglycate acts by inhibiting the release of histamine and other mediators from mast cells.

Type II. Cytotoxic type of hypersensitivity

Antigen forming part of a cell or attached to the surface of a cell reacts with antibody (usually IgG or IgM). Damage is caused by the lytic action of complement or by mononuclear cells.

Transfusion reactions

People normally possess antibodies against those antigens of the ABO blood group system which are absent from their own red cells, e.g. a person of blood group A has group A cells and anti-B antibodies. These 'natural' antibodies are usually IgM and probably arise through immunization by antigens arising from the gut flora. In mismatched transfusions the patient's antibodies react against the incompatible red cells.

Haemolytic disease of the newborn (rhesus disease)

When a rhesus-negative (Rh−ve) mother has a Rh+ve (usually RhD+ve) baby it is common for some of the baby's red cells to gain access to the mother, e.g. through a placental bleed at the time of birth. These red cells stimulate the mother to produce antibodies. IgG antibodies, unlike other immunoglobulins, can cross the placental barrier and are liable to damage the red cells of a Rh+ve baby in any subsequent pregnancy. Recently delivered Rh−ve mothers are normally given an injection of anti-D immunoglobulin. This destroys any RhD+ve cells in the maternal circulation and thereby suppresses formation of anti-D antibodies.

Type II drug reactions

A drug can sometimes function as a hapten by coupling to the surface of a cell and stimulating production of antibodies which are cytotoxic for the drug-cell complex. Some cases of drug-induced haemolytic anaemia, agranulocytosis and thrombocytopenic purpura are caused in this way.

Autoimmune disease

Many human diseases are associated with the production of auto-antibodies, i.e. in certain circumstances the body produces antibodies against antigenic constituents of its own tissues (p. 109).

Stimulatory hypersensitivity

An antibody sometimes reacts with an antigen on a cell surface and causes stimulation rather than damage. Thus 'long-acting thyroid stimulator' is an autoantibody which acts on thyroid cells and causes increased secretion of thyroid hormone.

Type III. Complex-mediated hypersensitivity

Antigen reacts with antibody (usually IgG or IgM) in the blood or tissue spaces to form antigen-antibody complexes ('immune complexes'). Damage is caused by local or systemic deposition of complexes in blood vessel walls and cell basement membranes.

These complexes cause acute inflammation and activation of the complement system and mechanical disturbance of normal function.

Local form (Arthus phenomenon)

Repeated injection of an antigen at intervals of a few days may produce progressively more severe reactions at the sites of successive injections until necrosis and ulceration occur. The reaction requires a high level of precipitating antibodies. The antigen-antibody reaction takes place at the site of injection. Damage is localized because the immune complexes are rapidly precipitated and exert a toxic effect on local tissue cells. The walls of blood vessels suffer the greatest damage. The Arthus phenomenon is only rarely seen in man.

Arthus-type reactions

Extrinsic allergic alveolitis. Several very similar human respiratory diseases represent intrapulmonary Arthus-type reactions arising in response to inhalation of antigens in organic dusts, e.g. 'farmer's lung', 'bird-fancier's lung' and hypersensitivity to spores of *Aspergillus fumigatus*. In Norwich, well-known for its association with canaries, we had a case of 'canary-fancier's lung'!

Infections. Local formation of complexes is probably responsible for much of the damage caused by filarial worms, e.g. *Wuchereria bancrofti* in the lymphatics and *Onchocerca volvulus* in the eye.

Systemic form (serum sickness)

A single injection of a large amount of foreign serum may produce toxic effects in individuals who have not been previously sensitized. Symptoms appear about ten days after injection and include fever, widespread urticaria and oedema, pain and swelling in the joints and enlargement of lymph nodes. The symptoms persist for two or three days. Serum sickness depends on the fact that sufficient foreign serum persists in the body to cause a reaction with the antibodies produced after the usual latent period. The reaction takes place in the blood. Damage is widespread because complexes circulate in the blood and are deposited at sites throughout the body, particularly in blood vessel walls and cell basement membranes. Foreign serum is now seldom used in treatment and serum sickness proper has become a rare disease.

Reactions of serum sickness type

Infections. Widespread deposition of complexes from the circulation is common in microbial infections and may cause tissue damage, e.g. polyarteritis in hepatitis B virus infection, petechiae in infective endocarditis, bleeding and shock in dengue haemorrhagic fever, and such lesions as cutaneous vasculitis, polyarteritis nodosa and erythema nodosum which arise in various infections. However, the greatest damage usually occurs in the kidneys (see below).

Nephritis. The glomerular basement membrane of the kidney is highly susceptible to damage by immune complexes. Many types of nephritis are caused by damage of this sort, e.g. nephritis associated with *Streptococcus pyogenes* infection, infective endocarditis, systemic lupus erythematosus, *Plasmodium malariae* malaria and the 'shunt' nephritis resulting from *Staphylococcus epidermidis* colonization of ventriculo-venous shunts used to treat children with hydrocephalus.

Drug reactions. Continued medication with drugs such as penicillin and sulphonamides will sometimes produce the same symptoms as serum sickness.

Type IV. Delayed type of hypersensitivity

Antigen reacts with sensitized T-lymphocytes bearing specific antigen-binding receptors on their surface. Antibodies (immunoglobulins) play no part. Damage is caused by liberation from the lymphocytes of factors ('lymphokines') which cause infiltration with mononuclear cells and, if the antigen forms part of a virus-infected cell or a transplant, by transformation of lymphocytes into blast cells ('killer cells') which kill cells bearing the particular antigen.

Infective allergy

In the course of microbial infections hypersensitivity reactions of types I to III often play an important role in the pathogenesis of disease. However, in most infections the body also develops a delayed type of hypersensitivity in which antibodies play no part. The phenomenon has been extensively studied in relation to tuberculosis and is often referred to as the *tuberculin type* of hypersensitivity. Some workers restrict the term allergy to this type of hypersensitivity.

Koch's phenomenon (1891)

Subcutaneous injection of living *Mycobacterium tuberculosis* into the thigh of a guinea-pig gives rise in about two weeks to a hard, slowly growing nodule which gradually breaks down and forms a discharging ulcer. This never heals. Meanwhile the inguinal and other glands become caseous and ultimately the infection spreads to produce a fatal generalized disease.

If about six weeks after the first injection a similar injection is given into the opposite thigh the reaction is different. Within 24—48 hours the skin at the site of this injection becomes intensely inflamed. The area soon becomes necrotic and a shallow ulcer is formed. This heals rapidly. No nodule forms beneath the skin and the local lymph nodes are not involved. Meanwhile the original infection runs its course.

The altered reactivity appears about ten days after the first injection but is not fully developed for about six weeks. Koch showed that dead tubercle bacilli or an extract of tubercle bacilli (*old tuberculin*) produced a similar reaction in tuberculous guinea-pigs. If a small dose of old tuberculin is injected into a tuberculous guinea-pig there may be inflammation and necrosis at the site of injection (*local reaction*), capillary dilatation and leucocytic infiltration around the existing lesions (*focal reaction*), and fever and constitutional upsets which may prove fatal (*general reaction*). In a normal animal the same dose may produce no reaction. On a less dramatic scale this reaction is the basis of an important clinical test, the tuberculin test.

Tuberculin tests

Purified protein derivative (PPD) is now usually preferred to old tuberculin. It is introduced into the skin of the forearm by intradermal injection (Mantoux test) or by multiple puncture (Heaf and similar tests).

Mantoux test. To avoid severe reactions in highly sensitive persons it is usual to start with a small dose and proceed to higher doses if the results are negative, e.g. 1, 10 and 100 tuberculin units of PPD in 0.1 ml of saline. The test is read at 48 to 72 hours (cf. a few minutes in skin tests for atopy). A positive result consists of an area of *induration* at least 5 mm in diameter. Erythema is usually present but by itself is of no significance. Induration persists for a week.

Heaf test. A concentrated solution of PPD and a special puncture instrument are used. The test is read at 3—7 days. The result is positive (grade I) if four or more of the six puncture sites show *indurated papules* at least 1 mm in diameter; stronger reactions (grades II, III and IV) produce more extensive induration.

Disposable multiple-puncture tests. The *tuberculin ring test* using liquid PPD gives results comparable to those found with the Mantoux test. The *tine test* using tines (prongs) coated with dried tuberculin not infrequently gives false negative results.

A positive tuberculin test indicates that the individual is suffering from tuberculosis or has had the disease, or BCG inoculation, in the past. A negative result usually excludes tuberculosis, but false negative results are sometimes found in acute forms of the disease, e.g. tuberculous meningitis, miliary tuberculosis, and in some other conditions, e.g. AIDS, Hodgkin's disease, sarcoidosis, steroid treatment. The results may be negative in early tuberculosis before hypersensitivity develops.

Other infectious diseases

Delayed hypersensitivity can arise in almost all acute or chronic infectious diseases. In many diseases caused by bacteria, viruses, fungi, protozoa and worms delayed (tuberculin-like) skin reactions can be used to provide evidence of past and present infection. However, as well as producing lymphocyte-mediated delayed hypersensitivity these infections also stimulate production of antibodies (humoral immunity) and for diagnostic purposes it is usually more satisfactory to measure these antibodies using conventional serological techniques.

Passive transfer

Delayed hypersensitivity can be transferred to a normal individual by injection of lymphocytes from blood, lymph glands, spleen and peritoneal exudate. It cannot be transferred by serum. If the serum transfers anything it is always an immediate-type hypersensitivity. Delayed hypersensitivity cannot normally be transferred by means of dead cells or cell antigens, but in man transference has been achieved for various antigens, including tuberculin, using a cell-free *transfer factor* extracted from human leucocytes. Transfer factor has a molecular weight of less than 10 000 daltons. Its mode of action is obscure. It has been used clinically in attempts to establish normal immunological responses in patients with defects of cell-mediated immunity, e.g. it is of value in the treatment of chronic mucocutaneous candidiasis.

Mechanism of antigen recognition

T-lymphocytes have specific antigen-binding receptors on their surface which enable them to recognize antigens. These receptors are similar to the antigen-binding regions of immunoglobulins but have additional peptides by which the T-cell recognizes antigens of the major histocompatibility complex. Combination of an antigen with the receptors of a previously sensitized T-lymphocyte causes liberation from the lymphocyte of complex soluble factors known as *lymphokines* which interact directly with the antigen or indirectly through macrophages. Antibodies (immunoglobulins) play no part in the reactions. Individuals with agammaglobulinaemia cannot produce antibodies, yet they can develop delayed hypersensitivity and their cells will transfer this hypersensitivity to normal subjects.

Contact dermatitis

Drugs and other non-antigenic substances may produce immediate types of hypersensitivity (anaphylaxis, atopy, etc.), but the most common response is a delayed type of hypersensitivity known as contact dermatitis, a chronic inflammatory condition often with vesiculation.

Sensitization occurs only when contact with the allergen takes place via the skin. Prolonged or repeated contact is usually required. Skin tests, commonly a 'patch test' in which the allergen is held in contact with the skin, give typical tuberculin-like responses. The tissue reactions and basic mechanisms are the same as those found in infective allergy, e.g. hypersensitivity can be transferred by lymphocytes. The allergens which may cause contact dermatitis are almost limitless and include sulphonamides and penicillin (which should never be applied to the skin), all manner of organic chemicals used in the home and in industry, substances present in plants such as poison ivy and primrose, and simple elements such as iodine, nickel and mercury.

Allograft reaction

The reaction of an animal to a graft from an animal of the same species but different genetic constitution is basically a delayed hypersensitivity reaction. Accelerated rejection of allografts can be transferred to normal animals with suspensions of lymphocytes (but not serum) obtained from an animal that has already received an allograft. The importance of lymphocytes in the allograft reaction is also shown by the ability of antilymphocytic sera to delay graft rejection. Thus antilymphocyte immunoglobulin, prepared by immunizing horses with human spleen cell suspensions, has been used in human organ transplantation. Monoclonal antibodies against particular subsets of T-lymphocytes have also been used.

Sterilization and Disinfection

I will kill thee a hundred and fifty ways.
Shakespeare

Sterilization implies the destruction or removal of all living organisms in or on an object. Sterility is an absolute term, i.e. an object is either sterile or it is not.

Disinfection implies the destruction or removal of pathogenic organisms so as to render the object non-infective. The process may amount to sterilization, or there may be survival of organisms, e.g. non-pathogens and spores.

Physical agencies

Heat

Heat is rapid, certain and controllable. It offers one great advantage over nearly all chemical methods, namely that when sterilization is complete no harmful substances remain.

Dry heat

Destruction by fire. Wire loops, etc., are sterilized in the laboratory by heating in a flame. Contaminated dressings, infected animals, used swabs, disposable plastic culture plates, etc., are best burnt. Many sterilizing and disinfecting procedures in hospitals can be avoided by using commercially prepared disposables which are burnt after use. This is often the cheapest and safest arrangement.

Hot air ovens (160°C for 1 hour) are used for sterilizing dry glassware, metal instruments, assembled all-glass syringes used for special purposes, and greases, oils and lubricants such as liquid paraffin and glycerol.

Moist heat

Pasteurization (65°C for 30 minutes or 72°C for 15 seconds) kills all bacterial pathogens likely to be present in milk (p. 65), but leaves a few unimportant heat-resistant vegetative organisms and spores.

Some viruses, such as hepatitis B virus, may survive. After pasteurization the milk is immediately cooled to discourage bacterial
growth.

'Ultra heat treated' (UHT) milk (132°C for 1 second) is heated
by steam infiltration in a special apparatus and is dispensed
aseptically into sterile containers. It contains very few organisms
and has a shelf-life of several months.

Relatively low temperatures (e.g. 60°C for 1 hour) are used to
kill vegetative organisms when it is desired to alter their properties
as little as possible, e.g. in vaccine production.

Boiling (100°C for 5 minutes) kills all vegetative organisms, but
a few spores may survive. Some spores will survive boiling for
many hours. Freely exposed vegetative organisms are in fact
killed in a few seconds, but a wide margin of safety is desirable
to cover exceptional circumstances, e.g. articles contaminated by
food, secretions, pus or blood. Boiling is satisfactory for disinfecting
contaminated cups, plates and cutlery but is not safe for instruments used in surgical and dental procedures. Sterility cannot
be guaranteed and instruments should be autoclaved or obtained
ready-sterilized from a central sterile supply department (CSSD)
or a commercial supplier. A small modern self-contained autoclave
is suitable for family doctors and dentists in general practice.

Laundering of sheets, cotton blankets, towels, handkerchiefs,
etc., is usually carried out at temperatures near 100°C and freshly
laundered articles are almost entirely free from organisms.

Intermittent steaming or 'tyndallization' (100°C for 30 minutes on
three consecutive days) can be used to sterilize culture media
which would be damaged by autoclaving. The first steaming kills
vegetative organisms but may leave spores. In the interval before
the next steaming the medium is kept warm (usually at room
temperature) to induce any spores to germinate into the more
vulnerable vegetative forms. These are killed at the second steaming. The third steaming is a traditional precaution.

Steam at subatmospheric pressure. Exposure to steam at 70–80°C
for 15 minutes in a special autoclave can be used for disinfection
(pasteurization) of cystoscopes and similar articles. In combination
with formaldehyde, low temperature steam can be used for sterilization (p. 162).

Steam under pressure (the autoclave). This is the usual method of
sterilizing surgical instruments, dressings, gowns, towels and
culture media. An autoclave consists of a closed chamber in
which objects can be subjected to steam at pressures greater than
atmospheric and therefore at temperatures greater than 100°C.
Steam is a much more efficient sterilizing agent than air at the
same temperature. If air is present not only will the temperatures
achieved be lower for a given pressure but pockets of air may

prevent penetration of the load by the steam. The air must therefore be removed.

In modern *high-vacuum autoclaves* over 98% of the air is removed by a powerful pump capable of producing an initial vacuum of less than 2 kPa of absolute pressure (10^5 Pa = 10^5 N/m^2 = 1 bar = 14.7 lb/in^2). Steam penetrates the load almost instantaneously and rapid sterilization of dressings and packs is possible, e.g. 3 minutes at 134°C (200 kPa or 30 lb/in^2).

In *downward-displacement autoclaves* the air is normally removed in two stages. A preliminary vacuum produced by a steam ejector or an electric pump is used to remove 30–50% of the air. This partial vacuum is sometimes drawn two or more times, steam being admitted between each vacuum. The remaining air is then removed by downward displacement (air is more dense than steam). Steam is admitted at the top of the chamber and residual air and condensed water are driven out at the bottom. The discharge pipe is fitted with a temperature-sensitive valve known as a *steam trap* which is set so that it remains open until all the air has been removed and pure steam at the desired temperature is emerging. The steam trap automatically ensures that sterilization is effected by an atmosphere of pure steam. In an efficient downward-displacement autoclave the *minimum* exposure times required for sterilization of instruments are 15 minutes at 121°C (100 kPa or 15 lb/in^2) or 10 minutes at 126°C (150 kPa or 20 lb/in^2). Bulky dressings and surgical packs may require exposure times two or three times as long.

When sterilization is completed the chamber is evacuated and sterile air is admitted through a filter. To avoid the risk of explosion when sealed containers of liquid are being autoclaved, the chamber door must not be opened until the temperature of the contents is less than 80°C. Most autoclaves have a steam-heated jacket to accelerate the drying of the load.

Failure to produce a sterile load may be due to:

1 Faults in the autoclave and the way it is operated, e.g. poor quality (wet) steam, superheating due to excessive jacket temperature, failure to remove air and condensate, faulty gauges, faulty timing, leaking door seals.
2 Errors in loading, e.g. excessive layers of wrapping material, impervious wrapping material, over-large packs, containers that are completely closed (hermetically sealed bottles containing aqueous fluids need not be opened), overpacking of the autoclave.
3 Recontamination after sterilization, e.g. inadequate air filter, leakage into the chamber, wet or torn packs, unhygienic handling, incorrect storage.

Control of sterilization is essential. Methods used include:

1 Automatic dial recording of temperatures and times of each sterilizing cycle.
2 Heat-sensitive tape fixed to the outside of each pack.
3 A chemical indicator placed in the most inaccessible part of each load, e.g. routine use of Browne TST strips or Browne tubes which change colour when an adequate temperature has been maintained for an adequate time.
4 For high-vacuum autoclaves, daily tests in an otherwise empty chamber with a standard test pack consisting of heat-sensitive tape fixed in the form of a cross to a sheet of paper and placed in the middle of a pile of 24–36 folded huckaback towels. If all air has been removed the tape shows a *uniform* colour change; if air remains, the colour change is incomplete at the centre (Bowie-Dick test).
5 Daily checks for leaks by evacuating the chamber and confirming that the leak rate does not exceed 1.3 kPa over a period of 10 minutes.
6 Heat-resistant spores as an occasional absolute check on sterility, e.g. use of paper strips impregnated with spores of *Bacillus stearothermophilus.*
7 An unprotected sterile swab as an occasional check on the possibility of recontamination.
8 Thermocouple measurements inside loads (special circumstances only).

Radiation

Direct sunshine kills vegetative organisms fairly rapidly, but spores are much more resistant. The disinfecting properties mainly reside in the ultraviolet range. Ordinary glass is impervious to these rays.

Ultraviolet light produced artificially has powerful germicidal properties, but its powers of penetration are so slight that its practical usefulness is limited. It is used for disinfecting the inside of inoculation cabinets. The air supply of operating theatres can usually be purified more simply by other means.

Ionizing radiations. Two types are available in special centres: gamma radiation from radioactive isotopes, such as cobalt-60 and caesium-137, and high energy electrons from a machine. Gamma rays are very penetrating and can be used to sterilize articles which are up to 0.5 m thick. The penetrating power of electrons depends upon the energy to which they are accelerated, but is normally very much less. Under most conditions 2.5×10^4 gray (2.5 Mrad) is a sterilizing dose with an adequate margin of safety. The method cannot induce radioactivity in the material irradiated.

Ionizing radiations can be used to sterilize a wide range of prepacked, heat-sensitive articles including bone grafts, surgical sutures, plastic arterial prostheses, disposable plastic dialysis equipment, syringes, catheters, Petri dishes and rubber gloves. Many pharmaceutical products including hormones, antibiotics and enzymes can be satisfactorily sterilized but others lose their potency.

In some countries irradiation is used to preserve certain food-stuffs. Some foods develop unpleasant flavours and unacceptable changes of colour and texture. The whole subject is still highly controversial.

Filtration

Bacterial filters are used for sterilizing injection fluids and bac-teriological media containing heat-sensitive substances (e.g. serum, delicate sugars, certain drugs); separating bacteria from their enzymes and toxins; and for removing bacteria from suspensions containing viruses.

Bacterial filters can be made of earthenware, sintered glass, asbestos, cellulose esters or other inert polymers. Those commonly used retain bacteria but allow viruses to pass through into the filtrate. Membrane filters made of mixed cellulose esters are the most useful for bacteriological work. They provide a high rate of filtration and are less absorptive than other filters. Retained bac-teria can be cultured by placing the membrane on the surface of a solid medium. Membrane filters can be prepared with a specific and highly uniform pore size and ultrafiltration can be used for measuring the size of viruses.

Water for human consumption is usually filtered in large filter beds consisting of a layer of sand 0.5−1.5 m thick, supported on gravel and clinker. The main filtering agent is a slimy coating of algae, protozoa and bacteria which forms on the surface of the sand. In some processes alum is added to the water before filtration to hasten deposition of suspended matter. These filters cannot be relied on to remove all bacteria and the water is later chlorinated.

Air filtration is required for operating theatres. The air is nor-mally passed through a coarse filter of glass wool to remove large particles of dirt and then through finer filters of disposable fabric. Some air purifiers use fine sprays of water to humidify the air but these are not recommended because of the dangers of *Legionella* infection. Electrostatic precipitators are efficient in removing very small particles which are difficult to trap with ordinary filters.

High efficiency particulate (hepa) filters are used when freedom from air-borne contamination is essential. They are fitted in laminar flow cabinets and clean rooms used for bacteriological, pharmaceutical and industrial purposes and in units dealing with patients who are unusually susceptible to infection, e.g. those undergoing immunosuppressive therapy.

Cotton-wool is an effective air filter for bacteriological work. It must be kept dry. It can be used as an air filter for autoclaves, but there are advantages in using filters consisting of folded sheets of glass-fibre paper. These need changing only every year or so.

Chemical methods

A vast number of chemical substances will kill or inhibit microbes. In practice different objects and circumstances impose limitations on what can usefully be employed as sterilizing or disinfecting agents. There is certainly no such thing as an ideal general purpose disinfectant. In assessing a disinfectant the following general points should be considered:

1 *Is a disinfectant really necessary?* It is cheaper, safer and more effective to use heat whenever this is possible. Disinfectants are not a substitute for cleanliness. Hot water, soap or detergent and a scrubbing brush used with vigour is often all that is required.

2 *Organisms killed.* Spores are highly resistant and only a few disinfectants, e.g. formaldehyde, glutaraldehyde, halogens and ethylene oxide, have any effect at the concentrations usually employed. *Mycobacterium tuberculosis* is more resistant than most vegetative organisms, e.g. although it is fairly sensitive to phenols and alcohols it is resistant to mineral acids, alkalis and halogens. Gram-negative organisms are often more resistant than gram-positive organisms. *Pseudomonas aeruginosa* is especially resistant. Viruses tend to be more resistant than vegetative bacteria. Most viruses are sensitive to halogens, oxidizing agents, formaldehyde and glutaraldehyde and only slightly sensitive to phenols.

3 *Organisms inhibited.* It is important to know that organisms are killed and not merely inhibited. Thus high dilutions of mercury salts have a bacteristatic or inhibitory effect on bacteria, but their bactericidal or killing effect is weak and very slow. With the aid of an appropriate neutralizer it can be shown that most of the bacteria are still alive after many hours. Other antiseptics show a much smaller ratio between bactericidal and bacteristatic concentrations. Some, such as formaldehyde, glutaraldehyde, halogens and ethylene oxide, are almost exclusively bactericidal.

4 *Rate of action.* Some powerful chemicals are effective in a few seconds, but most disinfectants take minutes, hours or even days. A higher temperature, a higher concentration of dis-

infectant and a smaller number of organisms to be killed decreases the time required. Some disinfectants are most active in acid, others in alkaline environments. Most disinfectants show little activity in the absence of moisture. All disinfectants are to some extent neutralized by organic matter such as blood, pus and faeces; marked neutralization occurs with mercury salts and halogens. The power of penetration is important in enabling a disinfectant to reach organisms protected by organic matter, grease, etc. Surface activity, ability to dissolve fats, solubility in organic solvents and miscibility with soaps and detergents may assist penetration.

5   *Side effects.* Suitability for a given purpose may be limited by toxicity, possession of an irritating vapour, corrosive and destructive effects on instruments and fabrics, unwanted staining properties, difficulties in handling, poor keeping qualities and cost.

6   *Standardized in vitro tests.* No single quantitative measurement can possibly indicate the value of a disinfectant for all purposes. *Use-dilution tests* designed to show at which dilution a particular disinfectant should be used for some particular purpose are more realistic but still have many limitations.

7   *In-use tests.* It is important to check that a disinfectant is effective under real-life conditions. This can often be achieved by taking samples from trolley tops, equipment and so on after disinfection. To confirm that a particular dilution of a disinfectant is suitable for a particular purpose various in-use tests have been devised in which the liquid phase of disinfection systems is examined for viable bacteria. Samples that can be tested include fluid wrung from mops, bucket contents after cleaning procedures, fluid used to store and disinfect brushes, mops and instruments, and stock bottles of dilute disinfectants. A satisfactory use-dilution yields only an occasional positive culture. Use-dilutions intended for rapid disinfection can be accepted only if the disinfectants are freshly made up from concentrations known to be self-sterilizing and if all containers, mops and brushes are frequently decontaminated by boiling, autoclaving or putting through a washing machine. Regular in-use tests provide a check on procedural errors and draw attention to excessive bacterial contamination or the presence of organisms of unusual resistance.

Chemical disinfectants

Salts

Many simple salts in high concentration inhibit bacteria though they may not kill them. Sodium chloride is used in the preservation of fish and meat. *Staphylococcus aureus,* enterococci and *Vibrio parahaemolyticus* tolerate higher salt concentrations than other human pathogens.

Mercuric chloride and oxycyanide are very toxic and inactivated by organic matter. They are largely bacteristatic and their bactericidal activity is negligible under most conditions. Organic mercury compounds such as thiomersal and mercurochrome are less toxic, but they too have very slight bactericidal activity.

Silver nitrate solution and silver sulphadiazine cream are used in the treatment of burns.

Acids and alkalis

Vinegar (acetic acid), sulphur dioxide and benzoic acid are used for preserving foods. A solution of acetic acid (0.25%) is sometimes used for bladder washouts in intractable urinary tract infections. Many strong mineral acids and alkalis are powerful germicides, but are not suitable for use as disinfectants.

Halogens

Halogens in very low concentration kill bacteria (*M. tuberculosis* is resistant), viruses, fungi and spores. They combine readily with organic matter and lose their germicidal activity.

Chlorine and substances which liberate it (*hypochlorites, chloramines* and *organic chloroisocyanurates*) are used for disinfecting water. Sufficient chlorine is added to saturate the demands of any organic matter and leave a small amount (0.2−0.5 parts per million) of residual chlorine. In swimming baths continuous chlorination is necessary to maintain the level of free chlorine. Very strong solutions of hypochlorites (e.g. 10% Chloros or Domestos, equivalent to 10 000 ppm of available chlorine) are used for disinfecting articles and surfaces contaminated with blood. This treatment is effective against the viruses causing hepatitis B and AIDS. Weaker solutions (0.2−1.0%) are valuable for disinfecting relatively clean articles such as feeding bottles, baths, dairy and catering equipment. Solutions of hypochlorites (eusol) are satisfactory for local treatment of bed sores and ulcers of the legs. Sodium dichloroisocyanurate in granular form is used to deal with spilt blood in wards, ambulances, etc. The granules are sprinkled on the blood. They soak it up, prevent it spreading and release chlorine which kills any organisms present.

Iodine as a 2−5% aqueous or ethanolic solution in potassium iodide is a very effective method of disinfecting intact skin before surgical operations. On rare occasions iodine causes severe skin reactions. *Iodophors* (e.g. Betadine), complexes of iodine with surface-active agents such as polyvinylpyrrolidone, do not stain or irritate the skin. They are effective for preoperative skin preparation and for the surgical scrub.

Oxidizing agents

These are active against viruses as well as bacteria.

Potassium permanganate is used in the tropics for disinfecting drinking water, fruit and vegetables.

Hydrogen peroxide is used for cleaning and disinfecting wounds.

Ozone is a powerful germicidal agent. It is highly toxic and is too expensive and inconvenient for routine use. It has been used for disinfecting water and for preserving food. It leaves no toxic residue.

Ether

Ether has little antibacterial activity. Viruses which possess an envelope are very sensitive. Others are almost completely resistant.

Alcohols

Ethanol kills vegetative bacteria and some viruses fairly rapidly if it is used at a concentration of about 70%. It is active against *M. tuberculosis*. It has poor penetrating power and is of little use in the presence of much organic matter. Pure ethanol has almost no antibacterial activity. Ethanol is used for preparing the skin prior to injections and for disinfecting trolley tops and other clean surfaces in high-risk areas.

Isopropanol has greater activity. At a concentration of 70% it is used for disinfecting the skin, thermometers, trolley tops and other work surfaces.

Soaps and detergents

Soaps have slight germicidal activity. *Streptococcus pneumoniae, Str. pyogenes, Haemophilus influenzae* and influenza virus are killed in a relatively short time, but *Staph. aureus, M. tuberculosis* and most gram-negative bacilli are unaffected. The main function of soap is the mechanical removal of organisms. The results inevitably fall far short of sterility. Organisms recently acquired by touching patients, etc., are removed more readily than those resident in the skin. In fact, washing commonly causes an increase in bacterial counts from the skin of the hands and fingers. The washing process appears to facilitate the escape to the surface of the resident flora which usually consists of harmless organisms but which in a few individuals includes *Staph. aureus*. There are advantages in using soap containing hexachlorophane; most other germicidal soaps are of no value.

Anionic detergents, such as sulphated long-chain fatty alcohols, are excellent cleansing agents for floors, walls, ledges, furniture, trolleys, crockery and cutlery. They have little germicidal activity but can be used in combination with phenolic disinfectants. In this form they are used in operating theatres and other high-risk areas.

Cationic detergents include the quaternary ammonium compounds, e.g. cetrimide (Cetavlon) is cetyltrimethylammonium bromide. Their surface-active properties make them excellent cleansing agents for intact skin, wounds and burns as well as for inanimate objects. The quaternaries are active against most gram-positive bacteria but less active against gram-negative bacteria. Their action is mainly bacteristatic. *Ps. aeruginosa* is relatively resistant and *M. tuberculosis,* spores and viruses are highly resistant. Their activity is readily neutralized by organic matter. It is important to guard against inactivation by soaps and anionic detergents, e.g. adding cetrimide when cleansing the skin with soap. The quaternaries have no place in environmental disinfection in hospitals.

Non-ionic detergents, such as ethylene oxide condensates, are excellent cleansing agents but have almost no germicidal activity. They can be used in conjunction with many disinfectants.

Phenols

Phenol ('carbolic acid') came into prominence with the introduction of the antiseptic (literally 'counteracting putrefaction') system of surgery by Lister. It is used as a preservative for materials for injection but is no longer used as a general disinfectant.

Substituted phenols. By introducing various chemical groups into the phenol nucleus substances of higher bactericidal activity are obtained. These include the cresols (methyl phenols), xylenols (dimethyl phenols) and the chloroxylenols. Mixtures of such substances form the basis of many proprietary disinfectants. The most useful disinfectants for general purposes are the *clear soluble phenolic fluids* (e.g. Clearsol, Hycolin, Stericol and Sudol) and the *white phenolic fluids* (e.g. Izal). These have a wide range of antibacterial activity and are only slightly inactivated by organic matter. Lysol consists of cresols in emulsion with soap; it is effective for disinfecting faeces, bed-pans, lavatories, floors and laboratory equipment but it is caustic and poisonous and a less dangerous disinfectant (e.g. Sudol) is preferred. Dettol contains a chloroxylenol; it is effective against gram-positive bacteria but has less action against gram-negative bacteria. *Ps. aeruginosa* is more resistant than other bacteria. Dettol is greatly inactivated by organic matter but it has low toxicity and can be used on the skin and tissues.

Hexachlorophane is a complex chlorinated phenolic compound. It has weak bactericidal activity, but very high dilutions exert a bacteristatic effect which is not easily reversed. Like many complex phenols it is more active against gram-positive than against gram-negative bacteria. *Staph. aureus* is very susceptible. Hexachlorophane can be mixed with soaps and some detergents without loss of activity and is a useful disinfectant for the preoperative surgical scrub. It is retained on the skin for long periods and repeated washing progressively reduces the bacterial flora of the skin. Hexachlorophane is also used in the form of dusting powders and creams and as an addition to bath water in attempts to control staphylococcal infections. Repeated exposure of infants to high concentrations causes brain damage. In 1972 at least 30 infants died in France after use of a talcum powder containing excessive hexachlorophane.

Triclosan resembles hexachlorophane in its activity. It is used for the surgical scrub and as a general skin disinfectant. It is not toxic for the newborn.

Diguanide compounds

Chlorhexidine (Hibitane) is bactericidal at high dilutions for a wide range of bacteria. It is moderately active against *Ps. aeruginosa*. Spores and viruses are resistant. *M. tuberculosis* is killed only by alcoholic solutions. It has very low toxicity and retains moderate activity in the presence of organic matter. It can be used for burns, wounds and other surgical conditions. Chlorhexidine (0.5%) in 70% ethanol or isopropanol is satisfactory for preoperative disinfection of the skin. Aqueous chlorhexidine digluconate (0.02% for 30 minutes) or ethanolic chlorhexidine (0.5% for 3 minutes) can be used for disinfecting cystoscopes, but the process is not reliable and heat treatment is preferred. Chlorhexidine used in conjunction with cetrimide has greater activity than chlorhexidine alone. The combination (Savlon) can be used for the surgical scrub, preoperative treatment of the skin, cleaning wounds in accident departments, adding to bath water as an antistaphylococcal agent, and for various other surgical and obstetric procedures. The surface activity of the cetrimide is an advantage for most purposes, but has a deleterious effect on the cement of optical instruments such as cystoscopes. Aqueous solutions of chlorhexidine and chlorhexidine-cetrimide mixtures are liable to become contaminated with *Pseudomonas* spp. and should be issued sterilized in sachets or other small containers for use on one occasion only.

Formaldehyde

This irritant gas is active against bacteria (including *M. tuberculosis*), fungi, viruses and, more slowly, spores. Solutions of formaldehyde (formalin is a 40% aqueous solution) are used to destroy anthrax spores in imported wool, hair and hides. They can be used to treat boots and shoes infected with the fungi of athlete's foot. Dilute solutions are used to kill motile bacteria in such a way as to preserve their H antigens. Formaldehyde (and glutaraldehyde) solutions can cause skin irritation and contact dermatitis.

The combination of low temperature steam and formaldehyde can be used to sterilize books, toys, clothing, plastic articles, electrical leads, cystoscopes and other surgical equipment that cannot withstand high temperature steam. An initial vacuum is used to remove air. To ensure penetration the load is subjected to several pulses of steam plus formaldehyde at 70–80°C. After a suitable holding period the chamber is evacuated to assist removal of the formaldehyde. Long narrow tubes such as arterial and ureteric catheters can be sterilized by this method but it is important to pack the articles in such a way that any residual moisture can drain away.

Gaseous formaldehyde in a chamber is sometimes used for disinfecting clothing, blankets, pillows, mattresses, toys and similar articles. The process is not reliable. Formaldehyde vapour liberated into a small container from tablets of paraformaldehyde is occasionally used to sterilize small heat-sensitive articles. It will sterilize the outside of articles but will not diffuse into long narrow tubes.

Formaldehyde is the most satisfactory agent for disinfecting a room and its contents. Cracks in windows and ventilators are sealed with tape, water is sprayed on the floor and walls to raise the relative humidity, and formaldehyde is generated by boiling a solution or adding formalin to potassium permanganate. The door is closed and sealed and the room is left until the next day.

Glutaraldehyde

Glutaraldehyde, like formaldehyde, is active against bacteria (including *M. tuberculosis* and *Ps. aeruginosa*), spores, viruses and fungi. A 2% aqueous solution buffered to pH 7.5–8.5 (e.g. Cidex) is useful for disinfecting cystoscopes, anaesthetic equipment and surgical instruments, but heat treatment is preferable. Vegetative bacteria (other than mycobacteria) and viruses (including hepatitis B virus and human immunodeficiency virus) are killed in 10 minutes, *M. tuberculosis* in 1 hour and spores in 10 hours.

Ethylene oxide

Ethylene oxide is active against organisms of all types, including spores. It is a gas at room temperature, but provided that it does not exceed 12% by weight there is no risk of explosion when it is mixed with inert gases such as carbon dioxide or a fluorocarbon. It is normally used in a closed chamber which can be evacuated before admission of the gas. Ethylene oxide diffuses rapidly through paper, fabrics and many plastics. It can be used for sterilizing heart-lung machines; artery and bone grafts; plastic articles such as dialysis equipment, transfusion sets and disposable syringes; surgical instruments such as cystoscopes and catheters; clothing, bedding, books and toys; bacteriologial media and vaccines; pharmaceutical products; and foodstuffs.

Liquid ethylene oxide (BP 10.7°C) can be used for sterilizing liquid media, vaccines and small objects such as graft tissues and plastic articles which can be immersed in fluid.

Ethylene oxide is toxic for man. It is also one of the most powerful mutagenic agents known. The liquid has a vesicant action on the skin. Rubber and plastic articles retain ethylene oxide for long periods and must not be handled immediately after sterilization. Anaphylactic reactions associated with antibodies against ethylene oxide have been reported in patients undergoing regular dialysis using equipment sterilized with this agent.

Beta-propiolactone

This has properties very similar to ethylene oxide. Unfortunately it is a potent carcinogen. In aqueous solution it can be used for sterilization of grafts, sera and vaccines.

Examination of Clinical Specimens

...routine urine-testing in the wards emerges as a marginally more exact science than palmistry, but not one which could fairly be compared to an intelligent game of noughts and crosses.

The Lancet, 1962

We sanguinely hope that the laboratory will answer our questions with a dogmatic 'yes' or 'no': its usual answer is 'perhaps'. Patients do not fit neatly into the specialties of medicine. Infection is often just one aspect of a wider problem and symptoms suggestive of infectious disease may be due to other pathological conditions, e.g. sore throat may be due to blood diseases, urinary symptoms may occur in diabetes, fever may be associated with neoplasm. It follows that the microbiologist must be prepared to let his mind wander to the other branches of clinical pathology.

If the technical procedures of the laboratory are to be used intelligently adequate clinical information is essential. Thus the age of the patient, the nature of the illness, source of the specimen, previous antibiotic therapy, etc., may influence the methods used and the attention that is paid to particular organisms.

The following diagnostic procedures are available:

1 Macroscopic examination of specimen (blood, pus, etc.).
2 Microscopic examination (organisms, cells, gram film, etc.).
3 Direct identification of organisms and their nucleic acids, antigens and products (DNA hybridization, fluorescent antibody staining, capsule swelling, gas-liquid chromatography, countercurrent immunoelectrophoresis, etc.).
4 Isolation and identification of organisms:
   a Cultural characteristics (conditions of growth, type of colonies, haemolysis, etc.).
   b Microscopic appearances (gram film, special stains, motility, etc.).
   c Biochemical properties (fermentation reactions, end-products, enzymes, etc.).

d   Antigenic properties.
e   Pathogenicity tests in animals.
f   Other tests (phage-typing, drug sensitivity, etc.).
5   Demonstration of antibodies in the patient's serum.
6   Other investigations (skin tests, response to treatment, histology, white cell count, etc.).

The relative importance of these procedures varies in different diseases. It is always more satisfactory if the organisms can be cultured and properly identified, but this is not always possible. The precise media and methods used in different laboratories vary greatly.

Urine

Catheterization carries a risk of infection. In men a mid-stream specimen is requested. In women a catheter specimen is often requested as a routine. This is not necessary. A properly instructed ambulant patient can usually produce a clean specimen which is satisfactory for bacteriological purposes. When infection with *Mycobacterium tuberculosis* is suspected three consecutive early morning specimens of urine should be sent to the laboratory.

Specimens must not be left at room temperature because bacterial growth will occur and the results will be unreliable. If the specimen cannot be examined immediately it should be refrigerated at 4°C. Boric acid (0.5 g in a 28 ml container) is a satisfactory preservative when delay is inevitable, e.g. for postal specimens.

Routine examination

The naked-eye appearance is noted and a sample is taken for culture. The specimen is tested for albumin and sugar and is examined under the microscope (wet preparation) for cells, organisms, casts and crystals.

Cultures are made on uncentrifuged urine so that semiquantitative results can be obtained. Bacterial counts made by inoculating plates with serial dilutions of urine are time-consuming and mainly used for special purposes, e.g. standardizing other methods. Counts of sufficient accuracy for routine purposes can be made (1) by using standard strips of sterile filter paper bent at one end to form a foot (6 × 12 mm) which is dipped in the urine, held for a moment and then pressed on to the surface of a plate of CLED medium or MacConkey medium; (2) by using a standard loop (e.g. 5 mm) which is removed vertically from the urine and plated out on the same media; or (3) by using slides coated with nutrient medium ('dip slides') which are dipped in the urine, drained, sent by post to the laboratory and incubated on arrival. Direct sensitivity tests should be set up if large numbers of organisms are seen in the direct film. The plates are incubated aerobically at 37°C for 18—24 hours and gram-stained films are made of representative colonies. *Escherichia coli* and some other organisms can usually be recognized without further investigation. Other colonies are picked off for subculture and identification. By reference to standard curves the bacterial count can be calculated from the numbers of colonies growing on the inoculated area, e.g. 25 colonies with the filter paper test or 50 colonies using a 5 mm loop correspond to approximately 100×10^6 organisms/litre.

Microscopy is frequently performed on the centrifuged deposit from 10—15 ml urine, the results being expressed as the number of cells per high power field. However, it is quicker, cheaper and just as reliable to perform microscopy on *uncentrifuged* urine. In one method a micropipette fitted with a disposable tip is used to deliver a small standard volume of urine into one of the flat-bottomed wells of a plastic tray. Red and white cells are counted under the medium power ($\times$ 20) lens of an inverted microscope and, by reference to a standard curve, the results can be expressed semiquantitatively as cells $\times$ 10^6/litre.

Examination for M. tuberculosis

The pooled deposit of three early morning specimens (300—500 ml) is examined. Films are stained by either the Ziehl-Neelsen (ZN) or the fluorescent (auramine) method and are examined for acid-fast bacilli. The rest of the deposit is treated to destroy contaminating organisms, e.g. with 4% NaOH followed by neutralization with HCl. It is then cultured on Löwenstein-Jensen slopes.

Results

1   *Organisms*. Urine is normally sterile but is often contaminated during collection and a small number of organisms can be ignored. Bacterial counts of more than 100×10^6/litre indicate urinary infection; counts less than 10×10^6/litre are usually due to contaminants; intermediate counts are equivocal. A pure culture is more likely to be significant than a mixture of organisms.

E. coli is the cause of 80—90% of cases of acute or 'primary' urinary infections. *Proteus mirabilis* and *Staphylococcus saprophyticus* account for many of the remainder. The bacteria are usually present in pure culture and are sensitive to the antibacterial agents used in treating urinary infections.

In chronic or 'secondary' infections associated with failed therapy, anatomical abnormalities, surgical operations, indwelling catheters, etc., *E. coli* is the commonest cause, but a variety of other bacteria are encountered including *Proteus, Klebsiella,* other coliforms, *Pseudomonas aeruginosa, Streptococcus faecalis, Staph. aureus* and *Staph. epidermidis.* Mixed cultures are common and the organisms are more likely to be resistant to antibacterial agents. Acute urinary infections may be superimposed on underlying infection caused by *M. tuberculosis.*

2   *Pus cells.* Urinary infections are associated with an increase in the number of leucocytes ('pus cells') in the urine. In a random specimen the pus cells do not normally exceed 2×10^6/litre (about 2 cells per high power field in the centrifuged deposit); slightly higher counts are sometimes found in normal women. In urinary tract infections the counts usually exceed 50×10^6/litre but may be very much higher.

Abacterial pyuria

The urine contains an excess of pus cells but routine culture is sterile. This is very common when the patient is excreting anti-bacterial drugs, but a rarer cause which must always be excluded is infection by *M. tuberculosis.* Abacterial pyuria occasionally occurs as an obscure condition of unknown aetiology.

Bacteriuria without pyuria

Large numbers of bacteria without pus cells are sometimes found in early pregnancy and in diabetes. Although the patient may have no urinary symptoms, persistent bacteriuria should not be ignored as many of these patients later develop frank urinary infection.

White cells are rapidly destroyed by strongly alkaline urine and in *Proteus* infections they may not be detectable if examination is delayed.

Urethral syndrome

Urine specimens from about 50% of women complaining of fre-quency and dysuria show no significant bacterial growth on routine culture. In general the cause of the symptoms is unknown, but some cases may be due to fastidious bacteria which are not picked up by ordinary methods.

Faeces

The faeces are passed into a clean container and a small sample is obtained with a disposable spoon. A rectal swab is satisfactory in the case of young children.

Macroscopic appearance

The colour, consistency and presence of blood, pus or mucus are noted.

Microscopic appearance

1   *Wet preparation*. A suspension in saline is examined for ova, cysts and parasites. The presence of large numbers of pus cells is a useful indicator of bowel inflammation. Motile *Entamoeba histolytica* will be seen only if the specimen is examined soon after it has been passed.

2   *Gram-stained film*. This is normally of no value since salmonellae and shigellae cannot be distinguished from *E. coli*. In the extremely rare condition, *Staph. aureus* enterocolitis, the faeces contain vast numbers of staphylococci and pus cells and an immediate diagnosis can be made.

Culture and further investigation

The faeces are plated out on deoxycholate citrate agar and a heavy inoculum is made into a liquid enrichment medium (tetrathionate or selenite F broth). If staphylococcal enterocolitis is suspected a plate of MacConkey medium or salt nutrient agar is also inoculated. The cultures are incubated aerobically at 37°C. Special techniques are used for isolation of vibrios (p. 287), *Yersinia enterocolitica* (p. 292) and campylobacters (p. 302).

Day 1. The plates are examined for non-lactose-fermenting (colourless) colonies, i.e. possible salmonellae or shigellae. A well-isolated colony is picked off and inoculated into peptone water and urea medium. When there is more than one type of non-lactose-fermenting colony each type must be investigated. If the organism splits urea in 2−4 hours (change of colour of indicator) it is *Proteus* and can be ignored. If it does not split urea the peptone water culture is (1) tested for motility, (2) inoculated into a set of 'sugars' and onto an agar slope and (3) plated out on MacConkey agar as a check on the purity of the culture.

Meanwhile a sample from the enrichment medium is plated out on MacConkey agar. If the original deoxycholate citrate plate is negative it is reincubated.

In staphylococcal enterocolitis an almost pure growth of *Staph. aureus* is found on the MacConkey plate.

Rapid methods. Special tests have been devised to speed up the provisional biochemical identification of non-lactose-fermenting organisms. These tests employ (1) composite media in which two or more reactions can be observed at the same time, (2) micromethods in which heavy suspensions of organisms are added to small volumes of reagents and (3) biochemical tests in which the reagents are contained in tablets or impregnated paper strips. Rapid tests are mainly of value in laboratories dealing with very large numbers of faecal specimens. The ONPG (*o*-nitrophenyl-β-D-galactopyranoside) test is of more general value. Potential lactose-fermenting organisms which take several days to produce acid in ordinary media ('late-lactose fermenters') can be rapidly identified by their ability to produce β-galactosidase as shown by the hydrolysis of ONPG on overnight incubation.

Day 2. The non-lactose fermenters are investigated further.

1 *Biochemical reactions.* The peptone water culture is tested for indole and the fermentation reactions are recorded. If rapid methods are used the results are noted. If the reactions suggest salmonellae or shigellae (p. 272) the organism is investigated by agglutination reactions; otherwise it is ignored.
2 *Agglutination reactions.* The agar slope culture is tested by slide agglutination using standard diagnostic sera. Positive results are confirmed by tube agglutination. It is possible to do agglutination reactions on colonies from the primary cultures (Day 1), but the results are apt to be misleading.

Shigellae. The sera used are: a composite serum against smooth and rough phases of *Shigella sonnei*; polyvalent sera against *Sh. flexneri* and *Sh. boydi*, followed by type-specific sera if the results are positive; and individual specific sera against the different types of *Sh. dysenteriae*.

Salmonellae. A positive reaction with a polyvalent *Salmonella* O antiserum is provisional evidence that the organism is a salmonella.

O antigens. The organism is tested with separate antisera against the main O groups and is assigned to a particular group (A, B, C, etc.). The Vi antigen of *S. typhi* may mask the O antigen and the organism should be also tested with a Vi serum.

H antigens. Some organisms show diphasic variation of their flagellar antigens. The organism is therefore tested with a polyvalent H (phase 1 + phase 2) serum and a polyvalent H (phase 2) serum. If, as is usually the case, the organism is in phase 1 (i.e. reacts with phase 1 + phase 2 serum but not with phase 2 serum) it can be identified by systematic testing with specific H phase 1 sera against organisms of the appropriate O group. If the organism is in phase 2 (i.e. reacts with H phase 2 serum) it cannot be identified until it has been obtained in phase 1. In Craigie's method a small tube open at both ends is inserted vertically into semi-solid medium containing anti-serum against phase 2. The culture is inoculated down the tube. Phase 2 organisms are agglutinated, whereas the few phase 1 organisms always present in such a culture remain fully motile and spread through into the medium outside the tube. They can then be identified with specific sera.

3   Non-lactose-fermenting colonies appearing in subculture from the enrichment medium or from further incubation of the original plates are investigated.

Infantile gastroenteritis

In children under three years of age additional tests are made for enteropathogenic strains of *E. coli*. The colonies do not differ from normal *E. coli*. They grow on MacConkey agar, but an additional blood agar plate is inoculated to improve the chances of isolation and to ensure that the colonies remain in the smooth phase. Some 5—10 colonies including all morphological types are tested for slide agglutination with polyvalent *E. coli* antiserum and, if the results are positive, with individual type sera. The results are confirmed by tube agglutination.

Diarrhoea in children is frequently caused by rotaviruses and a specimen of faeces should be examined by one of the rapid methods available for detecting rotavirus antigens.

Wounds, burns, abscesses, pus

Samples taken with a cotton-wool swab are usually adequate but it is always preferable to send a *large* sample of pus, e.g. to provide adequate material for full investigation for *M. tuberculosis*, to increase the chances of finding 'sulphur granules' in actino-mycosis, and to facilitate the isolation of anaerobes.

Direct films

A gram-stained film is always made. It shows whether pus cells are present or not, i.e. whether there is evidence of inflammation, and it indicates the type of organisms involved and provides a check on the organisms subsequently recovered in culture. A film is stained by the ZN or auramine method when the lesions are chronic and tuberculosis is a possibility.

Culture

The material is routinely plated out on (1) blood agar, (2) blood agar incubated anaerobically and (3) MacConkey agar. Additional media can be inoculated for special purposes, e.g. sensitivity agar for direct antibiotic sensitivity tests; selective media for *Neisseria gonorrhoeae*; Löwenstein-Jensen medium for *M. tuberculosis*.

The plates are inspected after incubation at 37°C for 24 hours. Gram-stained films are made of each type of colony present. If both blood agar plates show a pure culture and the appearances of the films are identical it is reasonable to assume that the organisms on the two plates are the same and only one plate need be investigated. If several types of colony are present and the colonies on the anaerobic plate do not obviously correspond with those on the aerobic plate, isolated colonies from the anaerobic plate must be subcultured aerobically and anaerobically to ensure that no organisms, particularly anaerobes, are overlooked. If the primary plates show no growth they are reincubated for a further 24 hours or longer if it is suspected that some slow-growing organism is present.

The MacConkey plate assists in the preliminary identification of many organisms. The medium inhibits swarming by *Proteus* and it is often possible to recover organisms from a mixed culture when the blood agar plates have been overgrown.

Results

Interpretation of the bacteriological findings can be difficult. Scanty growth of skin flora, together with *Staph. aureus* and coliforms, usually represent contamination and colonization rather than infection. Heavy growth of a single organism, particularly if associated with large numbers of polymorphs in the films, is more likely to have clinical significance. Foul-smelling pus suggests infection with anaerobic bacteria of which *Bacteroides* are the most commonly encountered. Overall, *Staph. aureus* is the commonest cause of wound infection; *E. coli* in association with *Bacteroides* is the next most important. Other organisms commonly encountered include *Streptococcus pyogenes*, *Klebsiella*, *Proteus*, *Ps. aeruginosa*, *Staph. epidermidis*, diphtheroids, various species of aerobic and anaerobic streptococci and *Cl. perfringens*. In abscesses similar organisms are found; other organisms sometimes encountered include *M. tuberculosis*, *Actinomyces israeli*, neisseriae and salmonellae.

Infections of the female genital tract

In puerperal sepsis and septic abortion a high vaginal or cervical swab is taken. The swab is examined in the same way as wound swabs. An additional plate of special medium for *Mycoplasma hominis* is inoculated and examined for 'fried egg' colonies after incubation for 6 days. *Str. pyogenes* is rarely found in the healthy vagina and the presence of only a few colonies is usually significant. *Cl. perfringens*, *E. coli*, *Str. faecalis*, *Staph. aureus* and *M. hominis* are usually important when they are present in large numbers, but a few colonies may have no significance. Anaerobic streptococci are frequently present in the healthy vagina. Their presence is usually significant when numerous streptococci are seen in direct films and the culture gives a heavy growth of anaerobic cocci, particularly when these are *Str. putridus*. In all cases the direct films should be examined for gram-negative intracellular diplococci suggesting *N. gonorrhoeae* and additional cultures should be put up if necessary.

Lactobacilli, diphtheroids, non-haemolytic streptococci, small gram-negative bacilli (*Gardnerella vaginalis*) and anaerobic gram-negative bacilli (*Bacteroides*) are often isolated from the vagina. On the whole these are normal inhabitants but *Bacteroides* sometimes assume a pathogenic role. Mixed infections of *G. vaginalis* and various anaerobes are associated with 'non-specific vaginitis' (anaerobic vaginosis). Films of vaginal secretion characteristically show 'clue cells', epithelial cells coated with large numbers of small gram-negative bacilli. Polymorphs are absent.

In infections such as acute cervicitis, vaginitis, urethritis and chronic vaginal discharge the same general procedures are followed, but it is important to exclude the following:

1 *Trichomonas vaginalis.* A drop of discharge obtained with a pipette is examined in a drop of saline for motile, flagellated protozoa. Swabs are satisfactory provided they are examined at once or sent to the laboratory in transport medium.

2 *Candida albicans.* Numerous yeasts are seen in the gram film. The organisms grow on blood agar.

3 *N. gonorrhoeae.* Samples from the urethra and cervix are examined for gram-negative intracellular diplococci and are plated out *without delay* on previously warmed plates of 'chocolate' agar or special selective media (p. 241) which are incubated in air with $5-10\%$ CO_2. If delay is inevitable, swabs should be sent to the laboratory in transport medium. A patient with gonorrhoea may also have syphilis (and *vice versa*) and serological tests for syphilis must be done. If a suspected syphilitic chancre is present the lesion is cleaned with saline, squeezed vigorously and rubbed with sterile gauze until it begins to bleed. The lesion is wiped clean and a drop of clear tissue fluid is collected with a capillary pipette and examined for spirochaetes under dark-ground illumination.

4 *Herpes simplex virus.* If genital herpes is suspected a swab is broken off into a bottle of viral transport medium for subsequent inoculation of tissue cultures.

In pelvic inflammatory disease, including salpingitis and pelvic abscess, samples of pus should be sent to the laboratory. *Chlamydia trachomatis* is the commonest cause of pelvic inflammatory disease and a major cause of tubal occlusion and infertility in women. Special methods are used to detect the organisms (p. 321). In routine cultures *Bacteroides,* alone or in association with other organisms, is usually the most significant organism. Cultures for *N. gonorrhoeae* should be set up in all cases.

Infections of the male genital tract

Gonorrhoea and syphilis must be excluded. The procedures for examining a urethral discharge or a suspected chancre are the same as those used in women (see above). If there is no obvious urethral discharge pus can sometimes be obtained by prostatic massage. *Trichomonas vaginalis* occasionally causes urethritis in men.

Throat

A swab is firmly rubbed on the tonsils or the tonsillar bed. If there is any exudate or membranous material this should be obtained.

Direct films

These are not made as a routine because commensal streptococci present in the throat are microscopically indistinguishable from *Str. pyogenes.* Similarly, diphtheroids closely resembling *Corynebacterium diphtheriae* are commonly present. Nevertheless if membranous material is obtained a film should be made because in rare cases a provisional diagnosis of diphtheria can be made; negative results should be disregarded. When Vincent's angina is suspected a film is essential. It is stained with crystal violet (or carbol fuchsin) and examined for spirochaetes and fusiform bacilli. The presence of large numbers of yeasts (*Candida albicans*) in stained films is diagnostic of thrush.

Culture

The swab is plated out on (1) blood agar and (2) blood agar incubated anaerobically. If there is any reason to suspect diphtheria the swab is also inoculated on (3) blood tellurite agar and (4) Loeffler serum medium.

The plates are examined after 24 hours and gram-stained films are made. If organisms resembling *C. diphtheriae* are found films are stained for metachromatic granules by Albert's or Neisser's methods.

Str. pyogenes. Both blood plates are examined for streptococci showing β-haemolysis. *Str. pyogenes* usually causes haemolysis under both aerobic and anaerobic conditions, but 5–10% of strains only show obvious haemolysis on the anaerobic plate. Samples are taken for Lancefield grouping. For routine purposes streptococci which show obvious β-haemolysis and are sensitive to bacitracin and penicillin can be assumed to belong to group A. *Str. pyogenes,* usually in small numbers, may be present in 5–10% of healthy throats.

C. diphtheriae. The tellurite plate is examined for characteristic black colonies. The microscopic appearances of *C. diphtheriae* are not typical on this medium. The characteristic morphology is best seen on the Loeffler slope, but many other organisms grow well on this medium and subculture will be necessary before *C. diphtheriae* can be obtained in pure culture. Any suspicious colony is picked off the tellurite plate and the blood plates for full investigation, i.e. fermentation reactions in serum sugars; colonial appearance on a fresh tellurite plate; microscopic appearances on a fresh Loeffler slope; and tests for toxin production. The original cultures are incubated for a further 24 hours before they are discarded.

Other organisms. These are investigated if their presence is thought to be abnormal. Viridans streptococci, non-haemolytic streptococci, *Branhamella catarrhalis* and diphtheroids are almost invariably present. *Streptococcus pneumoniae, Haemophilus influenzae, Staph. aureus* and *Candida albicans* are often present in small or moderate numbers, but may be significant if they are the predominant organism. *E. coli, Klebsiella* and other coliform organisms are frequently found in the throats of patients who are being treated with antibiotics.

Sputum

Sputum is collected in a wide-mouthed jar or carton provided with a close-fitting lid. Infants and young children swallow their sputum and a throat swab is examined instead. Special methods are used in suspected whooping cough (p. 298). When examination for *M. tuberculosis* is required specimens of sputum are collected on three consecutive mornings. If the patient does not produce sputum, laryngeal swabs or early morning gastric washouts may be examined. Bronchoalveolar lavage, in which saline washings are taken from the lower respiratory tract, is a valuable procedure for investigating pulmonary infiltrates in immunosuppressed patients.

Direct films

Purulent portions of the sputum are chosen. Films are stained by Gram and ZN methods. The fluorescent (auramine) modification of the ZN method is time-saving when large numbers of specimens have to be examined.

Culture

The specimen is plated out on two blood agar plates incubated aerobically and anaerobically. A plate of 'chocolate' agar can be inoculated to improve the chances of isolating *H. influenzae*. Special media are used for *Legionella pneumophila* and *Mycoplasma pneumoniae*. If a virus is suspected the specimen is examined for viral antigens by immunofluorescent techniques and tissue cultures are inoculated. Cultures for *M. tuberculosis* are set up in special cases. The sputum is treated to destroy contaminants and inoculated on Löwenstein-Jensen medium. The blood plates are examined after incubation for 24 hours and representative colonies are stained by Gram's method. Organisms are investigated and their sensitivities determined if their presence is abnormal.

When a pathogen such as *Str. pneumoniae*, *Staph. aureus* or *H. influenzae* is the predominant organism it is significant. The presence of large numbers of *E. coli* or other coliform organisms is usually due to previous antibiotic treatment. A moderate increase in the numbers of *Str. pneumoniae* and *H. influenzae* is often seen in acute exacerbations of chronic bronchitis. In many respiratory tract infections the organisms isolated do not differ in type or in numbers from those found as normal commensals of the throat, e.g. despite the scepticism of clinicians, a mixed growth consisting mainly of viridans streptococci and *B. catarrhalis* may be the only finding in the sputum of a patient seriously ill with bronchopneumonia.

Nose

It is usually sufficient to sample the anterior nasal mucosa with a dry swab. The swab is investigated as for throat swabs. Nasal swabs are often taken from patients and hospital staff with the sole object of detecting carriers of *Staph. aureus* or *Str. pyogenes*. In patients with purulent nasal discharge, etc., full investigation of all organisms is required. It is important to exclude the presence of *C. diphtheriae*.

Ear

Acute infection of the middle ear arises as an extension of infection occurring in the nasopharynx. In chronic ear infections invasion by yeasts and fungi is common and investigation for these organisms should supplement other procedures.

Eye

Some of the organisms which cause conjunctivitis are extremely delicate, e.g. *N. gonorrhoeae*, *H. influenzae* and *Moraxella lacunata*. The chances of isolating such organisms are increased if samples are taken with a wire loop and plated out at once on blood agar or 'chocolate' agar which is then incubated in air with 5–10% CO_2.

Cerebrospinal fluid

The cerebrospinal fluid (CSF) is collected in two or more sterile bottles. The colour and the presence of turbidity or clot are noted. If clot is present it is removed for microscopy. A white cell count is performed on the specimen least contaminated with blood, i.e. usually the second bottle taken. The CSF is then centrifuged. The deposit is used for direct films and culture; the supernatant fluid for investigation of cells, protein, serological tests for syphilis, chloride and glucose. Estimation of chloride and glucose and bacteriological examination can often be omitted if the CSF is crystal clear and the cell count is normal, i.e. up to 5×10^6/litre, all lymphocytes.

Direct films

Cells and bacteria are most readily found in the fine 'spider-web' clot which sometimes forms in the CSF before centrifugation. If there is no clot the centrifuged deposit is examined. Films are prepared and stained by Gram's method for bacteria and Leishman stain for a differential cell count. If there is an excess of lymphocytes and tuberculous meningitis is suspected a film is stained by the ZN method for acid-fast bacilli. A gross excess of polymorphs accompanied by a lowering of CSF glucose concentration usually indicates acute meningitis and the gram film may show organisms resembling *Str. pneumoniae* (lanceolate diplococci), *N. meningitidis* (gram-negative diplococci) or *H. influenzae* (small gram-negative coccobacilli with occasional filamentous forms). Neonatal meningitis is commonly caused by *E. coli* or group B streptococci. Other organisms encountered include various gram-negative bacilli and *Listeria monocytogenes*. In tuberculous meningitis the predominant cells are lymphocytes, though up to 30% of the cells may be polymorphs. The search for acid-fast bacilli should be thorough as the results of culture will not be available for several weeks. A lymphocytic reaction is found in multiple sclerosis, syphilis of the nervous system, leptospiral meningitis and viral infections. In poliomyelitis the cellular reaction is often of mixed type and polymorphs occasionally predominate, particularly in the early stages.

Culture

The deposit is streaked out on a plate of blood agar or 'chocolate' agar which is incubated aerobically with $5-10\%$ CO_2. Anaerobic plate culture is not necessary as a routine but may be desirable in special circumstances, e.g. for neurosurgical patients. The deposit is also inoculated into cooked meat medium. Any surplus CSF is incubated in its original bottle. When tuberculosis is suspected the deposit is streaked out directly on Löwenstein-Jensen medium. If a viral infection is suspected some of the CSF is added to viral transport medium for inoculation of tissue cultures.

The plates are inspected after incubation for 24 hours. In acute meningitis a pure growth of the pathogen is usually obtained. If the plates show no growth they are reincubated. Subcultures are made from the cooked meat medium and from the incubated CSF.

Rapid methods

Countercurrent immunoelectrophoresis or the use of antibody-coated latex particles can sometimes be used for rapid detection of bacterial antigens in the CSF, e.g. *N. meningitidis*, *H. influenzae*, *Str. pneumoniae* and *M. tuberculosis*. The results may be positive when routine methods are negative, e.g. because the patient has had previous antibiotic treatment. The *Limulus* lysate test can be used for rapid diagnosis of meningitis caused by gram-negative bacteria.

Blood culture

The number of organisms in the blood is likely to be very small and direct plating out of a drop of blood is of no value.

Medium

A large volume, 50 ml, of nutrient broth is used to prevent clotting and to reduce the bactericidal action of the blood. Broth containing Liquoid (sodium polyanethol sulphonate), an anti-coagulant which inhibits bactericidal action, can be used in smaller quantities. Thioglycollate broth is satisfactory for strict anaerobes. *Para*-aminobenzoic acid is incorporated in the media to neutralize the effect of sulphonamides, and penicillinase may be added to destroy penicillin.

Culture

Positive results are more likely if a *large* volume of blood is cultured. About 20 ml of blood is distributed at the bedside into three bottles of broth which have been warmed to 37°C. The bottles are incubated (1) aerobically, (2) aerobically with 5–10% CO_2 and (3) anaerobically. Thioglycollate broth has its own reducing properties and is incubated aerobically. The time taken for organisms to grow is variable; in brucellosis it may be as long as 2–3 weeks.

The bottles are inspected daily. Positive cultures usually show a growth of colonies on the surface of the sedimented red cells or turbidity of the supernatant fluid. Subcultures on to blood agar plates are made when growth is apparent. If there is doubt, subcultures can be made at intervals, e.g. 24 hours, 48 hours, 7 days and, in special cases, 3 weeks. Subculturing may introduce contaminants and if daily inspection of the bottles reveals no growth it is sufficient to rely on a single subculture before the bottle is discarded. Media containing glucose labelled with carbon-14 can be used to provide early evidence of bacterial multiplication. With positive cultures release of radioactive CO_2 can often be detected within a few hours.

Organisms can sometimes be grown from the blood by *clot culture*, e.g. from the clot left over after the serum has been removed for a Widal reaction in suspected enteric fever.

Results

The results are significant when (1) the same organism is isolated from all three bottles and (2) the same organism is isolated on more than one occasion. Confirmatory evidence is provided when (3) the organism is present in large numbers (e.g. more than 5/ml of blood as determined in special plate counts) and (4) the patient produces a high titre of antibodies against the particular organism.

If the organism proves to be *N. meningitidis*, a salmonella or a brucella, even a single positive bottle is significant. But if an organism such as *Staph. aureus, Staph. epidermidis,* a viridans streptococcus, *Str. faecalis* or *E. coli* is isolated from a single bottle interpretation is difficult. Such organisms occasionally gain access to the blood of normal individuals or they may contaminate the culture at the time the blood is taken or during subculture in the laboratory. No organism should be lightly dismissed as a contaminant. In difficult cases the proper course is to repeat the blood culture, if necessary several times a day.

In recent years there has been an increase in severe bacteraemic states caused by gram-negative bacilli and 'non-pathogenic' organisms such as *Staph. epidermidis.* The mortality rate of bacteraemia increases from about 20% at the age of 20 to about 70% at the age of 70. Elderly patients are often dead before a bacteriological diagnosis is established.

Marrow culture

In diseases such as enteric fever and brucellosis the causative organisms can sometimes be isolated from bone marrow when ordinary blood cultures are negative. In obscure fevers any bone marrow in excess of that required for microscopic examination should be inoculated into a blood culture bottle.

Viral diseases

Virus diagnostic laboratories undertake the investigation of diseases caused by viruses, rickettsiae, chlamydiae and mycoplasmas. Many of the investigations are time-consuming, expensive and require special facilities. The diagnosis may be obvious clinically and the results of investigation may not be available for several days or weeks. Full clinical details are essential and should include the date of onset of the illness and whether or not the patient has recently had live polio vaccine.

Specimens

1 *Viral isolation.* Attempts to isolate viruses are often futile unless the specimen is taken in the early stages of illness, preserved in viral transport medium, kept at 4°C but not frozen, and transported to the laboratory without delay. A few viruses are relatively stable, e.g. the enteroviruses (polio, coxsackie and echoviruses) will survive in faeces for 24 hours at normal temperatures. The advice of the virus laboratory should be sought before the specimen is taken. Faeces, nose and throat

swabs and CSF are usually required in viral meningitis; sputum, nose and throat swabs or garglings in respiratory tract infections; vesicle fluid or scrapings from skin lesions in infections caused by poxviruses (vaccinia, cowpox, milker's nodes and orf) and herpesviruses (herpes simplex, herpes zoster and chickenpox).

2 *Demonstration of antibodies.* When viral infection is suspected an 'acute' sample of serum should be obtained at the time of admission. If the patient remains undiagnosed a second 'convalescent' sample is obtained 10–21 days later. Comparisons can be made more easily if the paired sera are examined at the same time.

Investigations

Investigations vary with different diseases and in different laboratories but involve one or more of the following:

1 *Microscopic examination.* Rapid detection of viral particles in clinical specimens can be made by electron microscopy in infections with poxviruses, herpesviruses, hepatitis B virus and rotaviruses. Examination of stained films with the light microscope is of value in detecting the chlamydiae causing trachoma, inclusion conjunctivitis and lymphogranuloma venereum (LGV). It is also possible to see large viruses, e.g. poxviruses. Histological changes in affected tissues are sometimes characteristic, e.g. lymph nodes in LGV, the brain in rabies, and biopsy and post-mortem material in cytomegalovirus infection.

2 *Direct detection of viral nucleic acid.* Nucleic acid hybridization techniques ('DNA probes', etc.) can be used for specific identification of viral DNA or RNA in clinical material.

3 *Direct detection of viral antigens.* Fluorescent antibody techniques are widely used for the rapid identification of viruses in specimens such as sputum, nasopharyngeal secretions, faeces and CSF. Enzyme-linked immunosorbent assay (ELISA) is used for detecting rotaviruses in faeces, hepatitis B virus in blood and *C. trachomatis* in swabs from the genital tract. An agglutination test using antibody-coated latex particles is used to detect rotaviruses. In poxvirus and herpesvirus infections viral antigens can be detected in fluid or extracts from the skin lesions by precipitation (gel-diffusion), complement fixation and fluorescent antibody techniques.

4 *Viral isolation.* Suitable material is inoculated into tissue cultures, developing eggs or animals. The type of tissue, age of animal, route of injection, etc., depends on the type of virus likely to be present. Tissue culture techniques are usually the simplest

and are used if possible. The presence of virus is shown by various reactions: in tissue culture, cytopathic effects, pH changes, production of haemagglutinins; in eggs, death, tissue lesions, pock-formation on the chorio-allantoic membrane; in animals, death, a particular symptom or histological changes. The effects may be sufficiently characteristic to identify the virus, but usually it must be identified by serological means, e.g. neutralization of viral activity, including haemagglutination, by specific antisera; demonstration of viral antigens in infected tissue cultures by immunofluorescent techniques.

5 *Detection of antibodies.* Tests for antibodies are more easily carried out than the procedures involved in viral isolation but are less useful in diagnosis. The complement fixation reaction and fluorescent antibody techniques are the most generally useful serological procedures. Neutralization tests are more laborious, but have to be used for detection of antibodies against some viruses. Thus antibodies against enteroviruses are usually determined by neutralization of cytopathic effects in tissue culture. The virus used is preferably the strain isolated from the particular patient, but if necessary tests can be made with the more common stock strains of living virus. Antibodies can also be detected by precipitation (gel-diffusion), agglutination, haemagglutination-inhibition, radioimmunoassay (RIA) and ELISA techniques. IgM and IgG antibodies can be distinguished by RIA, ELISA, sucrose density gradient centrifugation (separation of antibodies by the size of their molecules) and by use of fluorescent anti-human IgM and IgG sera in indirect immunofluorescent tests.

6 *Non-specific tests.* These include a white cell count and the Paul-Bunnell test (or modern screening test) in infectious mononucleosis, the Weil-Felix test in rickettsial infections and the cold agglutinin test in mycoplasmal pneumonia.

Significance of results

Isolation of a virus does not necessarily mean it is responsible for the patient's symptoms, e.g. normal individuals may excrete enteroviruses in their faeces and carry herpes simplex and adenoviruses in their throat. On the other hand, isolation of a virus from the blood or CSF is highly significant. Similarly, neutralizing antibodies against many common viruses are frequently found in healthy adults. Complement-fixing antibodies and IgM antibodies tend to persist for shorter periods and are better indicators of current or recent infection.

The most convincing evidence of viral infection is provided when a virus is isolated and antibodies against it appear or increase during the illness. A four-fold rise in antibody titre is usually significant. Provided that there is clinical evidence of recent infection a high level of antibodies in a single specimen may be sufficient to make a diagnosis. In the complement fixation test the following minimum titres are consistent with a clinical diagnosis: any titre for lymphocytic choriomeningitis virus; 160 for influenza, respiratory syncytial virus, adenovirus, varicella-zoster, measles, mumps (160 for V antigen and 20 for S antigen), *Coxiella burneti*, psittacosis and LGV; 320 for *Mycoplasma pneumoniae* (but false-positives are a problem); 640 for cytomegalovirus. No titre by itself is acceptable for parainfluenza, herpes simplex, polio, coxsackie or echoviruses.

Control of Hospital and Community Infections

It may seem a strange principle to enunciate as the very first requirement in a hospital that it should do the sick no harm.

Florence Nightingale, 1859

Congregation of sick people in a hospital inevitably increases the risk of transmitting infection from one patient to another. A hundred years or so ago the incidence of sepsis and death following surgical operations and childbirth was appalling. Important landmarks in the struggle to overcome this problem were the emphasis on the contagious nature of puerperal fever by Oliver Wendell Holmes (1843) in Boston, the demonstration by Semmelweis (1847) in Vienna that the incidence of this disease could be dramatically reduced by insisting that students coming from the post-mortem room should wash their hands in a solution of chlorinated lime before examining the women, and the introduction by Lister (1864—8) of antiseptic (germ-destroying) methods of surgery, the forerunners of modern aseptic (germ-excluding) methods. In more recent times the advent of antibacterial drugs has helped to decrease the seriousness of many types of infection, particularly streptococcal infection. In the case of infections caused by *Staphylococcus aureus* and the 'coliform' group of gram-negative bacilli the results have been less satisfactory. Hospital-acquired infections (nosocomial infections) caused by these organisms still present serious problems.

Methods used to control hospital infection

General principles

The prevention or control of any infectious disease, whether in hospital or outside, depends on three lines of attack:

1 Removing the source of infection.
2 Interrupting the route of transmission.

3   Increasing the resistance of the individual.

The relative importance of these measures, the methods used and the success achieved in practice vary greatly with different diseases.

Routine surveillance

An Infection Control Officer, usually a clinical microbiologist, assisted by an Infection Control Nurse, ideally a senior nurse who has the ability to communicate tactfully and effectively with staff at all levels, should be responsible for maintaining up-to-date records of all infections occurring in the hospital. The records are compiled from two main sources:

1   Laboratory records of the more important organisms isolated.
2   Information acquired (a) in the course of routine visits to all wards and departments, (b) from the Occupational Health staff, Theatre Superintendent, Catering Officer, etc., about infections occurring in members of the medical, nursing and domestic staff and (c) from family doctors and the Community Physician about members of the staff who are treated at home and patients who develop infections after they have left hospital.

Epidemiological survey

When an outbreak occurs or is threatened more detailed records are required. Useful information includes: name, age, sex, disease; ward and date of admission, nature of operation and date; name of surgeon, assistant surgeons, nurses and anaesthetist; nature of minor surgical procedures in the ward, date and staff involved; type of sepsis (deep or superficial) and date of onset; date of swabs, pathogens isolated, antibiotic sensitivities and results of typing procedures.

From the results of the epidemiological survey and the bacteriological investigations it is often possible to decide whether an outbreak has its origin in the wards, the operating theatres or some other part of the hospital. The survey may draw attention to a particular operating theatre, surgical team, type of operation, ward, ward procedure or even an individual surgeon, nurse or patient. Appropriate measures can then be taken to look for carriers of the offending organism and to sample relevant parts of the hospital environment and check for defects in theatre and ward procedures.

Bacteriological studies of the environment

The presence of an Infection Control Officer engaged in questioning, swabbing and sampling provides a reminder that cross-infection matters. Valuable visual evidence is provided if the nursing staff and others are allowed to see the plates after they have been incubated. The main object, however, is to carry out investigations which will give answers to specific questions, e.g. is contaminated air being pumped into the theatre? The following are some of the technical methods used:

Air. For most purposes bacterial contamination can be measured by exposing culture plates ('settle plates') to the air for 30–60 minutes. Colony counts are made after the plates have been incubated. More rapid sampling can be achieved with a slit-sampler, an apparatus which draws air at high velocity through a narrow slit to impinge on the surface of a slowly revolving culture plate. Minute-by-minute changes in the degree of air contamination can be measured by this method. Air currents can be studied by measuring the dispersal of nitrous oxide by infrared absorption methods or by creating an aerosol of an easily recognizable organism such as *Streptococcus salivarius* which produces large mucoid colonies on sucrose agar, and finding where the organisms get to by exposing culture plates. The dense white smoke produced by titanium tetrachloride on exposure to air is convenient for determining the direction of air currents through doors, windows and ventilators.

Blankets, sheets, clothes, etc. Adequate samples of fluff and debris can usually be obtained by the sweep-plate method, i.e. an open plate of culture medium is moved to and fro across the surface of the fabric. Smooth fabrics are best sampled by the press-plate method, i.e. the fabric is pressed against the nutrient medium with a large rubber bung or similar object.

Ledges, equipment, dust, etc. A swab moistened with broth is usually adequate. It can be streaked out directly on plates of nutrient medium.

Disinfectants, lubricants, irrigation fluids. Large samples, preferably in their original containers, are usually required. Special procedures may be necessary to dilute or neutralize the effects of the disinfectant.

Hygiene in operating theatres

Ventilation

The air supply should be properly filtered. The air pressure in the theatre should be greater than in surrounding parts of the

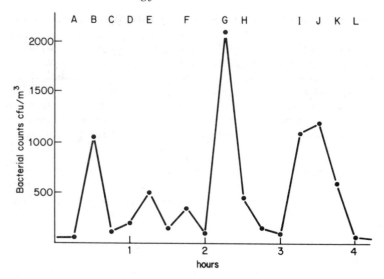

Fig. 28 Activities in an operating theatre. The air is sampled at 15 minute intervals and bacterial counts are expressed as the number of contaminated particles (colony-forming units) per cubic metre of air (cfu/m^3). A, Empty theatre. B, Patient brought in. C, House surgeon starts operation. D, Consultant arrives. E, More instruments, extra blood, X-ray apparatus and radiographers arrive. F, Medical student faints. G, Consultant complains of heat: ventilation turned off in error. H, Ventilation turned on again. I, Plastering and check X-rays. J, Patient taken out. K, Theatre cleaning. L, Empty theatre.

hospital to ensure that contaminated air cannot gain admittance through doors, windows, corridors, lift shafts or ventilators. The theatre sister should check that nobody interferes with the ventilation (Fig.28G). In an empty operating theatre with the ventilation plant running normally, the incoming air should contain not more than 35 bacteria-carrying particles/m^3 (1.0/ft^3). During quiet operating the bacterial counts should not exceed 150/m^3 (4.2/ft^3) and preferably should be below 50/m^3 (1.4/ft^3). Counts as low as 2/m^3 (0.06/ft^3) can be achieved with special systems of directed air-flow ventilation.

Sterilization

Tests on autoclaves and hot-air ovens should be made as a routine and whenever there is any suspicion of failure (p. 153). Sterilized materials must be stored so that there is no possibility of recontamination. Pharaoh's ants can carry pathogenic bacteria and it is

important to check that these and other insects do not invade
dressing packs, surgical equipment or clean laundry. Special
attention should be paid to disinfectant solutions. The arrangements made for cleaning and preparing trolleys should be checked.
Bacteria are liable to grow in ordinary corks and these should
never be used. Eye drops should be dispensed in single dose
containers.

Preparation of patient

Beds, blankets and other potentially contaminated materials
from the wards should not be allowed into the theatre. The
patient should be covered with a freshly laundered gown, sheet
or cotton blanket before entering the theatre. The solution used
to disinfect the skin should be suitable for the purpose and used
at the correct strength.

Surgical procedures

The surgical team should scrub up adequately, preferably using
a disinfectant. Contrary to what might be expected, there are
objections to taking a shower immediately before duty, as most
people shed more bacteria into the air after a shower than before
it. This effect lasts for an hour or so. The practice of putting on
freshly laundered clothes before putting on a gown should be
encouraged, for, although carriers of *Staph. aureus* still disperse
organisms when dressed in this way, the numbers of organisms
liberated are less than when a gown is worn over everyday
clothes. Everyone in the theatre should be dressed in cap, mask,
gown and theatre shoes. Unnecessary walking about and all
rapid movements should be discouraged. The number of individuals in the theatre should be kept to the minimum. Conventional surgical masks are inefficient and casual conversation should
be avoided.

General cleanliness

The theatre should be cleaned after every surgical list and when
necessary between individual cases. Attention should be paid to
dust traps such as the tops of lights, ledges and shelves. Septic
cases should be kept to the end of the list or dealt with in a
separate theatre. Precautions should be taken to minimize contamination caused by blood, pus and soiled dressings. Cupboards,
packs, apparatus, etc., should be kept in ancillary rooms whenever
possible. Anaesthetic equipment should be disinfected regularly.
Care should be taken that contamination is not introduced into
the theatre on X-ray and anaesthetic machines and on non-sterile

materials such as boxes, boards, plaster and cotton-wool. Un-authorized persons should not be allowed to wander into the theatres between lists.

Ward routine

Wound dressing

Wounds should be exposed to the atmosphere for the shortest possible time on the fewest possible occasions. The procedures are best carried out in a properly equipped and properly venti-lated theatre or dressing room. When this is not available a time is chosen when activity in the ward is at a minimum, i.e. bed-making, dusting, sweeping, drawing of curtains and unnecessary traffic should cease at least 15 minutes before the wound is dressed. All wounds should be inspected and dressed with full aseptic precautions. Hands should be washed, masks and gowns should be worn and a sterile trolley should be available with adequate sterile forceps. Casual lifting of soiled dressings with the fingers and prodding the skin around the wound with bare hands is indefensible. Contaminated materials must be disposed

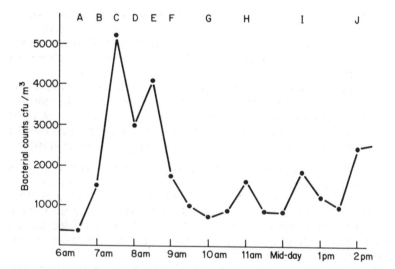

Fig. 29 Activities in a surgical ward. The air is sampled at 30 minute intervals and bacterial counts are expressed as the number of contami-nated particles (colony-forming units) per cubic metre of air (cfu/m³). A, Patients sleep. B, Tea and bed-pan rounds. C, Washing and bed-making. D, Breakfast. E, Ward cleaning. F, Doctors' rounds. G, Wound dressing. H, Patient with cardiac arrest. I, Lunch. J, Visitors arriving.

of safely, e.g. soiled dressings should be placed in a paper bag for incineration.

General procedures

Facilities for hand washing should be readily available and the supply of paper towels should be adequate. These facilities must be used between cases and whenever contaminated material has been handled. Disinfectant hand creams or rinses should be available. Gloves and gowns should be worn when handling heavily infected articles.

Isolation nursing

Patients do not take kindly to being labelled 'infectious' or 'dangerous' and the need for isolation must be explained to them with tact. Highly restrictive measures should not be used unnecessarily.

Precautions that are essential against one disease may be irrelevant against another. There are therefore advantages in dividing isolation procedures into different types, each to be used for specified diseases. One such scheme recognizes four types of isolation:

1 Strict isolation for serious infectious diseases which spread very easily, e.g. infantile gastroenteritis and diphtheria.
2 Stool-urine-needle isolation for infectious diseases which are spread by one or more of these routes, e.g. salmonella infections and viral hepatitis.
3 Standard isolation for most other infectious diseases, e.g. *Streptococcus pyogenes* infections and pulmonary tuberculosis.
4 Protective isolation for highly susceptible patients who need protection against infection, e.g. patients with severe uninfected burns and those undergoing immunosuppressive therapy.

A list is provided for ward sisters showing which type of isolation is appropriate for different diseases and organisms. Detailed instructions lay down the precautions to be observed for each type of isolation, together with additional measures that are required for particular diseases. Coloured notices fixed to the door of the patient's room provide a reminder of the precautions that must be applied.

Certain general measures apply to most types of isolation. The patient should be nursed in a single room and should leave this room only in exceptional circumstances. Gowns and aprons should be available within the isolated area and used by all who attend the patient, masks should be worn, hands should be washed before and after leaving the infected area and articles used by the patient should as far as possible be kept within the area. Crockery, bed-pans and other articles which are brought out of the area must be disinfected. When the patient is discharged the room and its contents are cleaned and disinfected. Ideally nurses looking after infected cases should not attend non-infected cases. Protective isolation requires rather different arrangements, e.g. there is no risk of infecting other patients and the ventilation system must ensure that organisms do not *enter* the isolation room.

Nursing of infants

This should be similar to isolation nursing even when the infants are healthy. Nurses should not handle infants unnecessarily. Each nurse should be responsible for only a small number of infants. Communal use of any article should be avoided. Napkin-changing, washing, weighing, dressing and feeding should preferably be done by the mother. The umbilical stump is a wound and use of an antiseptic dusting powder discourages bacterial colonization.

Disinfection and sterilization

Baths, lavatories, bed-pans and urinals should be regularly cleaned and disinfected. The methods used to sterilize and store instruments should be checked.

Ward cleaning

No part of the ward or ward equipment should be visibly dirty. Sweeping and dry-dusting raise clouds of organisms and should not be allowed. Wet-mopping and use of a damp cloth is less dangerous and more efficient. Modern vacuum cleaners which are fitted with special filters and collect dust in a paper bag are safe, but some of the older types are powerful disseminators of organisms.

Laundry arrangements

Each patient is entitled to clean bed clothes which are changed frequently. Boilable cotton blankets should be used. Used linen must not be sorted in the wards or in rooms from which contaminated air might reach the ward. Bags and baskets used for soiled laundry must not be used for clean laundry. Clean laundry must be stored where it cannot become contaminated by dust or insects such as Pharaoh's ants.

Ward ventilation

Special systems of ventilation such as those fitted in burns units should be checked to see that they are functioning properly. In wards without air-conditioning it is important to see that contaminated air is not gaining access from septic wards or laundry sorting rooms.

Infections caused by Staphylococcus aureus

Staph. aureus is widely distributed among patients and hospital staff and extensive contamination of the hospital environment is usual (p. 67). Opportunities for cross-infection are frequent and hospitals have become breeding grounds of dangerous antibiotic-resistant strains. *Staph. aureus* is responsible for 30—40% of all cases of sepsis occurring in surgical wounds. The incidence of staphylococcal infection of clean operation wounds is often 5% and sometimes much higher. Serious sepsis in maternity departments is less frequent, but the incidence of breast abscesses is commonly 2—3% and of sticky eyes and skin lesions in babies is often 10—20%. In the UK at least five hundred people die each year of staphylococcal infection acquired in hospital. In addition a large number of patients are permanently invalided because operations have failed to achieve their object or because infection has involved such structures as growing bones and joints.

Typing of organisms

It is essential to find out at the earliest possible moment whether or not the patients are infected with the same strain of organism. Antibiotic sensitivity patterns often give useful provisional information, e.g. organisms showing major differences in their sensitivities do not belong to the same strain. However, dissimilar strains often have very similar antibiotic patterns and for proper investigation phage-typing is essential. As this is not a routine procedure all strains of *Staph. aureus* isolated in the hospital should be preserved for 3 to 6 months. Selected strains can be typed without delay if an emergency arises.

Epidemiological survey

A careful survey always yields more useful information than any amount of undirected swabbing of staff or the environment.

Deep-seated sepsis developing within a few days of an operation and before the wound has been dressed indicates a theatre infection. The survey may direct attention to a particular theatre, type of operation, surgical team, surgeon or nurse. An outbreak involving several surgical teams and a variety of phage types may indicate some general failure of theatre hygiene and sterility.

Ward infections are often more superficial and follow the dressing of wounds and burns in the ward or some minor postoperative procedure such as changing a catheter. Infection developing in sites unconnected with the operation, e.g. boils, sticky eyes, etc., is usually acquired in the ward. The survey may direct attention to a particular ward, nurse, or some defect in ward procedure.

Isolation of infected patients

All patients with *Staph. aureus* infection should be isolated. Strains of methicillin-resistant *Staph. aureus* (MRSA) must be regarded as particularly dangerous. Barrier nursing in an open ward does almost nothing to prevent air-borne spread of staphylococci. Success is greater if the patient can be nursed in a separate side-ward. If the number of infected cases is large a ward can be set aside to be used exclusively for patients with *Staph. aureus* infection. Despite normal methods of control staphylococcal infection may become widespread and serious. Sometimes the only solution is to close the infected ward and disinfect and clean it and all its fittings, furnishings and equipment. When the ward is reopened care is taken that no patients or staff carrying the epidemic strain are readmitted.

Infected members of the staff should be banished from operating theatres and surgical wards until they are cured.

Search for carriers

If phage-typing shows that the infections are caused by a mixed collection of strains there is usually no point in looking for carriers. If a single phage-type is responsible for the outbreak a search is made for carriers among all individuals who are a possible source of infection. Swabs are taken from the nose, throat and skin (wrist and fingers) and from minor septic spots, pimples and styes. When there are special reasons to suspect that an individual is a dangerous carrier, swabs are taken from other skin areas, in particular the perineum and axillae, and the clothing is sampled by the sweep-plate method. Dangerous dispersers of *Staph. aureus* can be detected by exposing culture plates while the individual undertakes mild exercise, e.g. 'marking time' for 5 minutes.

Treatment of carriers

Individuals who carry the offending strain and who are a likely source of infection should be taken off work. If they are patients they should be isolated. Attempts are made to eliminate the organisms from the nose by local treatment with antibacterial preparations such as mupirocin in soft paraffin or a cream (Naseptin) containing chlorhexidine and neomycin, and from the skin by the use of hexachlorophane soap. Systemic antibiotic treatment is not justifiable.

Carriers of non-epidemic strains are usually best left alone. Inevitably a high proportion of the staff will be carriers. The incidence of carriers among the patients may also be very high, e.g. among infants in a maternity department carrier rates often approach 100%. A systematic attack on all carriers of *Staph. aureus*, e.g. routine use of an antiseptic nasal cream, may sometimes help to diminish the incidence of cross-infection, but on the whole the results are disappointing. A danger of local nasal treatment is that if a relatively harmless staphylococcus is removed the individual may subsequently pick up a more dangerous strain.

Infections caused by gram-negative bacilli

Gram-negative bacilli are responsible for 40–50% of all cases of sepsis occurring in surgical wounds but many coliform infections represent contamination and colonization rather than true infection. Often there is an underlying infection caused by an easily overlooked anaerobe such as *Bacteroides* acting synergistically with *Escherichia coli*. The remaining cases are infected with *Pseudomonas aeruginosa*, *Klebsiella*, *Proteus* and miscellaneous coliforms in roughly equal proportions. The alarming frequency with which coliforms in the hospital environment acquire resistance to antibiotics, particularly by the mechanism of transmissible drug resistance, and the fact that the antibiotics to which they remain sensitive are often highly toxic, has made coliform infections at least as serious a problem as staphylococcal infections.

Burns frequently become infected with coliforms and *Ps. aeruginosa* in particular may cause outbreaks resulting in delayed healing, failure of grafts and sometimes generalized infection terminating in death. Extensive outbreaks of coliform infection are also common in urological departments. Newborn infants, especially when premature, are very susceptible to coliform infections and may develop pneumonia, meninigitis and bacteraemia. *Ps. aeruginosa* has caused outbreaks of eye infection leading to loss of sight in newborn infants and in adult patients in eye departments. In recent years, probably because of increasing use of antibiotics, steroids, immunosuppressants and cytotoxic drugs, there has been an increase in serious coliform infections including bacteraemia, empyema and meningitis.

Typing of organisms

The methods currently available for typing the organisms are unsatisfactory. In special centres strains of *E. coli, Klebsiella* and *Proteus* can be subdivided into a large number of serological types on the basis of their antigenic structure. Strains of *Ps. aeruginosa* can be identified by a combination of phage-typing, pyocin-typing and agglutination reactions. Recognition of multi-resistant coliforms often indicates which patients require isolation. Typing of R plasmids may provide valuable epidemiological information.

Sources of infection

Most of the gram-negative bacilli responsible for infection are part of the normal intestinal flora. Others are free-living organisms which grow in moist places in the hospital environment.

Intestinal organisms

E. coli is invariably present in large numbers in the normal adult intestine. *Klebsiella* and *Proteus* are found in about a third of normal people. Only about 5% of normal adults carry *Ps. aeruginosa.* Normal people seldom carry coliforms in sites outside the intestine. In patients in hospital other sources of coliforms are common, e.g. the respiratory tract of patients being treated with broad-spectrum antibiotics and the urine of patients with urinary tract infections. However, coliforms are sensitive to drying and usually do not survive long in the air, on bed clothes or in dust. Most coliforms are soon killed by contact with human skin but *Klebsiella* may survive for several hours.

Free-living organisms

Many species of coliforms have very simple requirements and can multiply at room temperature in moist surroundings such as the water in humidifiers of ventilators and incubators, 'sterile' solutions and weak disinfectants. *Ps. aeruginosa* is especially successful in gaining a footing in such seemingly unpromising surroundings and has been described as the nearest thing there is to spontaneous generation. Other free-living coliforms which have caused human infection after environmental contamination include *Klebsiella*, other species of *Pseudomonas*, e.g. *Ps. cepacia*, and many less well-known coliforms.

Modes of infection

The incidence of wound infections caused by coliforms varies greatly with the type of operation. Coliform infections are particularly common following operations on the intestinal tract, e.g. appendicectomy, and it is probable that in such cases the organisms are derived from the patient's own intestines. However, coliforms often infect clean operation wounds in other parts of the body. It seems likely that most of these cases are due to cross-infection.

The epidemiology of infection is complicated by the fact that patients acquire new strains of coliforms after admission to hospital. For instance, certain serological types of *E. coli* are relatively rare in the faeces of patients outside hospitals but appear with increasing frequency during a stay in hospital. Such 'hospital strains' account for a disproportionately large number of urinary tract and wound infections acquired in hospitals. Colonization of the intestines with new strains of *E. coli* can result from consumption of food contaminated with these organisms, e.g. because of inefficient washing-up.

Little is known about the routes of patient-to-patient infection. In burns units the patients are highly susceptible to infection and any infected patient is likely to be a prolific source of organisms. When patients are infected with *Ps. aeruginosa* it is usual to find the organism in large numbers on the surface of dressings and in smaller numbers on nurses' hands, in floor dust and on articles of ward equipment. Infection spreads mainly by contact but spread by airborne particles is also important. In outbreaks of this kind the strains of *Ps. aeruginosa* isolated from the patients and the environment usually belong to the same type. Similar environmental contamination by a particular species or strain of coliform sometimes occurs in the course of extensive outbreaks in urological wards. Infections caused by *Klebsiella* are spread mainly by contact and nurses' hands are an important vehicle of infection.

In contrast, the mode of infection is often, in retrospect, only too obvious in those types of common-source outbreaks in which coliforms contaminate an article of hospital equipment or a fluid used in treatment, multiply in this environment and are then transferred directly to a number of patients. The results may be disastrous. Thus there have been frequent reports of respiratory and other infections caused by growth of coliforms in the water of humidifiers of mechanical ventilators and babies' incubators.

Supposedly 'sterile' solutions and lotions have been responsible for a great variety of infections. Severe eye infections with *Ps. aeruginosa* have been caused by contaminated eye drops. Disinfectants themselves are far from blameless: not only may they fail to destroy bacteria, which in itself is an important cause of coliform infection, but they sometimes provide a medium in which coliforms, especially *Ps. aeruginosa*, can multiply. This provides a dangerous situation in which the disinfectant itself becomes the vehicle by which organisms are spread to the patient. Outbreaks of coliform infection have also been traced to infected sources such as suction apparatus, tracheal catheters, anaesthetic apparatus, local anaesthetics, aerosol sprays, mouthwashes, lubricants, hand-creams, ointments, drugs and fluids (including blood and blood products) given intravenously, water-baths used for thawing frozen plasma, shaving brushes, corks of bottles, dripping taps, sinks and sink traps, washing bowls, liquidizers used for preparing nasogastric feeds, defective ice-making machines, buckets used for soaking plaster bandages, anti-static operating-table mattresses, humidifiers of operating theatre ventilation plants and medical leeches used in plastic and reconstructive surgery.

Control of infection

This depends mainly on strict adherence to correct theatre and ward hygiene. The tendency of coliforms to survive and multiply in moist surroundings emphasizes the importance of regular checks on the sterility of potential vehicles of infection such as the humidifiers of babies' incubators, the need for regular in-use tests on disinfectants and the desirability of eliminating disinfectants altogether when sterilization can be achieved by more certain methods such as heat.

Streptococcal infections

Group A haemolytic streptococci (*Streptococcus pyogenes*) are no longer a major plague of hospitals, but the dangers of these organisms should not be underestimated. Infection is a fairly common and serious complication of burns and plastic operations. *Str. pyogenes* is the one organism that almost always causes the complete failure of grafts. Small outbreaks of wound sepsis and puerperal fever still occur and deaths are by no means rare. Haemolytic streptococci of other groups are relatively unimportant, but groups C and G occasionally cause small outbreaks in hospitals.

Str. pyogenes consists of a number of serological types and it is usually necessary to type the strains in order to trace the spread of infection. In searching for carriers, nose and throat swabs should be taken from patients and staff. Nasal carriers are rare but are more dangerous than throat carriers. They should be excluded from surgical and obstetric wards until they are cured. Throat carriers should be excluded if they have a sore throat or other symptoms of respiratory tract infection. Symptomless throat carriers are often relatively harmless: in general they should be excluded at times of epidemics, but at other times they may be allowed to work. Routine screening of nurses and midwives to exclude carriers is not usually necessary. *Str. pyogenes* is invariably sensitive to penicillin and systemic penicillin can be used to treat dangerous carriers. In practice, it may be ineffective in eradicating *Str. pyogenes* if the individual is also a carrier of penicillin-resistant (β-lactamase-producing) *Staph. aureus* or *Bacteroides*.

Urinary tract infections

A regrettably large proportion of urinary tract infections seen in hospitals are the result of hospital procedures. About 75% of cases are associated with the use of catheters, which makes this instrument the most important cause of hospital-acquired infection. The organisms responsible include *E. coli*, *Klebsiella*, *Proteus*, other coliforms, *Ps. aeruginosa*, *Str. faecalis*, *Staph. aureus* and *Staph. epidermidis*. It is not sufficiently realized that urinary infections often constitute a clear-cut outbreak. If the organisms are identified with precision it is usual to find that a number of cases in a ward or unit are infected with the same strain. Sometimes the outbreaks are extensive.

In attempting to control outbreaks of urinary infection it is important to check that cystoscopes are properly sterilized, catheters are used only when essential and always with full aseptic precautions, closed systems of bladder drainage are used for patients with indwelling catheters, urine collection bottles are properly sterilized, and irrigation fluids, disinfectants and catheter lubricants are sterile.

Diarrhoea and vomiting

Outbreaks of diarrhoea and vomiting are not uncommon when people eat communal meals in schools, factories, hospitals and at banquets, weddings and fêtes. The majority are bacterial in origin.

Staphylococcal food poisoning is due to consumption of pre-formed toxins of enterotoxin-producing strains of *Staph. aureus*. *Clostridium perfringens* food poisoning is caused by ingesting a large dose of the organisms which then form toxins in the gut. The condition is not infective for others. Infective diarrhoea may be due to salmonellae (*S. typhimurium*, *S. enteritidis*, etc.), shigellae (particularly *Sh. sonnei*), *Campylobacter jejuni* and, in the case of infants, rotaviruses and enteropathogenic strains of *E. coli*. Rare causes of gastroenteritis include *Bacillus cereus*, *B. subtilis*, *Vibrio parahaemolyticus* and *Yersinia enterocolitica*. The role of the gram-negative bacilli *Aeromonas hydrophila* and *Plesiomonas shigelloides* in causing gastrointestinal symptoms is controversial. Other causes of food poisoning should not be overlooked, e.g. scom-brotoxin poisoning due to histamine in smoked mackerel prepared from fish grossly contaminated with bacteria; sushi poisoning due to nematode larvae in raw fish; paralytic poisoning due to the neurotoxin of certain planktonic dinoflagellates in shellfish; poisoning from toxins in raw or under-cooked red kidney beans; cadmium poisoning resulting from storage of acid fruit juices in unsuitable metal containers.

Epidemiological survey

A record should be made of the total population at risk, the number of affected cases, the time of onset of symptoms, the nature of the symptoms and the meals taken in the previous 48 hours with precise details of the foods and drinks consumed or not consumed by both well and ill people.

Outbreaks of staphylococcal and clostridial food poisoning have an explosive onset with the majority of the individuals affected at roughly the same time, usually a few hours after consumption of the affected food, e.g. 2−6 hours with *Staph. aureus*, 6−12 hours with *Cl. perfringens*. The symptoms may be severe but rarely last more than a day. Prostration is common but pyrexia does not occur. Vomiting is unusual in *Cl. perfringens* food poisoning.

Outbreaks of infective diarrhoea are of two sorts:

1 Explosive outbreaks resembling food poisoning are not very common. They are usually due to salmonellae and the survey and subsequent investigations will indicate the particular food involved. The onset of symptoms is more scattered in time than in staphylococcal and clostridial food poisoning and is usually about a day after eating the affected food. Severe initial prostration is unusual. The symptoms may persist for many days and pyrexia is common.

2 Most outbreaks due to salmonellae, shigellae, *E. coli* and rotaviruses take the form of a spreading infection extending over days or weeks. There is usually no evidence to connect the outbreaks with food, but this possibility must be investigated. The routes of transmission include faecal contamination of the hands and widespread contamination of dust, towels, bed-clothes and objects such as crockery, eating utensils, feeding bottles and teats.

Investigation of foodstuffs

Immediate steps should be taken to secure samples of foods, including 'left-overs', likely to be a source of infection.

Staphylococcal and clostridial food poisoning can occur only when these organisms have been able to multiply in the food, i.e. because the food has been kept for several hours in a warm place. Large numbers of the organisms will be seen in gram films of the affected foods and culture will often yield a pure growth. Direct demonstration of toxins in food and faeces by enzyme-linked immunosorbent assay (ELISA) techniques can be used for rapid diagnosis. Staphylococcal food poisoning is commonly due to the growth of the organisms in custard, trifle, synthetic cream and in meat dishes such as cold ham, tongue and meat pies. The organisms are usually derived from a food-handler who may be a healthy carrier or an individual with a septic lesion. Clostridial food poisoning is invariably associated with meat dishes such as stews, minced meat (a routine laboratory medium for anaerobes!), cooked sliced meat and gravy. The organisms are probably derived from the meat itself.

Salmonellae can be conveyed in a variety of foods. Cakes and pastries and various milk and egg dishes are often incriminated. Foods of this kind are only lightly cooked and the temperature inside the article may not rise sufficiently to kill the bacteria. A further hazard is provided by the frothy nonsense with which cakes and puddings are often filled and adorned. Several severe outbreaks have been traced to symptomless excreters in hospital bakeries. More commonly, the food is already contaminated with salmonellae on arrival at the kitchen. Cattle, sheep, pigs, hens, ducks and turkeys are often infected and the organisms may contaminate meat and meat products. Deep-frozen poultry is particularly dangerous unless properly thawed and adequately cooked. Over 75% of all chickens sold in the UK are contaminated with salmonellae. Other foods which may contain salmonellae include unpasteurized egg products, duck eggs and shredded coconut. Rats and mice are frequently infected and may contaminate stored foods. Salmonellae have been found in powdered infant milk feed, pancreatic preparations used for therapeutic purposes and in contaminated marijuana. Tracing salmonella infections back to their source and instituting appropriate control measures is a specialized branch of microbiology. *S. typhimurium* is widely distributed but is most frequently associated with a bovine source. Other species such as *S. hadar* are associated with chickens and turkeys; the prevalent species vary from time to time. A common finding is that infected animal feeding stuffs such as imported bone or fish meal have been fed to pigs and poultry. Sterilization of feeding stuffs, good animal husbandry and hygienic food handling are important in preventing infection.

Investigation of patients and carriers

Samples of faeces and vomit should be obtained from all affected patients. In outbreaks of infective diarrhoea a search is also made for symptomless excreters among patients, ward staff and food-handlers. Faecal specimens are normally all that are required. Serological tests are occasionally helpful in detecting chronic intermittent excreters of salmonellae.

The identity of strains isolated from various sources can sometimes be proved by special techniques, e.g. phage-typing and plasmid profile analysis of *S. typhimurium*, colicin-typing of *Sh. sonnei* and serotyping of *Cl. perfringens*. Phage-typing of *Staph. aureus* and determination of the antigenic type of enterotoxin by gel-diffusion tests may confirm that an individual is a possible source of the organism, but the information is of little value since the prevention of staphylococcal food poisoning is essentially a matter of food hygiene and not the treatment of carriers.

Individuals who have been infected with salmonellae or shigellae can usually be pronounced clear of infection when three consecutive specimens of faeces have given negative results. The specimens should be collected at intervals of 2 or 3 days, at a time when chemotherapy is not being given.

Hygiene in kitchens

An outbreak of gastroenteritis calls for a check that proper routine hygienic precautions are being observed. All individuals with intestinal symptoms should report sick and be sent off work (with pay) until they have been cleared bacteriologically. Individuals with septic lesions should also be excluded. The supply of wash-basins and paper towels must be adequate. It is important to check that these facilities are used, particularly after use of the lavatories. Cooked and perishable food must not be allowed to stand about in the warm: it must either be very hot so that the.

organisms are killed or very cold so that they are unable to multiply. Refrigerators should be checked from time to time, especially in a heat wave, to see that shelf temperatures are maintained at a safe level, usually 4°C. Hot food should be eaten within $1\frac{1}{2}$ hours; otherwise it must be refrigerated. 'Meals-on-wheels' and food in heated trolleys should be in transit for the shortest possible time. As far as possible, meat should be eaten on the day it is cooked and not reheated. Food that is reheated must reach boiling point throughout. Sample meals should be retained in a refrigerator for 48 hours. Raw and cooked foods must be processed and stored separately. Mincers and similar equipment must be dismantled and washed in very hot water and detergent after each use. The kitchen as a whole should be cleaned regularly. Mice, flies, ants and cockroaches must be exterminated. Pharaoh's ants sometimes infest heated food-trolleys and drink-vending machines.

Poor hygiene in hospital kitchens has been responsible for many outbreaks. In 1984 over 400 patients and staff in a psychiatric hospital in Wakefield were infected with *S. typhimurium*. At least 19 frail, elderly patients died. In 1986 *S. typhimurium* infected more than 90 individuals at the British Diabetic Association meeting in Cardiff and 28 doctors were admitted to hospital!

Ward hygiene

No special precautions need to be taken with patients suffering from food poisoning. Patients with infective diarrhoea as well as any symptomless excreters should be isolated. Chemotherapy tends to prolong the carrier state and is best avoided.

Infective diarrhoea in infants is liable to spread with alarming rapidity. Cases and excreters should be looked after by special nurses who take no part in the care of healthy infants. Feeds should be prepared with full aseptic precautions. Feeding bottles should be sterilized using hypochlorite or the milk should be heat-sterilized in the final bottle. Feeds should never be prepared by nurses who handle infected infants. If the outbreak shows signs of spreading there should be no hesitation in stopping admissions, sending healthy infants home and closing and disinfecting the ward.

Notification

Food poisoning, dysentery and salmonella infections are notifiable diseases. Quite apart from any statutory duties the cooperation of the hospital and public health authorities is important. The Community Physician should be notified by telephone. The forms can follow later.

Viral hepatitis

Hepatitis may occur in a variety of viral diseases including infectious mononucleosis, herpes simplex, cytomegalovirus infection, group B coxsackievirus infection, rubella and yellow fever. However, viral hepatitis usually refers to infection caused by hepatitis A virus (infective hepatitis), hepatitis B virus (serum hepatitis) or non-A, non-B hepatitis viruses.

Hepatitis A is endemic in the community and small outbreaks may occur in schools and in institutions for the mentally handicapped. The virus is excreted in the faeces and infection is acquired by mouth. Control of outbreaks mainly depends on hygienic measures to prevent faecal spread of the disease. Contamination of food or water by faeces must always be considered. Human normal immunoglobulin will protect close contacts and is occasionally of value in family or institutional outbreaks.

Hepatitis B is also widespread in the community as judged by the presence of hepatitis B surface antigen (HBsAg) in sporadic cases of hepatitis and by detectable levels of hepatitis B antibody (anti-HBs) in about a third of the population in some areas. Infection by the parenteral route is of prime importance and in the past the medical profession played a regrettably large part in spreading this disease. Before the risks were properly appreciated, hepatitis was a major risk when patients with chronic renal failure were treated in haemodialysis units. There were several deaths, particularly among doctors, nurses and technicians.

Prevention of hepatitis B depends essentially on preventing the transfer of infected blood. A separate needle and syringe must be used for each individual patient. Instruments used for other invasive procedures must be sterile, e.g. sterile disposable needles should be used for taking blood by finger prick. Blood for transfusion must be screened to exclude HBsAg. All persons giving a history of jaundice in the previous year or whose blood has produced jaundice in a recipient must be excluded as blood donors. Small pools of not more than ten donors must be used in preparation of plasma. Blood products must be sterilized whenever possible. Human immunoglobulin as currently prepared is safe.

In haemodialysis units, scrupulous precautions must be enforced to avoid contamination from the patients, their excreta and, most particularly, their blood. The staff and all visitors to the unit must be properly briefed on the risks and precautions. Patients and staff should be screened for HBsAg before admission and at regular intervals thereafter. Isolation facilities must be available. Staff turnover should be minimized and patients should not be transferred to other units. Patients should be trained to undertake their own dialysis and when possible should do this at home. Blood transfusions should be reduced to the minimum and renal transplantation should be carried out at the earliest opportunity. Patients with acute renal failure should be treated in a separate unit.

Contaminated equipment should be autoclaved whenever possible. Maximum use should be made of disposable articles which can be incinerated. Other equipment and surfaces should be treated with very strong hypochlorite for surfaces contaminated with blood, and 2% glutaraldehyde for metal objects.

Routine laboratory investigations should be kept to a minimum. Blood samples should be taken wearing gloves and protective clothing. Specimens should be transported to the laboratory in sealed plastic bags labelled 'Danger of Infection'. Laboratory staff must take special precautions, e.g. cuts and abrasions should be covered with waterproof dressings; gloves and protective clothing, including a vizor or safety spectacles if there is a danger of splashing, must be worn when handling specimens; needles should be covered when not in use; sharp-pointed instruments should be avoided; glassware should be replaced by plastic equivalents whenever possible; procedures likely to cause aerosols or spillage must be carried out in a properly ventilated protective cabinet; post-mortem examinations must be carried out with special care.

Hepatitis B vaccine should be offered to people at special risk. Human normal immunoglobulin is ineffective against hepatitis B, but human anti-HBsAg immunoglobulin can be used for protection of non-immune people who have been accidentally inoculated with HBsAg-positive material or, in serious outbreaks, for general protection of patients and staff. Infective jaundice of any type is a notifiable disease.

AIDS

The acquired immunodeficiency syndrome (AIDS) is caused by infection with human immunodeficiency virus (HIV). The virus is transmitted principally by sexual intercourse, predominantly by male homosexuals, and by transfusion or inoculation of blood and blood products. There has been a steady increase in cases of AIDS among female sexual partners of HIV-infected men and in children born to infected mothers. There is no evidence that the virus is spread by normal social contact, by food or by air-borne routes. For instance, antibody-positive children should not be excluded from ordinary schools.

Infected persons and those at special risk such as homosexuals, haemophiliacs and drug addicts should be advised against multiple sexual partners. Anal intercourse and intimate kissing should be avoided. The use of condoms may reduce transmission of infection. Women who are antibody-positive should be advised not to become pregnant.

Blood for transfusion must be screened for HIV antibody. Blood products such as factors VIII and IX should be heat-treated to destroy the virus. Persons infected with HIV and those at special risk should not donate blood, plasma, tissues, organs or sperm. Needles, syringes and other articles which come into contact with blood should be disposable. If this is not possible they should be sterilized in an autoclave. Intravenous drug abusers who will not give up the habit should be provided with a personal supply of sterile needles and syringes. Domestic articles such as razors, scissors, sewing needles and toothbrushes which could become contaminated with blood should not be shared. Surfaces contaminated with blood should be cleaned with strong hypochlorite solutions.

The risk of transmission to health care staff is very small but precautions similar to those used in the prevention of hepatitis B must be taken. Individuals who are aware that they are HIV antibody-positive should inform their doctors and dentists before undergoing further blood tests or surgical procedures. Patients with AIDS should be nursed in an isolation unit. Gloves and a disposable gown should be worn when taking blood samples. Specimens should be sent to the laboratory only by prior arrangement. They must be in leak-proof containers clearly labelled 'Danger of Infection'. Laboratory procedures should be carried out under conditions complying with laboratory containment level 3 (separate laboratory, ventilated safety cabinet, etc.) as defined by the Advisory Committee on Dangerous Pathogens (1983). Contact with the bodies of patients who have died of AIDS should be kept to a minimum.

Fear of AIDS has produced near panic in some circles. It is important to stress that AIDS is not highly infectious and that the chance of acquiring AIDS in the course of normal social and medical contact is remote. Proper counselling and support of AIDS patients and their contacts is essential. AIDS is not a notifiable disease but it is advisable to report all cases in confidence to the Communicable Disease Surveillance Centre (CDSC) at Colindale.

Chemotherapy

One of the first duties of the physician is to educate the masses not to take medicine.

William Osler

Chemotherapy is the treatment of infectious disease by the administration of drugs which are lethal or inhibitory to the causative organisms. The essential requirement of such a drug is that it should have *selective toxicity*, i.e. under the conditions of use it must be more poisonous to the microbes than it is to the host. Disinfectants and antiseptics will kill bacteria, but they are highly toxic to tissue cells and are unsuitable as chemotherapeutic agents.

Ehrlich developed methods by which many subsequent chemotherapeutic agents have been obtained: he discovered a substance of limited activity and then set about the synthesis and comparative study of related compounds. In 1907 he synthesized an organic arsenic compound, arsphenamine, active against the spirochaete of syphilis. This was the first time that organic chemistry had provided a remedy for a human infectious disease.

Domagk (1935) reported the successful treatment of streptococcal infections with the dye Prontosil. Other workers soon showed that the activity of this compound depended on the liberation in the body of sulphanilamide (p-aminobenzenesulphonamide), the forerunner of a large series of sulphonamides subsequently synthesized.

An antibiotic is an antimicrobial substance produced by a living micro-organism and active in high dilution. However, the term is now widely used for any antimicrobial chemotherapeutic agent, whether naturally produced or synthetic. Pasteur and Joubert (1877) noted that a culture of anthrax bacilli was killed if it was contaminated by common air-borne organisms. They realized that a phenomenon of this kind might well have therapeutic possibilities.

Fleming (1929) noted that the products of a mould, *Penicillium notatum*, were strongly active against a wide range of pathogens but were non-toxic to mammalian cells. Attempts to concentrate the active agent (penicillin) were not successful.

In 1940 Chain and Florey and their co-workers at Oxford suc-
ceeded in obtaining penicillin preparations of high antibacterial
activity. These preparations were highly effective in controlling
experimental infections in animals. The remarkable clinical
potentialities of penicillin were quickly demonstrated.

Most antibiotics are produced by species of *Streptomyces*. A few
are produced by *Bacillus* spp., actinomycetes and fungi. Several antibiotics are semi-synthetic in origin, e.g. cloxacillin and ampicillin
are prepared from naturally produced 6-aminopenicillanic acid.

General properties of chemotherapeutic agents

Type of action

From their behaviour towards bacterial populations antibacterial
agents are divided into two classes:

1 *Bactericidal drugs* have a rapid lethal action, e.g. penicillins,
   cephalosporins, aminoglycosides and polymyxin. Erythromycin
   is sometimes bactericidal in high concentrations.
2 *Bacteristatic drugs* merely inhibit the growth of organisms, e.g.
   sulphonamides, tetracyclines and chloramphenicol.

The differences are not clear-cut and most drugs are to varying
extents both bactericidal and bacteristatic. What happens in particular circumstances depends on the drug, its concentration, the
number and type of organisms and other factors. The physiological
condition of the organism is often important, e.g. penicillin has
powerful bactericidal effects on rapidly growing organisms, but no
effect when they are in the resting stage, and so-called 'persisters'
may survive very high concentrations of penicillin.

Mode of action

The chemical structures of antibiotics and other chemotherapeutic
agents are diverse and the mechanisms by which they interfere
with bacterial metabolism or structure differ with each major
group.

Sulphonamides act by competitive inhibition of a bacterial
enzyme which normally has as its substrate the structurally similar
substance *p*-aminobenzoic acid, an essential metabolite for many
bacteria.

Trimethoprim is a powerful inhibitor of the bacterial enzyme dihydrofolate reductase but has little effect on the corresponding human enzyme. It interferes with folic acid metabolism and thereby inhibits bacterial DNA synthesis. Trimethoprim and sulphonamides act on separate steps of the same metabolic pathway.

Penicillins, cephalosporins, bacitracin, vancomycin and cycloserine interfere with cell wall synthesis and secondarily cause cell fragility and bacterilysis. The bacterial cell wall, by virtue of its unique structure and function, is an ideal point of attack by selectively toxic agents.

Chloramphenicol acts as a specific inhibitor of protein synthesis.

Tetracyclines also inhibit protein synthesis.

Streptomycin and other aminoglycosides bind to certain ribosomal subunits and inhibit protein synthesis.

Polymyxin becomes firmly bound to the cytoplasmic membrane and acts by damaging this structure.

Quinolones inhibit bacterial DNA gyrases (topoisomerases) which catalyse supercoiling of bacterial DNA.

Range of action

Antibiotics fall into three main categories:

1 Active mainly against gram-positive organisms, e.g. penicillins, erythromycin and lincomycin.
2 Active mainly against gram-negative organisms, e.g. polymyxin, mecillinam, aztreonam and nalidixic acid.
3 Active against both gram-positive and gram-negative organisms (broad-spectrum activity), e.g. the tetracyclines, chloramphenicol, ampicillin, cephalosporins and sulphonamides.

These are generalizations and there are many exceptions, e.g. neisseriae are gram-negative but are usually highly sensitive to penicillins and erythromycin; the natural susceptibility of a species may be altered by previous exposure to chemotherapeutic agents.

Mycobacteria are resistant to all the common antibiotics except rifampicin and streptomycin. They are sensitive to isoniazid and ethambutol which have little effect on other bacteria.

Rickettsiae, chlamydiae and mycoplasmas are susceptible to tetracyclines and chloramphenicol. *Chlamydia trachomatis* is also sensitive to sulphonamides. Some mycoplasmas are sensitive to erythromycin.

Viruses, yeasts, fungi and protozoa are unaffected by the common antibiotics.

Sensitivity tests

Tube methods

Serial dilutions of the drug are made in broth and a standard inoculum of the organisms is added. After incubation the lowest concentration of the drug which inhibits growth is recorded as the minimum inhibitory concentration (MIC). If tubes showing no visible growth are subcultured on to solid nutrient media the lowest concentration yielding no growth is the minimum bactericidal concentration (MBC). Tube sensitivity tests are used for special purposes, e.g. accurate determination of sensitivity of organisms in cases of infective endocarditis.

Plate methods

In one method ('break-point' sensitivity tests) the organism is inoculated on plates of solid medium containing known concentrations of antibiotics. After incubation the results are recorded as 'growth' or 'no growth' (Fig. 30). By using several plates containing different concentrations of the same antibiotic the MIC can be estimated. In other methods a plate is seeded with the culture, and filter-paper discs impregnated with suitable amounts of representative antibiotics are applied to the surface. After incubation the presence or absence of zones of inhibition is noted and the organisms are reported as 'sensitive' or 'resistant' by comparison with known sensitive strains. Several such methods

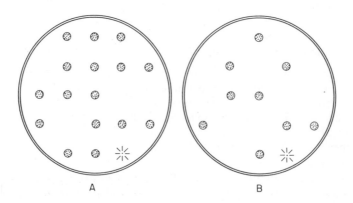

A   B

Fig. 30 Sensitivity tests using solid media containing antibiotics. Twenty different organisms have been inoculated on both plates using a mechanical inoculator. Plate A contains a low concentration of an antibiotic: 16 cultures show growth. Plate B contains a higher concentration of the same antibiotic: 9 cultures show growth.

are available: two techniques are illustrated in Fig. 31. Plate methods are satisfactory for routine purposes. Direct sensitivity tests on materials such as pus and urine have the advantage of speed. Indirect sensitivity tests on organisms obtained in pure culture entail some delay but tend to be more accurate. Indirect tests are often essential in the presence of mixed cultures. The Oxford strain of *Staphylococcus aureus* (NCTC 6571) is a widely used standard strain. Its MIC for benzylpenicillin is about 0.02 mg/litre.

Sulphonamides are antagonized by p-aminobenzoic acid and folic acid which occur in ordinary laboratory media. Special media free from antagonizers are required for sensitivity tests.

Tests for β-lactamases

Early recognition of β-lactamase-producing (penicillin-resistant) bacteria is often important in deciding treatment. Such bacteria can be identified in a few minutes by sampling a colony with a moistened paper disc or stick impregnated with a chromogenic cephalosporin which changes colour (yellow to red) when hydrolysed by β-lactamases.

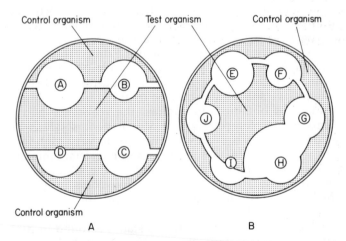

Fig. 31 Paper disc methods for testing antibiotic sensitivities. Plate A: the test organism has been spread across the middle of the plate and a control organism on either side. The test organism is sensitive to antibiotics A and C and resistant to B and D. Plate B: a mechanical rotator has been used to inoculate the test organism over the centre of the plate and a control organism round the periphery. The test organism is sensitive to antibiotics E, G and H and resistant to F, I and J.

Assay of antibiotics

The tube and plate methods of estimating sensitivities can be adapted to measure the concentration of antibiotics in blood and other biological fluids. Comparative tests are carried out using known concentrations of antibiotics and a sensitive organism. These biological methods are simple to perform but have the disadvantage that the results are not available for several hours. For this reason chemical and immunological methods of assay are often preferred. Blood assays are important when toxic antibiotics, particularly aminoglycosides, are being given to patients with impaired renal function.

A test of the bactericidal activity of the patient's serum against his own organism is useful in endocarditis. A common recommendation is that the dose of antibiotic or mixture of antibiotics should be large enough to ensure that the patient's serum will kill the organism when the serum is diluted 1 in 8 or more.

Drug resistance

If bacteria are repeatedly subcultured in the presence of gradually increasing subinhibitory concentrations of an antibiotic it is usually possible to obtain mutant organisms which will survive and multiply in concentrations which are lethal for the parent strain. The degree of resistance and the speed with which it develops varies with the organism and the drug. Thus the resistance of *Staph. aureus* to penicillin, chloramphenicol and the tetracyclines usually develops slowly in multiple small steps and many successive subcultures may be required before a high level of resistance is obtained. In contrast the resistance of various organisms to streptomycin and of *Mycobacterium tuberculosis* to isoniazid often rises suddenly in one step to very high levels.

While it is possible to select antibiotic-resistant mutants of most organisms *in vitro* this rarely reflects the situation *in vivo*. Thus naturally occurring strains of *Streptococcus pyogenes* have remained fully sensitive to penicillin in spite of the widespread use of the drug and it has not been possible to obtain resistant strains artifically. When antibiotic resistance is found in clinically derived strains of bacteria the mechanism of resistance often differs from that obtained by laboratory means. For example, penicillin-resistant *Staph. aureus* encountered in hospitals produce penicillinase (β-lactamase) whereas resistant mutants selected in the laboratory have a decreased ability to bind the drug. Likewise, many of the clinically isolated bacteria resistant to aminoglycosides produce plasmid-mediated antibiotic-inactivating enzymes, but resistant strains selected *in vitro* possess mutated ribosomal binding sites.

A third form of antibiotic resistance is known as 'drug tolerance'. Penicillin-tolerant strains of *Staph. aureus* are inhibited by low concentrations of penicillin but are resistant to the lethal (bactericidal) effects of the antibiotic. It has been suggested that tolerant organisms are deficient in autolytic enzyme activity which is necessary for cell lysis and the lethal action of penicillin. Penicillin tolerance is also common among streptococci, though not *Str. pneumoniae*.

Specificity

Resistance is specific in the sense that if an organism becomes resistant to penicillins its susceptibility to gentamicin, chloramphenicol, erythromycin, tetracyclines and sulphonamides is unaffected. When the antibiotics are similar cross-resistance occurs, e.g. an organism which becomes resistant to one of the tetracyclines also becomes resistant to the others of the group. If an organism which is resistant to one antibiotic is subsequently exposed to the action of a completely different antibiotic it may acquire resistance to the second as well. In this way organisms may become resistant to many antibiotics.

In the special case of transmissible drug resistance organisms may become *simultaneously* resistant to many antibiotics.

Mutation

The organisms responsible for the infection produce resistant mutants during treatment, i.e. the resistant organisms are direct lineal descendants of the original organisms.

Resistant mutants are particularly liable to arise during treatment with streptomycin. Sulphonamides, isoniazid, nalidixic acid and rifamycins are also serious offenders. Erythromycin is a moderate offender. Penicillin, cephalosporins, chloramphenicol and tetracyclines are relatively free from this defect. Commonly encountered examples are the development of resistance of gram-negative bacilli to nalidixic acid and sulphonamides, of *M. tuberculosis* to streptomycin and isoniazid, and *Staph. aureus* to fusidic acid and erythromycin when these drugs are used singly. The emergence of resistant mutants is encouraged by inadequate dosage, prolonged treatment and the presence of a closed focus of infection.

Transmissible drug resistance

This is a type of transferable or 'infective' drug resistance mainly found among intestinal bacilli. If a suitable strain of *Salmonella typhimurium* resistant to, say, ampicillin, streptomycin, tetracycline and sulphonamide is grown in a mixed broth culture with a suitable strain of *Escherichia coli* sensitive to these drugs, sub-culture on selective media will reveal that some of the *E. coli* have acquired simultaneous resistance to all four drugs. These resistant strains of *E. coli* can in turn be used to transfer the full pattern of resistance to suitable sensitive strains of *S. typhimurium*, other species of salmonellae, shigellae and other gram-negative bacilli. In such experiments the property of drug resistance is clearly contagious or infectious, and it can be shown that the phenomenon is due to transference of resistance (R) plasmids between the bacteria (p. 24). Plasmid-mediated resistance also occurs among many other organisms, e.g. penicillin resistance in *Neisseria gonorrhoeae* and ampicillin resistance in *Haemophilus influenzae* depend on plasmid-mediated β-lactamases. R plasmids capable of carrying resistance to as many as nine agents at one time have been described. When the genes for resistance to several different agents are carried on the same plasmid use of any one agent will select for strains resistant to all the others, e.g ampicillin will select for aminoglycoside-resistant organisms and so on.

Transmissible drug resistance is the most important mechanism by which drug-resistant organisms are produced in the community. Multiple drug resistance can be transferred by organisms multi-plying freely in the intestinal tract of experimental animals and there is good evidence that this process can occur under everyday conditions in farm animals and man.

Superinfection

The organisms originally responsible for infection are inhibited and are replaced by pre-existing antibiotic-resistant organisms present in the environment, i.e. the resistant organisms represent a fresh infection.

Superinfection is sometimes caused by the same species that caused the original infection. In infections caused by *Staph. aureus* a resistant strain of this organism appearing for the first time during treatment with penicillins, cephalosporins, chloramphenicol or tetracyclines is usually evidence of infection by a new strain acquired from someone else, e.g. the organisms usually belong to a different phage-type. Cross-infection with antibiotic-resistant strains is likely to occur when the lesions are superficial and the environment contains large numbers of resistant organisms as in hospitals.

A more general type of superinfection is the suppression of the normal flora and its replacement with drug-resistant organisms. This follows the use of any antibiotic but is seen in its most severe forms as a result of treatment with broad-spectrum antibiotics. Thus when tetracyclines are given, the normal coccal flora of the upper respiratory tract regularly becomes replaced by resistant coliform organisms and yeasts. Similarly the flora of the gut is disturbed with overgrowth of resistant coliforms, staphylococci, yeasts and clostridia such as *Clostridium difficile*. These changes in flora usually cause little harm though they may be responsible for such symptoms as sore tongue, sore lips and diarrhoea. In a few cases serious infection develops, e.g. generalized infection with coliforms or *Candida albicans*, staphylococcal enterocolitis or pseudomembranous colitis associated with the toxin of *Cl. difficile*.

Resistant strains in the community

The presence of resistant strains in the community is more serious than the occurrence of resistant organisms in an individual. With some organisms the prevalence of resistant strains is placing severe limitations on previously effective forms of treatment.

In hospitals it is common to find that of strains of *Staph. aureus* responsible for hospital-acquired infection 90% or more are resistant to penicillin and smaller percentages are resistant to other antibiotics. The figures vary in different hospitals and correspond roughly to the amounts of the different antibiotics that are used. Coliform organisms and strains of *Staph. aureus* showing multiple antibiotic resistance have become a major and intractable problem in most hospitals.

In the community at large the problem is less serious but cannot be ignored. Many staphylococcal infections encountered in general practice are still likely to respond to penicillin, but in some areas 50–75% of strains are penicillin-resistant.

Clinical use of antibiotics

The object of antibiotic therapy is to cure the patient with the minimum of complications and discomfort. At the same time it is important to discourage the emergence of drug-resistant organisms. The following principles should be observed:

1 Antibiotics should not be given for trivial infections.

2 They should be used for prophylaxis only in special circumstances (p. 226).

3 The availability of antibiotics active against all the common bacterial pathogens is no reason for adopting slipshod methods of asepsis in surgery or neglecting other methods of controlling cross-infection.

4 Treatment should be based on a clear clinical and bacteriological diagnosis. Suitable specimens should be sent to the laboratory before treatment is begun. It is frequently justifiable to start treatment without waiting for the final reports, though it may be advisable to modify treatment when these become available.

5 The choice of antibiotic is essentially a clinical matter. The laboratory report is not intended as a directive for treatment but it may be a useful guide. All antibiotics are potentially lethal substances. In general it is bad treatment to use broad-spectrum antibiotics when an infective condition can be treated with a more specific agent. Many antibiotics are extremely dangerous, particularly in renal failure.

6 Antibiotics for systemic treatment should be given in full therapeutic doses for an adequate period, e.g. usually a minimum of three days. If towards the end of this time there has been no obvious clinical response it usually means that the infecting organisms are resistant to the antibiotic. Further specimens should be sent to the laboratory. In other cases failure to respond may be an indication that the drug is failing to reach the microbes, e.g. because the patient is not taking the drug or the organisms are in an abscess cavity or a platelet thrombus. In the special case of penicillin therapy a fully sensitive organism may survive because the drug is being destroyed by β-lactamase-producing organisms such as penicillin-resistant *Staph. aureus* present in a mixed infection.

7 Combined therapy with two or more antimicrobial drugs should always be used in tuberculosis and certain other diseases.

8 In local treatment of superficial infections it is important to use either antiseptics or antibiotics which are rarely or never used systemically, e.g. mupirocin, bacitracin and polymyxin. Local treatment with some antibiotics such as penicillin may produce severe hypersensitivity reactions in addition to the dangers of infection with resistant organisms.

9 Antibiotic solutions and powders should not be liberated into the environment. They can cause hypersensitivity reactions and encourage development of antibiotic-resistant strains.

10 In an attempt to prevent the emergence of antibiotic-resistant strains hospitals may find it necessary to introduce an antibiotic policy, e.g. insisting on combined use of two antibiotics, keeping a particular antibiotic in reserve for desperately ill patients, using antibiotics in rotation.

Simultaneous use of antimicrobial agents

There is *in vitro* evidence that in special circumstances two or more antibiotics used together may be either synergistic or antagonistic in their action (Fig. 32). More commonly their inter-action is one of indifference. Synergism is usually seen when both agents are bactericidal, e.g. a penicillin plus an aminoglycoside (gentamicin, netilmicin, etc.). On the other hand, most bactericidal agents only kill rapidly multiplying cells and antagonism is liable to occur when a bactericidal agent is used with a bacteristatic agent, e.g. penicillin plus tetracycline. Sulphonamides do not appear to antagonize penicillin, possibly because their bacteristatic action is too slow. Polymyxin is an unusual bactericidal antibiotic in that it kills both resting and multiplying cells and is therefore not antagonized by bacteristatic agents.

How far synergisms and antagonisms matter in clinical circum-stances is obscure. Combined therapy is certainly recommended in a few specific diseases, particularly when the organisms are relatively inaccessible, e.g. penicillin (or ampicillin) plus an aminoglycoside in infective endocarditis caused by viridans streptococci or *Str. faecalis*. The addition of nystatin to prevent

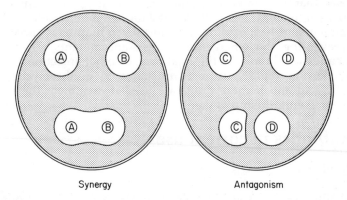

Synergy   Antagonism

Fig. 32 Synergy and antagonism. In the paper disc sensitivity test illus-trated, antibiotics A and B are synergistic and C and D are antagonistic.

candidiasis is of value when therapy with broad-spectrum anti-biotics has to be prolonged. In other cases the use of two anti-biotics may be justified because the patient is severely ill and not responding to a previously prescribed antibiotic and it seems likely that the infection is a mixed one or due to some organism the laboratory has failed to isolate. For blind antibiotic therapy in very ill patients flucloxacillin, piperacillin and gentamicin provide one of the widest bactericidal combinations.

When combined therapy is directed against a mixed infection there is usually no advantage in giving antibiotics with similar spectra of antibacterial action. Thus penicillin and erythromycin are active against an almost identical range of organisms, and the activity of chloramphenicol is much the same as that of the tetracyclines. On the other hand a combination such as gentamicin plus metronidazole covers the majority of gram-positive and gram-negative organisms, including anaerobes (particularly *Bacteroides*), and is very effective against mixed infections such as those resulting from escape of intestinal organisms.

One theoretical advantage of using two chemotherapeutic agents is that if a particular organism is sensitive to both drugs a mutant resistant to both of them is highly unlikely to arise during treatment. If the incidence of mutants resistant to any drug singly is, say, $1:10^7$ then the chances that a mutant will arise simultaneously resistant to two drugs are $1:10^{14}$ and to three drugs $1:10^{21}$. Whereas a total population of 10^7 organisms is usual in disease it is unlikely that populations as large as 10^{14} are ever reached. This is probably a simplification of the true state of affairs.

It has been clearly demonstrated in the chemotherapy of tuber-culosis that a standard regime of combined treatment with rifampicin, isoniazid and ethambutol for two months followed by rifampicin and isoniazid for a further seven months is successful in preventing the emergence of resistant mutants. The same principles may apply in the treatment of other infections. Thus staphylococci rapidly acquire resistance to erythromycin and fusidic acid and if these drugs are used in treatment there is a case for giving them together.

Antibiotics in current use

Penicillins

Penicillins, cephalosporins and certain closely related compounds, e.g. clavulanic acid, contain the β-lactam ring and are known collectively as β-lactam antibiotics. Penicillins are the most valuable of all the antibacterial agents. They may be classified into four groups:

1 Benzylpenicillin (penicillin G) and penicillins with similar activity, e.g. phenoxymethylpenicillin (penicillin V) and phenethicillin. This group is normally implied when one refers to 'penicillin'.
2 Penicillins with broad-spectrum activity, e.g. ampicillin, amoxycillin and carbenicillin.
3 Penicillins resistant to staphylococcal penicillinase (β-lactamase), e.g. methicillin, cloxacillin and flucloxacillin.
4 Penicillins more active against gram-negative bacilli than against gram-positive organisms, e.g. mecillinam.

Group 1

Benzylpenicillin is destroyed by gastric hydrochloric acid and is normally given by frequent intramuscular injections. The number of injections can be cut down by giving sparingly soluble forms such as procaine penicillin and benzathine penicillin. Penicillin V and phenethicillin are acid-resistant and can be given by mouth. Probenecid delays the excretion of most penicillins (and some cephalosporins) and can be used to maintain high blood levels.

Penicillin is the antibiotic of choice in infections caused by *Staph. aureus* (when sensitive), *Str. pyogenes*, *Str. pneumoniae*, *Clostridium perfringens* and other gas gangrene organisms, *Bacillus anthracis* and *Actinomyces israeli*. It is highly effective in the treatment of infections caused by Vincent's organisms and is used as the routine treatment for syphilis. It is extremely valuable in the treatment of sore throats, otitis media and many cases of bronchitis, bronchopneumonia and postoperative chest infections. *Corynebacterium diphtheriae* is sensitive and penicillin can be used to supplement antitoxin treatment and to treat carriers. *Neisseria meningitidis* is almost invariably sensitive. Penicillin penetrates the blood-brain barrier in only small amounts unless the meninges are severely damaged, but satisfactory cerebrospinal fluid (CSF) levels can be obtained by employing large doses systemically. *N. gonorrhoeae* is usually sensitive though moderately resistant strains are fairly common. Since 1976 some strains have acquired an R plasmid coding for penicillinase (β-lactamase) production and as a result are completely resistant to penicillin.

Group 2

Ampicillin is slightly less active than benzylpenicillin against gram-positive organisms with the exception of *Str. faecalis*. It has a special place in the treatment of endocarditis caused by this organism. It is inactivated by β-lactamases and so has no effect on penicillin-resistant *Staph. aureus*. Unlike benzylpenicillin, ampicillin is active against many gram-negative bacilli including salmonellae, shigellae, *E. coli*, *Proteus* and *H. influenzae*. Klebsiellae and *Pseudomonas aeruginosa* are resistant. It has been used for the treatment of urinary infections caused by *E. coli* and some strains of *Proteus* (especially *Pr. mirabilis*) and for wound infections, peritonitis and bacteraemic states caused by coliforms. *H. influenzae* is usually highly sensitive but completely resistant β-lactamase-producing strains have appeared since 1974. Ampicillin has a special place in the treatment of acute exacerbations of chronic bronchitis caused by this organism. In the treatment of most types of meningitis ampicillin used by itself in high doses is probably as effective as various combinations of penicillin, chloramphenicol and sulphonamides. Ampicillin is normally given by mouth. Talampicillin is an ester of ampicillin. Following oral administration it is rapidly hydrolysed to give high blood levels of ampicillin.

Amoxycillin closely resembles ampicillin in its activity but is better absorbed and produces higher blood levels.

Carbenicillin has an even wider range of activity against gram-negative bacilli. It is active against most strains of *Proteus* and, in high concentration, some strains of *Ps. aeruginosa*. It is given by intravenous infusion. Carfecillin is an ester of carbenicillin. Following oral administration it is hydrolysed and high concentrations of carbenicillin appear in the urine. Carfecillin should be reserved for urinary tract infections caused by *Ps. aeruginosa*. It is not suitable for systemic infections caused by this organism.

Ticarcillin, mezlocillin, azlocillin and piperacillin resemble carbenicillin in their range of activity. They are more active against *Ps. aeruginosa*.

Group 3

In the special case of penicillin-resistant *Staph. aureus* the resistance is due to production of penicillinase (β-lactamase) by an organism which is inherently sensitive to penicillin. Methicillin, cloxacillin and flucloxacillin are largely unaffected by this enzyme and originally nearly all strains of *Staph. aureus* were sensitive. By the 1980s methicillin-resistant *Staph. aureus* (MRSA) strains were causing serious problems in many hospitals. Cross-resistance between these antibiotics is complete. Use should be restricted to infections caused by penicillin-resistant *Staph. aureus*. They are less active than other penicillins against other organisms. Cloxacillin and flucloxacillin are usually given by mouth. Flucloxacillin is better absorbed than cloxacillin and produces higher blood levels.

Methicillin can be given only by injection and is now seldom used.

Group 4

Mecillinam, an amidinopenicillanic acid, has very unusual properties for a penicillin in that it is highly active against *E. coli* and other gram-negative intestinal bacilli but has only weak activity against gram-positive organisms. It is not absorbed when given by mouth but an ester, pivmecillinam, is well absorbed from the gut and is rapidly hydrolysed to liberate mecillinam.

Side effects

Penicillin is remarkably free from toxicity and massive doses can usually be given with safety though *only small doses can be given intrathecally*. Over the years there has been an alarming increase in the incidence of hypersensitivity reactions, some of which have been very severe and even fatal. In many cases hypersensitivity to penicillin is attributed to traces of a penicilloylated protein impurity arising in the production process. The incidence of reactions is greatly reduced when this impurity is removed. However, some people are hypersensitive to penicillin itself or to polymers which form when penicillin is stored. If a patient has had a severe reaction to penicillin on a previous occasion another antibiotic must be used. A patient hypersensitive to one type of penicillin is also hypersensitive to other penicillins. Most types of penicillin cause urticarial rashes in about 5% of patients. Ampicillin causes a distinctive maculopapular rash in about 10% of patients and, for unknown reasons, in nearly all cases of infectious mononucleosis. This ampicillin rash is not a contraindication to later penicillin therapy. Nevertheless penicillin, particularly in a highly purifed form, is still safer and less liable to produce undesirable side effects than any other antibiotic. Penicillin and other β-lactam antibiotics can be used in pregnancy.

Cephalosporins

Cephalexin, cephradine, cefuroxime, cefotaxime and ceftazidime contain the cephalosporin nucleus which is chemically related to the penicillin nucleus. Cefoxitin contains the cephamycin nucleus but behaves like a cephalosporin. Several other cephalosporins are in current use but offer no special advantages. Cephalosporins resemble penicillins in being bactericidal and of low toxicity. About 10% of patients who are hypersensitive to penicillin show hypersensitivity to cephalosporins. Cephalosporins have a broad spectrum of activity and can be used against streptococci (enterococi are resistant), staphylococci (including penicillin-resistant strains) and a wide range of gram-negative bacteria. Staphylococci resistant to cloxacillin and other β-lactamase-resistant penicillins show cross-resistance to the cephalosporins. Cefuroxime, cefoxitin, cefotaxime and ceftazidime are highly resistant to the β-lactamases of gram-negative bacteria and are often effective against strains of gram-negative bacilli resistant to other cephalosporins. Ceftazidime is highly active against most strains of *Ps. aeruginosa*. Cephalexin is given by mouth, cephradine by mouth and injection, and the others by injection only. Cefuroxime axetil, an ester of cefuroxime, is given by mouth.

Occasional patients are hypersensitive and develop rashes. High blood levels of some of the earlier cephalosporins were liable to cause renal damage but this is very rare with the cephalosporins listed here. However, the combination of a cephalosporin plus an aminoglycoside is probably best avoided, especially when there is impaired renal function.

Other beta-lactam antibiotics

Clavulanic acid, a naturally occurring β-lactam compound with little intrinsic antibacterial activity, is a powerful inhibitor of many bacterial β-lactamases. These enzymes inactivate β-lactam antibiotics (penicillins and cephalosporins) and are mainly responsible for the widespread resistance to penicillins shown by staphylococci and many gram-negative bacilli such as *E. coli* and *Klebsiella*. Amoxycillin used in combination with clavulanic acid is effective in the treatment of infections caused by amoxycillin-resistant (β-lactamase-producing) bacteria. The combination (Augmentin) is normally given by mouth.

Latamoxef is active against a wide range of gram-positive and gram-negative organisms. It is resistant to the β-lactamases of most gram-negative bacilli. It is given by injection. Hypoprothrombinaemia, interference with platelet function and thrombocytopenia may occur.

Aztreonam is active against a wide range of gram-negative organisms including β-lactamase-producing strains. It is given by injection. It is usually well tolerated by patients who are hypersensitive to penicillins and cephalosporins.

Aminoglycosides

This group of antibiotics includes streptomycin, neomycin, kanamycin, gentamicin, netilmicin, tobramycin, amikacin and framycetin. They are similar in chemical structure, antibacterial activity, pharmacological properties and toxicity. They are not absorbed by the gut and are normally given intramuscularly.

The aminoglycosides have a wide range of antibacterial activity. They show considerable activity against gram-positive organisms, although these will usually be more sensitive to other antibiotics. Their main activity is against gram-negative bacilli and they are particularly effective in severe infections caused by coliform organisms. Streptococci and anaerobes are resistant.

Streptomycin has been largely superseded for general purposes. Its most important specific use is as the major alternative to rifampicin in the treatment of tuberculosis. For this purpose it should always be used in conjunction with other chemotherapeutic agents. High blood levels of streptomycin are liable to cause severe disturbances of hearing and vestibular function. The drug should not be used in patients with impaired renal function.

Neomycin and *kanamycin* resemble streptomycin. Neomycin is given by mouth in the treatment of intestinal infections, e.g. infantile gastroenteritis due to *E. coli*, and as an intestinal antiseptic prior to operations on the bowel. Given intramuscularly both drugs are liable to cause deafness and renal damage. Neomycin is too toxic for systemic use but kanamycin can be used to treat severe infections caused by coliform organisms resistant to other antibiotics. A single large dose of kanamycin given by intramuscular injection is an effective treatment for gonorrhoea.

Gentamicin is the preferred aminoglycoside for general use. It is more active than kanamycin against gram-negative bacilli and is usually effective against *Ps. aeruginosa*. Most strains of *Staph. aureus* are highly sensitive. It is widely used in the treatment of severe infections caused by coliform organisms, but high blood levels can cause severe impairment of vestibular function.

Netilmicin is active against some gentamicin-resistant gram-negative bacilli.

Tobramycin resembles gentamicin but has greater activity against *Ps. aeruginosa*.

Amikacin, a derivative of kanamycin, resembles gentamicin. It is active against some strains of gram-negative bacilli that are resistant to gentamicin and tobramycin.

Framycetin is a form of neomycin. It is used for local treatment of infections of the ear, nose, eyes and skin.

Tetracyclines

The tetracycline group includes tetracycline, oxytetracycline, chlortetracycline, demeclocycline, clomocycline, doxycycline and minocycline. They are normally given by mouth. Members of the group are very similar in their antibacterial activity but differ slightly in their rates of absorption and excretion.

The tetracyclines are broad-spectrum antibiotics active against many gram-positive and gram-negative bacteria. In practice, most infections caused by gram-positive cocci and gram-negative bacilli can be treated more effectively with other antibiotics. Emergence of tetracycline-resistant strains has also been a problem. Tetracyclines remain the treatment of choice for most infections caused by rickettsiae (including Q fever), chlamydiae and mycoplasmas. They are used to treat exacerbations of chronic bronchitis because of their activity against *H. influenzae*. They are of value in *Brucella* infections. Tetracyclines in small doses over long periods are used to treat acne vulgaris.

Superinfection, particularly with tetracycline-resistant *Staph. aureus*, is a serious complication. Large intravenous doses can cause severe liver damage, particularly in pregnancy and associated pyelonephritis. Tetracyclines, other than doxycycline and minocycline, should not be given to patients with impaired renal function as they aggravate the condition. They markedly inhibit growth and development of bones and teeth in the developing fetus and in infancy. Teeth which are being mineralized in the fetus and in children up to the age of about eight may subsequently develop permanent unsightly staining. As far as possible tetracyclines should not be given to pregnant women or infants, and long-term administration should be avoided in young children.

Chloramphenicol

Chloramphenicol has a range of activity similar to that of the tetracyclines although it shows little or no cross-resistance with these antibiotics. It is normally given by mouth. Depression of bone marrow function is a rare but potentially fatal complication. The drug also causes severe shock and death in premature infants ('grey baby syndrome'). For these reasons *less toxic antibiotics should be used whenever possible*. Chloramphenicol is still the drug of choice in the treatment of typhoid fever although resistant organisms have appeared, e.g. chloramphenicol-resistant *S. typhi* caused extensive outbreaks in Mexico in 1972–3. There are few other indications for its use. It readily penetrates the blood-brain barrier and is of value in the treatment of meningitis caused by *H. influenzae*. However, ampicillin is usually an effective alternative. Severe respiratory tract infections which have shown little response to other antibiotics often respond dramatically to chloramphenicol, probably through its action on certain gram-negative bacilli such as *H. influenzae*, *Bordetella pertussis* and coliforms. The use of chloramphenicol should be restricted to short courses of treatment. A fall in the reticulocyte count is the earliest evidence of toxicity and blood counts should be performed daily. It is professional malpractice to give systemic chloramphenicol for minor infections but local treatment with chloramphenicol is valuable in eye infections.

Erythromycin

Erythromycin is a member of the macrolide group of antibiotics. It has the same general spectrum of activity as penicillin and is best reserved for patients who are hypersensitive to penicillin or are infected with penicillin-resistant organisms which cannot easily be treated in other ways. It is effective against *Mycoplasma pneumoniae, Legionella pneumophila,* chlamydiae and most strains of *Campylobacter*. It is of value in whooping cough, though chloramphenicol is usually preferred in life-threatening cases. It is used for long-term treatment of acne vulgaris. Some organisms such as *Staph. aureus* rapidly become resistant. It is normally given by mouth.

Minor gastrointestinal upsets may occur. Erythromycin estolate may cause jaundice and impaired liver function if treatment is prolonged.

Sulphonamides

All sulphonamides have much the same spectrum of activity and cross-resistance between them is complete. The choice of a particular sulphonamide is based on pharmacological grounds such as rate of absorption from the gut, rate of excretion in the urine and toxicity. The following are recommended: sulphadiazine and sulphadimidine for general infections; sulphadimidine, sulphafurazole and sulphamethizole for urinary infections. Sulphonamides are normally given by mouth.

In the treatment of infections caused by gram-positive organisms sulphonamides have been largely superseded by antibiotics, though they are very effective against sensitive organisms such as *Str. pyogenes* and *Str. pneumoniae. N. meningitidis* is often sensitive and the ability of sulphonamides to diffuse into the CSF gives them a special place in the treatment of meningitis caused by this and other sensitive organisms. Sulphonamides are also of value in the prophylaxis of meningococcal infections caused by sensitive strains. The main use of sulphonamides is in the treatment of urinary infections caused by *E. coli*. Hypersensitivity, particularly the occurrence of rashes, is common. Agranulocytosis and acute haemolytic anaemia are rare. Crystalluria is not common with the more soluble sulphonamides.

Trimethoprim

Trimethoprim is active against a wide range of gram-positive and gram-negative organisms. It is not active against *Ps. aeruginosa* or anaerobes and is only weakly active against neisseriae. It is normally given by mouth and is highly effective in acute exacerbations of chronic bronchitis and in acute infections of the urinary tract. Because of its anti-folate action it should not be given to patients with megaloblastic anaemia. A few patients experience rashes, nausea and vomiting.

Trimethoprim shows synergism with sulphonamides *in vitro* but there is doubt whether this occurs *in vivo*. Co-trimoxazole is a fixed ratio (1:5) mixture of trimethoprim and sulphamethoxazole. It is probable that most of the antibacterial activity of co-trimoxazole is due to trimethoprim and most of the side effects, including fatal bone marrow aplasia, are due to the sulphonamide. It is doubtful whether use of the combination discourages the emergence of resistant organisms.

Other antibiotics

Fusidic acid is a steroid antibiotic, mainly active against gram-positive organisms. It is normally given by mouth. It is of value only in the treatment of staphylococcal infections, but the organisms rapidly acquire resistance. It diffuses readily into abscesses and bone and is of low toxicity.

Lincomycin and its derivative *clindamycin* are mainly active against gram-positive organisms. They are normally given by mouth. Clindamycin is better absorbed, produces higher serum levels and has greater antibacterial activity. They are of value in the treatment of staphylococcal infections including septicaemia, osteomyelitis and sepsis following orthopaedic operations. Resistant strains may arise during treatment. The drugs are also effective in the treatment of infections caused by anaerobes, e.g. *Bacteroides*. Occasional patients develop severe pseudomembranous colitis and safer antibiotics should be used whenever possible.

Polymyxin B, *polymyxin E* (*colistin*) and their sulphomethyl derivatives are polypeptide antibiotics. Parenteral use of these drugs is liable to cause renal damage and neurological abnormalities, including respiratory paralysis in rare cases, and should be reserved for severe infections caused by *Ps. aeruginosa*. Intrathecal injection may be used in meningitis caused by *Ps. aeruginosa* and highly resistant coliforms.

Rifampicin is a derivative of the rifamycin family of antibiotics and is mainly active against gram-positive organisms. It is given by mouth and, in conjunction with other drugs, is used in the treatment of tuberculosis and leprosy. It is highly active against staphylococci and can be used in the treatment of endocarditis and other serious infections caused by *Staph. aureus* and *Staph. epidermidis*. It is effective in the treatment of legionnaires' disease and for prophylaxis of meningitis and other infections caused by *N. meningitidis* and *H. influenzae* type b. Rashes and transient disturbance of liver function are common. Severe hypersensitivity reactions and thrombocytopenic purpura occur occasionally. Rifampicin reduces the effectiveness of oral contraceptives.

Cycloserine is occasionally used in the treatment of tuberculosis. It is active against a wide range of other organisms, e.g. coliform organisms in the urinary tract, but is only rarely used. It can cause convulsions.

Spectinomycin is active against a wide range of organisms. A single large intramuscular injection is effective treatment for gonorrhoea.

Vancomycin is mainly active against gram-positive organisms. It is sometimes used in the treatment of endocarditis and other bacteraemic conditions caused by multi-resistant staphylococci (*Staph. aureus* and *Staph. epidermidis*) and in severe infections caused by gram-positive organisms in patients who are hypersensitive to penicillin. In these conditions it is given intravenously. High blood levels cause deafness. Thrombophlebitis is common. Oral vancomycin is effective in the treatment of antibiotic-associated pseudomembranous colitis.

Teicoplanin closely resembles vancomycin but is less toxic and has greater activity against most gram-positive organisms. It can be used in the treatment of endocarditis and other severe infections caused by enterococci and methicillin-resistant staphylococci. It is given by intramuscular injection.

Bacitracin and *gramicidin* are polypeptide antibiotics active against gram-positive organisms. They are too toxic for systemic use, but can be used for local treatment. For this purpose they are often combined with neomycin or polymyxin.

Mupirocin (pseudomonic acid) is mainly active against gram-positive organisms. It can be used for local treatment of skin infections.

Nitrofurantoin and *nalidixic acid* are used exclusively for urinary tract infections. They are given by mouth. Nitrofurantoin is active against a wide range of gram-positive and gram-negative organisms. Nalidixic acid is active only against gram-negative bacilli. *Cinoxacin* closely resembles nalidixic acid.

Norfloxacin, *enoxacin* and *ciprofloxacin* are members of the nalidixic acid family ('quinolones'). They are highly active against a wide range of organisms, including *Ps. aeruginosa*, and have been used in the treatment of many types of localized and systemic infections. They are given by mouth.

Hexamine mandelate liberates formaldehyde in an acid medium. It is given by mouth in enteric-coated tablets for long-term suppress-ive therapy in intractable urinary infections, e.g. *Ps. aeruginosa* infection in a patient with a permanent indwelling catheter.

Isoniazid and *ethambutol* are active only against mycobacteria. They are first-line drugs used in the treatment of tuberculosis, normally in conjunction with rifampicin. *Thiacetazone, pyrazinamide* and *p-aminosalicylic acid* are second-line drugs occasionally used in the treatment of tuberculosis, particularly against drug-resistant strains. *Dapsone*, a sulphone, and *clofazimine* are used in the treatment of leprosy.

Metronidazole is active against strict anaerobes and certain protozoa but not against aerobes, facultative anaerobes or micro-aerophiles. It is normally given by mouth and is effective in the treatment of infections caused by the *Bacteroides* group (including Vincent's organisms), anaerobic cocci and clostridia. It is of value in non-specific vaginitis, presumably because of its action on anaerobes. It has a special place in the prevention and treatment of anaerobic infections associated with major abdominal and pelvic surgery. It is also effective in trichomonal urethritis and vaginitis, amoebic dysentery and giardiasis. *Tinidazole* closely resembles metronidazole but has a longer plasma half-life.

Nystatin is active against *Candida albicans*. It is poorly absorbed from the gut and there are few cases of spontaneous or antibiotic-induced candidiasis in which oral treatment with nystatin is useful. It is most effective in intestinal candidiasis. Local treatment with nystatin is often valuable, e.g. in vaginal candidiasis.

Amphotericin B has been used for systemic treatment of severe generalized infections by yeasts and fungi, e.g. cryptococcosis and blastomycosis. It is toxic and may cause renal damage.

Griseofulvin is specific for dermatophyte infections and is given by mouth. It is concentrated in keratinized tissue and is valuable in the treatment of intractable ringworm. Treatment takes several months.

Miconazole and *ketoconazole* are active against a wide range of fungi and have been used to treat severe generalized fungal infec-tions. Ketoconazole can cause liver damage. *Hydroxystilbamidine* is a toxic drug used in the treatment of cutaneous blastomycosis. *Flucytosine* is used in cryptococcosis and generalized infections caused by *Candida* spp.

Chemoprophylaxis

Chemoprophylaxis is the prevention of infection by administra-tion of antimicrobial agents. The process inevitably entails risks, particularly the exposure of patients to the side effects of the antibiotics used and the selection and dissemination of resistant organisms. Indiscriminate 'routine' use of antibiotics is likely to do more harm than good. Prophylaxis should be restricted to individuals in whom the risk of infection is high and the drugs used should be active against the organisms likely to be responsible. It must be said that for most surgical procedures there is little clear-cut information about the effectiveness of different regimes. The following are the principal conditions for which prophylactic antibiotics are positively indicated.

Large bowel surgery. Infection by organisms of the normal flora, particularly *Bacteroides*, is very common. Metronidazole is effective. It is often combined with gentamicin or a cephalosporin such as cefuroxime.

Major orthopaedic and cardiac surgery. The effects of infection following total hip replacement, implantation of artificial cardiac valves, etc., can be disastrous. Flucloxacillin alone or flucloxacillin plus gentamicin or a cephalosporin alone are often used.

Amputations. There is serious risk of gas gangrene following amputation of an ischaemic leg. Penicillin is active against all clostridia and is the drug of choice. Erythromycin can be used in patients who are hypersensitive to penicillin.

Infective endocarditis. Dental procedures almost invariably introduce oral streptococci into the circulation. A single large dose of amoxycillin given immediately prior to dental treatment is recommended for patients with structural cardiac abnormalities. If the patient is already being treated with some form of penicillin the normally penicillin-sensitive streptococci will have been replaced by resistant strains and erythromycin can be given. To cover operations on the bowel or urinary tract amoxycillin can be supplemented with gentamicin.

Rheumatic carditis. Long-term prophylaxis with penicillin V is used to prevent *Str. pyogenes* infection in children who have had rheumatic fever. Monthly intramuscular injections of benzathine penicillin can be used instead of oral penicillin.

Meningococcal meningitis. It is important to prevent infection among close contacts, especially children. Rifampicin is commonly used but sulphonamides are effective if the strain of *N. meningitidis* is known to be sensitive.

Haemophilus meningitis. Rifampicin is also used for prophylaxis against meningitis caused by *H. influenzae,* type b.

Malaria. Chemoprophylaxis of malaria is extremely important. The drugs used (p. 386) must be active against the local strains of malaria parasite and treatment must be continued for 6 weeks after the last possible exposure.

Chemotherapy of viral infections

At present there is no specific treatment for the great majority of viral diseases, even in experimental animals. The intimate relationship between a multiplying virus and its host cell makes for major difficulties in devising effective antiviral therapy. Many substances can inhibit viral multiplication by specifically interfering with processes such as the synthesis of protein, deoxyribonucleic acid (DNA) or ribonucleic acid (RNA), but these inhibitors interfere with the same processes in tissue cells. At concentrations which will inhibit viruses, the drugs are toxic for normal cells and therefore unsuitable as chemotherapeutic agents. The fact that some viruses depend on newly synthesized enzymes not usually present in the cell may eventually lead to the discovery of drugs which inhibit these enzymes without harming the cell.

Another obstacle to effective therapy is that in many viral diseases viral multiplication may be coming to an end by the time the disease is first recognized. Future antiviral drugs may well be of more value in prevention than in treatment.

Antiviral chemotherapeutic agents

Acyclovir (acycloguanosine) is highly active against herpesviruses. It is of low toxicity and is of value systemic treatment of life-threatening localized or generalized infections with herpes simplex and varicella-zoster virus, particularly in patients having immuno-suppressive therapy. It is effective in herpes encephalitis if given before the onset of coma. Mutant viruses resistant to acyclovir may arise during treatment.

Vidarabine (adenine arabinoside) inhibits DNA viruses. It is a toxic drug but can be used for the systemic treatment of serious infections with herpes simplex virus, particularly encephalitis, and chickenpox and shingles in immunosuppressed patients.

Idoxuridine (iododeoxyuridine) also inhibits DNA viruses. It is too toxic for systemic use but can be used in the form of eye-drops for the treatment of herpetic keratitis, and for local treatment of herpes of the skin and mucous membranes.

Trifluorothymidine can be used to treat herpetic keratitis. It is active against strains of virus that are resistant to idoxuridine.

Methisazone and related thiosemicarbazones inhibit poxviruses. In the past methisazone was occasionally used for smallpox prophylaxis and for treating certain complications of vaccination.

Amantadine inhibits certain myxoviruses. Given by mouth it is moderately effective in preventing infection with type A influenza virus and it reduces symptoms if given within the first two days of illness.

Ribavirin is active against many DNA and RNA viruses. It has been used successfully in the form of an aerosol to treat infants with bronchiolitis or pneumonia caused by respiratory syncytial virus and other respiratory viruses. It reduces the mortality in Lassa fever.

Enviroxime is highly active against rhinoviruses and has been considered as a possible agent for use against common colds.

Zidovudine (azidothymidine or AZT) prolongs the life of AIDS patients suffering from *Pneumocystis carinii* pneumonia by inhibiting DNA synthesis by the reverse transcriptase of human immunodeficiency virus. Severe bone marrow depression with anaemia necessitating transfusion is a common complication.

Dideoxycytidine (DDC) is another nucleoside analogue which inhibits reverse transcriptase and which is undergoing trials in patients with AIDS.

Interferon is of low toxicity and as far as is known is active against all viruses affecting man. It will provide protection against experimental viral infection, but to exert a maximum effect must be administered several hours before the virus. Promising results have been observed in herpetic keratitis, chronic hepatitis B and infections such as shingles, chickenpox and cytomegalovirus in patients undergoing immunosuppressive therapy. Some cases of malignant disease have appeared to respond favourably, e.g. hairy cell leukaemia. Human interferons can be obtained from human leucocytes, from fibroblasts or lymphoblastoid cells grown in tissue culture and by recombinant-DNA techniques.

Gram-positive Cocci

Hospitals must be the Mecca of all truly virulent staphylococci.

S. D. Elek, 1959

Staphylococcus

This genus consists of catalase-positive gram-positive cocci arranged in grape-like clusters. Staphylococci can be classified into two groups on the basis of coagulase production, i.e. the production of a clot on incubating the organisms with plasma. The species *Staph. aureus* is coagulase-positive. All other staphylococci are coagulase-negative.

Staphylococcus aureus

Cultural characteristics

Colonies on solid media appear after 24 hours as large, 2—4 mm diameter, smooth, circular, shining domes which are characteristically opaque and golden. The intensity of pigmentation varies with different strains. A few strains have white colonies. A zone of haemolysis may be seen around colonies on blood agar.

Subdivisions

Phage-typing has proved of great value in epidemiological investigations. Staphylococcal phages are not specific for individual strains, but by exposing staphylococci to a battery of 20—30 different phages the pattern of susceptibility can be determined. Several hundred types have been recognized in this way, e.g. types 80 and 80/81 have caused many severe hospital outbreaks; types 47/53/75/77 and 52/52A/80 are common antibiotic-resistant strains; type 52A/79 has caused many outbreaks in maternity departments; type 71 is the most common cause of impetigo and exfoliative diseases. Epidemic methicillin-resistant (MRSA) strains are poorly typable with routine phages.

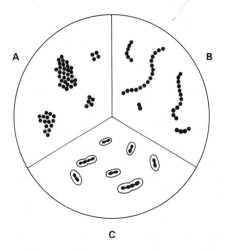

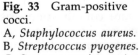

Fig. 33 Gram-positive cocci.
A, *Staphylococcus aureus.*
B, *Streptococcus pyogenes.*
C, *Str. pneumoniae*, stained to show capsules.

Toxins and enzymes

All strains produce coagulase and a heat-stable nuclease which like coagulase can be used as the basis for a specific test for *Staph. aureus.* Three distinct haemolysins are recognized, each causing lysis of a different range of animal red cells. Culture filtrates are lethal to animals on intravenous injection and cause necrosis on intradermal injection. Other products are a leucocidin which destroys white cells, hyaluronidase or spreading factor, and a weak fibrinolysin which dissolves fibrin. Certain strains which cause blister-like skin lesions (bullous impetigo and 'scalded skin syndrome') produce exfoliative (epidermolytic) toxins. Food poisoning strains produce an enterotoxin which causes diarrhoea and vomiting when ingested. Six antigenic types (A—F) of enterotoxin are recognized.

Infections

Staph. aureus is a human pathogen which lives as a commensal on the anterior nasal mucosa of 30—50% of the general population, with higher carrier rates among hospital staff and patients. It may also colonize the skin. It is the most common cause of acute pyogenic (pus-producing) infection in man. It has a marked predilection for the skin and surface structures and causes boils, carbuncles, pustules, septic fingers, styes, impetigo (often in association with *Streptococcus pyogenes*), pemphigus neonatorum and sticky eyes in babies. Acute osteomyelitis in children and young adults and breast abscess in lactating mothers are usually caused by *Staph. aureus.* It is the commonest cause of infection of wounds and burns. Staphylococcal infections tend to be more localized than streptococcal infections, but septicaemic states and formation of multiple abscesses are not rare. *Staph. aureus* septicaemia is a predominantly iatrogenic disease: over half the cases are associated with infections of vascular access sites or surgical wounds. *Staph. aureus* is an important cause of infective endocarditis, particularly in drug addicts and following cardiac surgery. Sometimes the organisms localize in a single focus, e.g. septic arthritis or a perinephric abscess. Staphylococcal pneumonia is a destructive type of bronchopneumonia particularly liable to occur as a complication of influenza. Staphylococcal enterocolitis is a rare complication arising from the use of broad-spectrum antibiotics. Staphylococcal food poisoning is not an infection, but is due to consumption of preformed enterotoxin in food. *Staph. aureus* is also responsible for a rare toxic shock syndrome (TSS) associated with high fever and a scarlatiniform rash with subsequent desquamation ('staphylococcal scarlet fever') occurring mainly in women using vaginal tampons but also found in a variety of staphylococcal infections. The organisms usually produce TSS toxin-1. Hospital infections caused by *Staph. aureus* are discussed in more detail elsewhere (p. 191).

Antibodies against *Staph. aureus* are present in the serum of all normal people. An antistaphylolysin (anti α-haemolysin) titre of more than 2 units/ml or an antinuclease titre of more than 4 units/ml, especially when the titres are rising, may be of value in the diagnosis of deep-seated infections, e.g. a bone abscess.

Coagulase-negative staphylococci

Staph. epidermidis (*Staph. albus*) is the name given to a heterogeneous group of coagulase-negative staphylococci which produce opaque white colonies on solid media. They are common commensals of the skin and are often isolated from clinical specimens. They are of low pathogenicity and can usually be regarded as secondary invaders of little importance. However, they sometimes cause urinary tract infections, particularly after instrumentation and when there are pre-existing abnormalities. They are an increasingly common cause of severe infections such as sepsis following total hip replacement, endocarditis following cardiac operations, sepsis associated with intravascular lines, colonization of the valves of ventriculo-venous shunts used in the treatment of hydrocephalus, peritonitis in patients undergoing continuous ambulatory peritoneal dialysis (CAPD) and bacteraemia in the newborn and in patients undergoing immunosuppressive therapy.

Staph. saprophyticus is an important cause of urinary tract infection in otherwise healthy young women.

Anaerobic cocci growing in clumps ('peptococci') are common inhabitants of the nose, throat and vagina. They may play a part in such infections as lung abscess and puerperal sepsis.

Other coagulase-negative cocci belonging to the genera *Staphylococcus*, *Micrococcus* and *Sarcina* are frequently encountered in water, dust and air. Many of them produce white or yellow colonies. They are usually harmless.

Micrococcus

This genus consists of gram-positive, coagulase-negative cocci growing in clusters. They can be distinguished from staphylococci by their G + C content and biochemical properties, e.g. micrococci oxidize sugars or do not attack them whereas staphylococci ferment sugars anaerobically. Micrococci are often isolated from clinical specimens. In general, they have the same medical significance as *Staph. epidermidis*.

Streptococcus

The genus *Streptococcus* consists of catalase-negative gram-positive cocci growing in chains. Chain formation is best seen in liquid cultures and in pus. On solid media the organisms may occur as short chains, pairs or single cocci. Unlike staphylococci, streptococci are often slightly oval and tend to be arranged end-to-end in pairs; the colonies are usually small, translucent and non-pigmented. The characteristics of most value in classification are:

1 *Changes produced on blood agar.* Three types of reaction are recognized:

   Alpha-haemolysis. The colony is surrounded by a narrow zone of partial (α) haemolysis and green ('viridans') discoloration of the medium, e.g. viridans streptococci and *Str. pneumoniae.*

   Beta-haemolysis. The colony is surrounded by a wide, clear zone of complete (β) haemolysis sharply demarcated from the unaltered cells in the surrounding medium, e.g. *Str. pyogenes* and other 'haemolytic streptococci'.

   No haemolysis. No change is produced in the medium, e.g. non-haemolytic streptococci, including most strains of *Str. faecalis.*

2 *Presence of specific carbohydrate haptens.* The carbohydrate or C substance of the organism is extracted in soluble form and identified by precipitation reactions with specific antisera. At least 17 of these *Lancefield groups* can be distinguished.

Group A includes the important human pathogen *Str. pyo-genes*. Group B (*Str. agalactiae*) is a common cause of bovine mastitis and is found in the vagina of 20—30% of pregnant women. It occasionally causes meningitis and other serious infections of human neonates. Group C causes disease in animals and is sometimes responsible for small outbreaks of sore throat and puerperal sepsis in humans. Group D includes the enterococci (*Str. faecalis*, etc.) and *Str. bovis* (another common bowel organism) and ranks next to group A as a cause of human infection. Group E is found in cow's milk and is not pathogenic for man. Groups F, G, H and K are commensals in the human throat: group F, which includes many strains of *Str. milleri*, is occasionally pathogenic, group G has caused small outbreaks of puerperal sepsis and sore throat, and groups H and K sometimes cause infective endocarditis. *Str. suis* are group D streptococci with additional 'group' antigens R, S or T. They cause disease in pigs and occasionally severe infections, including meningitis, in farmers, abattoir workers and butchers.

Lancefield grouping has been mainly applied to 'haemolytic streptococci', i.e. those showing β-haemolysis. Some α-haemolytic and non-haemolytic streptococci can be assigned to Lancefield groups, e.g. group D, *Str. bovis* and most strains of *Str. faecalis*.

3   *Oxygen requirements.* Most streptococci, including *Str. pyogenes*, *Str. faecalis*, *Str. pneumoniae* and viridans streptococci are facultative anaerobes. Many are anaerobes when first isolated. Some species of streptococci are strict anaerobes, e.g. *Str. putridus*.

4   *Other tests.* Fermentation reactions and biochemical tests are used in the identification of streptococci and in the finer differentiation of varieties, types and subtypes.

Streptococcus pyogenes

Str. pyogenes (Fig. 33B, p. 231) belongs to Lancefield group A.

Cultural properties

After 24 hours the colonies on blood agar are small, 1 mm diameter, dry, semi-transparent discs with a finely granular or matt surface. On further incubation the edges of the colony may curl up, producing a 'fallen leaf' appearance. Matt colonies are most frequently encountered, but some strains with a hyaluronic acid capsule produce large glistening mucoid colonies, and strains of low virulence which possess little or no M substance produce small glossy colonies.

The colonies are surrounded by a clear zone of β-haemoloysis. Some 5—10% of strains produce haemolysis only under anaerobic conditions. Very rarely, non-haemolytic group A streptococci are encountered: in other respects they are typical of *Str. pyogenes.*

Subdivisons

Many serological types each possessing a different protein antigen (M substance) can be recognized by agglutination and precipitation reactions. The M substances are associated with the antiphagocytic properties of *Str. pyogenes* and are essential for virulence.

Toxins and enzymes

Str. pyogenes produces a large number of biologically active substances including an erythrogenic toxin (pyrogenic exotoxin) which reproduces the rash of scarlet fever on injection, two haemolysins (streptolysin O and S), a leucocidin, probably identical with streptolysin O, which kills leucocytes and other tissue cells and has a toxic effect on the heart, fibrinolysin (streptokinase), deoxyribonuclease (streptodornase) and hyaluronidase. Not all these products are produced by every strain, e.g. the production of erythrogenic toxin depends on the possession of a particular prophage. It is tempting to think that fibrinolysin, deoxyribonuclease and hyaluronidase are responsible for the serous nature of streptococcal pus and the ability of streptococci to spread rapidly through the tissues, but in fact the role of these substances in pathogenicity is still obscure.

Infections

Some 5—10% of normal persons carry the organism in the throat. It is occasionally present in the nose. Streptococcal sore throat (acute tonsillitis) is the most common type of infection. Most sore throats are due to viral infections, but *Str. pyogenes* is by far the most important bacterial cause, being responsible for about 30% of all cases. Repeated attacks may occur because the different serological types do not provide cross-immunity.

Scarlet fever is streptococcal tonsillitis with the addition of an erythematous rash. Less commonly the rash accompanies streptococcal infection of other sites ('surgical scarlet fever'). The occurrence of the rash depends on infection with a strain which produces erythrogenic toxin and susceptibility of the individual to this toxin. The rash is probably the result of hypersensitivity to the toxin rather than a direct toxic effect. Individuals who possess antibodies against the toxin as a result of previous infection with a toxin-producing strain are immune to scarlet fever, but may develop sore throat with no rash if they are infected with a toxin-producing organism of a new serological type. There are three antigenic types of erythrogenic toxin. This may explain the occasional occurrence of second attacks of scarlet fever.

Str. pyogenes is responsible for severe infections of wounds and burns and is the most important cause of puerperal sepsis. Spread of infection through the tissues may produce cellulitis. Septicaemia is common. The organism is also responsible for erysipelas and (often in association with *Staph. aureus*) some cases of impetigo.

Delayed sequelae

Rheumatic fever and acute nephritis are characteristically preceded by streptococcal infection of the throat and have their onset after a latent period of 3 weeks. When there is no history of sore throat it is often possible to obtain serological evidence of streptococcal infection, e.g. nearly all cases of acute rheumatic fever have an antistreptolysin O titre above 200 units/ml. Rheumatic fever may follow infection with many serological types of *Str. pyogenes*, but acute nephritis is associated with a limited range of serological types of which type 12 is the most important. Streptococci are not present in the affected tissues and the diseases depend on immunological mechanisms. It is known for instance that antibodies produced in *Str. pyogenes* infections react with antigens of normal human heart muscle. In acute nephritis immune complexes containing a streptococcal polypeptide antigen (*endostreptosin*) are deposited in the glomerular basement membrane.

Enterococci

The enterococci belong to Lancefield group D. They include *Str. faecalis* and several less important species.

Cultural properties

Most strains are non-haemolytic, but α- and β-haemolytic varieties are common. Enterococci are more robust than other streptococci and will grow readily on media containing bile salts, e.g. MacConkey medium, or 6.5% sodium chloride. They will tolerate relatively high temperatures, e.g. 60°C for 30 minutes.

Infections

Enterococci are normal intestinal inhabitants. They are a common cause of acute infections of the urinary tract. Together with other organisms they are often responsible for wound infections, particularly following intestinal operations. They occasionally cause infective endocarditis.

Viridans streptococci

The name 'viridans streptococci' or 'Streptococcus viridans' is given to a group of α-haemolytic streptococci which vary greatly in their biochemical and antigenic properties. The group includes several species, such as Str. mitior (Str. mitis), Str. sanguis, Str. mutans and Str. milleri.

Cultural properties

The colonies on blood agar are usually small, 0.5–1.0 mm, transparent domes with a narrow surrounding greenish zone of α-haemolysis.

Occurrence

Viridans streptococci are invariable inhabitants of the normal human throat. They are also found in the tissues surrounding the teeth and may pass into the blood during extractions and other dental operations. Transient bacteraemia may occur during eating, particularly in patients with severe periodontal disease. In normal individuals the organisms are disposed of harmlessly but if there is a breach of the endothelial lining of the heart the organisms may set up infective endocarditis (subacute bacterial endocarditis). Endothelial damage may be due to congenital cardiac abnormalities, degenerative heart disease, cardiac surgery and previous rheumatic endocarditis. Infective endocarditis is a serious disease. Viridans streptococci (particularly Str. sanguis) are the commonest cause but in recent years other bacteria such as Str. faecalis, Str. bovis and Staph. aureus have been found with increasing frequency, especially in elderly patients. Patients with congenital cardiac defects, artifical heart valves or a history of rheumatic fever should be given an antibiotic (usually some form of penicillin) shortly before dental operations. Long preoperative courses of treatment must not be given as the normally sensitive viridans streptococci will be replaced by antibiotic-resistant streptococci.

Certain viridans and non-haemolytic streptococci are found in large numbers in dental plaque and play a major role in initiating dental caries and periodontal disease. Some species, e.g. Str. mutans, produce a gelatinous polysaccharide which causes the organisms to adhere to the surface of teeth. Streptococci, together with lactobacilli, ferment dietary carbohydrate and produce lactic acid which attacks the mineral component (hydroxyapatite) of enamel and dentine.

Str. milleri, unlike other viridans streptococci, is a common cause of abscess formation and bacteraemic states. It is a normal inhabitant of the mouth and bowel and is particularly associated with disease of the gastrointestinal tract. It is often isolated from deep-seated infections such as liver abscesses, appendix abscesses and purulent peritonitis.

Anaerobic streptococci

Strictly anaerobic, non-haemolytic streptococci ('peptostreptococci') are common commensals of the normal vagina. They are found in smaller numbers in the intestines and in the upper respiratory tract. *Str. putridus* can cause a severe form of puerperal sepsis. Anaerobic cocci of various kinds are often isolated from wounds and abscesses, usually in association with other organisms.

Streptococcus pneumoniae (Pneumococcus)

Pneumococci are a separate and well-defined group of streptococci. They are gram-positive lanceolate cocci arranged in pairs (diplococci) or short chains. They usually possess an obvious capsule (Fig. 33C, p. 231).

Cultural properties

They grow poorly on unenriched media but well on blood agar. Young colonies are smooth, glistening, transparent domes. Pneumococci readily undergo autolysis, and as the colonies increase in size the central part of each colony tends to sink. The final result is a colony with a thin raised outer rim and a flat depressed inner portion which may show a central papilla. These 'draughtsmen' colonies are very characteristic. The colonies are surrounded by a narrow green zone of α-haemolysis.

The smoothness of the colonies is due to the presence of capsular material. Strains with well-developed capsules (particularly type 3 pneumococci) produce large mucoid colonies. Naturally occurring non-capsulated strains and strains which have lost their capsules as a result of subculture have rough colonies and are non-virulent.

Subdivisions

Over 80 serological types are recognized on the basis of differences in their capsular polysaccharides. The organisms also possess M proteins which are often type-specific and a C or carbohydrate substance which is characteristic of the genus as a whole.

Infections

Pneumococci are present in the throat of a high proportion of normal people. Many of these strains are of low virulence.

Pneumococci are responsible for over 75% of all cases of bacterial pneumonia. Pneumococcal pneumonia is classically associated with lobar or segmental consolidation of the lung ('acute lobar pneumonia') but frequently there is patchy consolidation around terminal bronchi throughout the lungs (often described as bronchopneumonia). Occasionally the pneumococcus attacks apparently healthy individuals, but usually there are predisposing causes such as viral infections, particularly measles and influenza, bronchitis, debilitating illnesses and surgical operations. Strains of pneumococci isolated from 'primary' pneumonia mostly belong to a limited number of highly virulent serological types whereas strains from 'secondary' pneumonia often belong to types commonly encountered as commensals of the respiratory tract.

In pneumonia, infection may spread locally to involve the pleura and pericardium or the organisms may enter the blood and set up secondary foci of infection in the joints, meninges and endocardium. Pneumococci are an important cause of primary meningitis. They frequently infect the middle ear and the nasal sinuses and, together with *Haemophilus influenzae*, are sometimes responsible for acute exacerbations of chronic bronchitis. Primary pneumococcal peritonitis sometimes occurs, particularly in girls. Generalized pneumococcal infections are not uncommon following splenectomy and in patients with sickle-cell anaemia.

Countercurrent immunoelectrophoresis can be used for rapid diagnosis of pneumococcal infections. In pneumococcal pneumonia capsular antigens can be detected in the sputum. Their presence in the blood and urine usually indicates a poor prognosis.

Gram-negative Cocci

I protest I know nothing of the matter.
                    Louisa to Boswell, 1763

Neisseria

This genus consists of gram-negative aerobic cocci growing in pairs (diplococci) and small clumps. It includes the human pathogens *N. gonorrhoeae* and *N. meningitidis*, and various commensal species.

Neisseria gonorrhoeae (Gonococcus)

Morphology

The characteristic diplococcal form is best seen in pus. The cocci are oval or bean-shaped and are arranged in pairs with their long axes parallel (not in line as in the case of *Streptococcus pneumoniae*) and their contiguous sides flattened or concave.

Cultural properties

The organism is very delicate and an enriched medium is required for isolation. Heated blood ('chocolate') agar is satisfactory.

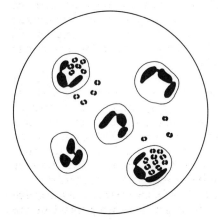

Fig. 34 *Neisseria gonorrhoeae* in pus.

Selective media containing colistin, vancomycin and nystatin are valuable in extricating gonococci from a mixture of other organisms. Gonococci are susceptible to cold and drying, and plates (preferably warm) should be inoculated immediately the specimen has been obtained. When this is impracticable swabs may be sent to the laboratory in transport medium. Incubation in 5–10% CO_2 greatly increases the chances of successful isolation. The colonies are slow to develop and cultures should not be discarded for 2 or 3 days. After 24–48 hours the colonies are usually translucent, colourless domes about 1 mm in diameter. Four types of colonies are recognized. Organisms of types 1 and 2 are virulent and possess pili which attach the organisms to the surface of epithelial cells.

A few colonies of gonococci can be detected in the presence of a heavy growth of other organisms by means of the oxidase reaction. The plate is flooded with a 1% solution of tetramethyl-*p*-phenylenediamine. Colonies of neisseriae rapidly turn purple, while those of most other organisms do not alter. The reagent kills the organisms in a few minutes. Before this occurs oxidase-positive colonies should be subcultured on to fresh media for further investigation.

N. gonorrhoeae is distinguished from other neisseriae by the fact that glucose is the only carbohydrate it ferments. Colonies of the organism can also be identified by fluorescent antibody staining.

Infections

N. gonorrhoeae is the cause of the sexually transmitted disease gonorrhoea. Man is the only host. The organism cannot survive for long outside the body and statements from patients that they have been infected from lavatory seats should be taken with reserve. It does not adopt a commensal existence although gonorrhoea may exist in a quiescent form for long perids. Asymptomatic females are a dangerous reservoir of infection. Asymptomatic males are comparatively rare. An attack of the disease provides little or no immunity to reinfection.

Gonorrhoea usually takes the form of an acute urethritis. In women the cervix is often infected in addition to the urethra. From the initial site of infection the organisms may spread to infect Bartholin's glands, uterus, fallopian tubes, ovaries and peritoneum, and in men, the prostate, seminal vesicles, epididymis and testes. Infection of the pharynx and rectum is not uncommon. Invasion of the blood may occasionally produce infection of joints and tendon sheaths: rarely there may be endocarditis.

Non-venereal infection is rare. Newborn infants may acquire gonococcal conjunctivitis when the organisms are present in the maternal birth canal at the time of delivery. Gonococcal conjunctivitis in adults is usually caused by transference of gonococcal pus to the eyes by the fingers.

Diagnosis

This mainly depends on finding gram-negative intracellular diplococci in films of pus. Not all the polymorphs are equally active at phagocytosis: in a typical film there are hundreds of polymorphs which do not contain any organisms and an occasional polymorph which has engulfed large numbers of them.

In acute gonorrhoea in males the films are usually so characteristic that the diagnosis is seldom in doubt. In females the films are very valuable in early cases, but their value decreases as infection continues. Gram-negative cocci, and fat gram-negative bacilli which sometimes look remarkably like diplococci, are often present in normal women; the organisms should be ignored if they are extracellular. In all cases an attempt should be made to culture the organisms. In chronic infections in women, cultures often give positive results when smears are negative.

A gonococcal complement fixation test (GCFT) using several strains of gonococci as a source of antigen is sometimes of value in the diagnosis of the late complications of gonorrhoea such as arthritis.

Neisseria meningitidis (Meningococcus)

The organisms closely resemble *N. gonorrhoeae* in their main morphological and cultural properties. Enriched media and an atmosphere containing $5-10\%$ CO_2 are usually required for isolation. They are less exacting than gonococci and growth tends to be more profuse and the colonies are usually larger. They can be distinguished from gonococci by their ability to ferment both maltose and glucose, but strains with atypical reactions are not uncommon. Virulent strains of meningococci possess a thin capsule which, although not visible under ordinary circumstances, can be detected by the capsule swelling reaction using specific antisera.

Subdivisions

Three main serological groups (A, B and C) are recognized on the basis of agglutination reactions. Group B is at present responsible for about 65% of cases of meningococcal infection in the UK and is the predominant organism isolated from healthy carriers. The three serogroups can be further subdivided into a number of serotypes.

Infections

Meningococci are found in the throat of about 5% of normal people, but at times the carrier rate may rise as high as 50—90%. The carrier rate of pathogenic strains associated with outbreaks, i.e. strains fully identified by serogroup and serotype, is usually only 1—2%. Infection occurs in three stages:

1 Growth of the organisms in the nasopharynx. This may produce mild local inflammation, but in most cases there are no symptoms. Most infections do not proceed beyond this stage.
2 Invasion of the blood. Development of petechial and purpuric rashes ('spotted fever') is characteristic. In many cases the disease does not proceed beyond this simple bacteraemic stage. Metastatic foci of infection occasionally arise in other sites such as joints or the endocardium. Chronic meningococcal septicaemia without meningitis may last for many weeks, but in the rarely encountered acute fulminating form the patient dies in a few hours of circulatory collapse due to adrenal cortical failure caused by haemorrhage into the adrenals (Waterhouse-Friderichsen syndrome).
3 Invasion of the meninges. Acute meningococcal meningitis (cerebrospinal fever) is produced. Epidemics are mainly associated with overcrowding, e.g. troops in barracks. Sporadic cases are most common in young children.

Diagnosis

In early cases gram-negative intracellular diplococci are found in the cerebrospinal fluid (CSF). In later stages the organisms are often very scanty. When no organisms can be seen the presence of meningococcal antigens in the CSF can sometimes be detected by serological methods. The diagnosis is confirmed by culturing the CSF and identifying the organisms by fermentation reactions and agglutination tests with specific antisera. In the septicaemic stage the organisms can often be cultured from the blood and skin lesions.

Other species of Neisseria

Non-pathogenic neisseriae are normal inhabitants of the mucous membranes of the upper respiratory tract and are often found on other body surfaces including the vagina.

N. flavescens is a serologically distinct species which has occasionally been responsible for outbreaks of meningitis.

Branhamella

B. catarrhalis differs from neisseriae in its G + C content and other biochemical properties. It is a very common commensal of the mouth and throat and is frequently isolated in large numbers in specimens from the respiratory tract. It probably plays a part in lower respiratory tract infections, particularly in patients with chronic chest disease.

Veillonella

This genus consists of small *anaerobic*, gram-negative cocci growing in masses. They are usually present in large numbers in the mouth and upper respiratory tract and are frequently found in the intestinal tract and vagina. They are sometimes isolated from suppurative lesions, usually in association with other organisms, but are of doubtful pathogenicity.

Gram-positive Bacilli

> ...*the bacilli which are present in the tuberculous substances not only accompany the tuberculous process, but are the cause of it.*
>
> Robert Koch, 1882

Bacillus

The genus *Bacillus* consists of gram-positive, aerobic, spore-bearing rods. The spores of most species, unlike those of the genus *Clostridium*, are the same width as the bacteria or slightly narrower and do not produce a bulge in the contour of the cell.

There is only one species pathogenic for man, *B. anthracis*, the cause of anthrax. Several species are insect pathogens. The remainder are common saprophytes of the soil and air, e.g. *B. subtilis*.

Bacillus anthracis

Morphology

B. anthracis is a large, square-ended, non-motile bacillus. In the tissues it occurs singly or in pairs, but in culture the bacilli adhere end-to-end to produce long chains. Capsules are formed in the tissues but are not usually seen in cultures unless the organism is grown in the presence of a high concentration of carbon dioxide. Spores are not found in the tissues but are produced readily in cultures.

Cultural properties

It grows readily on ordinary media, producing characteristic 'medusa head' colonies which are flat, greyish-white, felted structures with a wavy edge due to irregular outgrowths of long parallel chains of bacilli arranged like locks of hair.

Antigenic properties

Three main antigenic components are recognized: a capsular antigen consisting of a polypetide composed of 40 or more

A

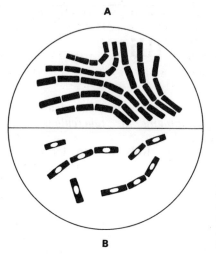

B

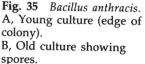

Fig. 35   *Bacillus anthracis.*
A, Young culture (edge of colony).
B, Old culture showing spores.

molecules of D-glutamic acid; a polysaccharide somatic antigen; and a protein somatic antigen which stimulates immunity and which is one of the components of a toxin produced when the organism is growing in the tissues. There is considerable antigenic overlap between *B. anthracis* and saprophytic species.

Anthrax

Anthrax is a septicaemic infection of animals, particularly sheep and cattle. Infected animals excrete large numbers of the organisms in their faeces, urine and saliva. The vegetative cells sporulate and the spores may persist in the soil for many years, infecting successive generations of animals. Anthrax spores liberated on Gruinard Island off the coast of Scotland during germ-warfare experiments in 1942 were still present in 1986 when attempts were made to decontaminate the island with formaldehyde. Anthrax is not common in the UK and many of the outbreaks which do occur are due to spores in imported winter feeding stuffs.

Anthrax in man is mainly found among farmers, veterinary workers, slaughterhouse men, dockers, and those whose work brings them into contact with bones, hides, skins, wool, hair and bristles.

Cutaneous anthrax (malignant pustule) is the most common form of the disease. It is due to implantation of spores in cuts and scratches, usually on the face, neck, hands or arms. It takes the form of an acute inflammatory lesion progressing to central necrosis and production of a ring of secondary vesicles. Generalized infection occurs in about 10% of cases.

Pulmonary anthrax (woolsorter's disease) is a severe form of bronchopneumonia which usually progresses to septicaemia and death. Infection is acquired by inhalation of infected dust.

Diagnosis

The presence of large gram-positive bacilli in films from a suspected malignant pustule is virtually diagnostic, but in all cases the diagnosis should be confirmed by culture. Non-pathogenic, aerobic, spore-bearing bacilli are often isolated from wounds, ulcers and other sites, but in most cases can readily be distinguished from *B. anthracis* by their morphological and cultural characteristics. *B. anthracis* can be positively identified by means of a specific phage.

Treatment

B. anthracis is almost invariably sensitive to penicillin. Recovery is usual if massive doses are given early in the disease.

Prevention

Pasteur (1881) showed that *B. anthracis* attenuated by growth at 42°C could be used for the immunization of animals. A naturally avirulent strain is now preferred. Infected animals must be promptly isolated, killed and disposed of by deep burial or cremation. Post-mortem examinations should never be performed. Rigid control of the methods used to clean and disinfect imported hides, hair and wool has greatly diminished the incidence of human anthrax in the UK.

Non-pathogenic species of Bacillus

B. subtilis is the most commonly encountered member of a large group of aerobic spore-bearing bacilli found in soil, water, dust and air. The organisms are important because their heat-resistant spores may contaminate culture media, injection fluids, etc., or cause spoilage in the food industry. Rarely they may cause food poisoning.

B. cereus is a not uncommon cause of food poisoning, e.g in Chinese restaurants when boiled rice has been kept at room temperature. Heat-stable exotoxins are responsible. On a few occasions highly toxigenic strains of *B. cereus* have caused septic conditions in man.

Clostridium

The genus *Clostridium* consists of gram-positive, *anaerobic*, spore-bearing rods. The spores, unlike those of most species of *Bacillus*, are wider than the bacteria and produce a distinct bulge.

Clostridia are mainly free-living inhabitants of the soil and play an important part in the decomposition of animal and vegetable matter. Many species are normal commensals of the intestinal tract of man and animals. Features used for differentiation include the colonial appearance, the shape and position of the spores, motility and a battery of biochemical tests. The pathogenic clostridia produce powerful exotoxins which are lethal to guinea-pigs and mice. Final identification is made by inoculating two animals one of which has been protected by specific antitoxin.

Clostridium botulinum

Cl. botulinum is a motile bacillus which produces oval, sub-terminal or central spores. It is distinguished from other clostridia by cultural and biochemical properties, but chiefly by its potent neurotoxin.

Seven main types (A–G) of *Cl. botulinum* are recognized. Each produces an antigenically distinct toxin. The toxins are proteins and, unlike most bacterial toxins, are toxic when taken by mouth. The toxins produced by the seven types have the same paralytic effect in animals. They cause no direct injurious effects and act by inhibiting the output of acetylcholine by parasympathetic and motor nerve endings. Their action is slow and death may not occur until several days after receiving a fatal dose.

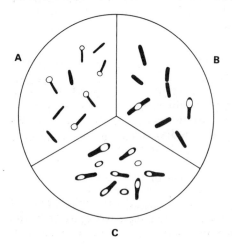

Fig. 36   Clostridia.
A, *Clostridium tetani*, sporing ('drumstick') and non-sporing forms.
B, *Cl. perfringens* (*Cl. welchi*), sporing forms rarely seen.
C, *Cl. sporogenes*.

Botulism

Botulism is a form of poisoning classically caused by the consumption of food containing preformed toxin of *Cl. botulinum*, but in infants (and very rarely in adults) the disease can arise from intra-intestinal toxin production. Botulism due to growth of *Cl. botulinum* in wounds has been described. The organism itself does not invade the body.

Cl. botulinum is a common inhabitant of the soil and often contaminates foods. If the food provides anaerobic conditions the organism can grow and produce its toxin. This is only likely to happen with preserved foods. Fresh foods (cooked or uncooked) are not a source of danger. In the past the foods mainly incriminated were canned meats, meat products, ham and sausages (Lat. *botuli*). The risk from these sources is now very much less, since in modern commercial canning the food is heated sufficiently to kill the spores. At present the greatest source of danger is home-canned and home-bottled vegetables such as peas, beans and corn. Home-preserved fruits are safe because their acidity inhibits growth of the organisms. A few cases of botulism (type E) have been traced to preserved fish. The foods usually show signs of spoilage but may appear normal.

Classical botulism is rare. In the UK less than a dozen episodes have been reported. The most serious was at Loch Maree in 1922 when eight people died after eating potted duck paste. In 1978 four elderly people in Birmingham acquired botulism from a can of salmon. The organisms were thought to have entered the can through a pinhole defect during the cooling process following sterilization. Infantile botulism is more common. Man is mainly affected by type A, occasionally by type B and rarely by the other types.

Symptoms

Botulism is a neurological disease and gastrointestinal symptoms are slight or absent. The effects include ocular and pharyngeal paralyses, dilatation of the pupils and loss of accommodation. General muscular weakness develops later. Classical botulism has a mortality of over 50%. Infantile botulism is less likely to be fatal but is a possible cause of sudden infant death syndrome ('cot death').

Diagnosis

Botulism is diagnosed on clinical grounds. Confirmation is obtained by demonstrating toxin in the suspected food or in the contents of the gut. It may also be possible to culture the organism.

Treatment

Polyvalent antitoxin is of little value once symptoms have developed. It may have prophylactic value for those who have consumed the affected food but who have not yet developed symptoms.

Clostridium tetani

Morphology

Cl. tetani produces round terminal spores which give the organism a characteristic 'drumstick' appearance (Fig. 36A, p. 248). Unfortunately this appearance is shared with certain non-pathogenic species, e.g. *Cl. tetanomorphum*.

Cultural properties

Under anaerobic conditions *Cl. tetani* spreads rapidly over the surface of moist solid media, producing a thin film of growth with an irregular rhizoid edge. If cultures or material from a wound are heated to kill non-sporing organisms and inoculated in the moisture at the bottom of a blood-agar slope which is then incubated anaerobically, *Cl. tetani* can often be recovered in pure culture from the film of growth which spreads up the slope. A few strains are non-motile and do not swarm. *Cl. tetani*, unlike *Cl. tetanomorphum*, does not ferment carbohydrates.

Toxins

Cl. tetani produces a powerful protein neurotoxin known as tetanospasmin. Ten types of *Cl. tetani* are recognized on the basis of their flagellar antigens, but they all produce the same toxin.

Occurrence

Cl. tetani is present in the intestinal tract of herbivores, particularly horses, and is widely distributed in the soil, especially when the land has been manured and cultivated. It may also be present in the dust of streets, houses and hospitals. It has occasionally been found in human faeces.

Tetanus

Tetanus occurs when a wound is contaminated with tetanus spores and the conditions are suitable for them to germinate. Spores alone are incapable of causing tetanus, but if they are injected with an agent which causes tissue necrosis (e.g. sterile soil, calcium salts, *Cl. perfringens* toxin, living *Staphylococcus aureus*), the oxidation-reduction potential of the tissues is reduced, the spores germinate, the organisms multiply, toxin is produced and tetanus results.

Tetanus toxin travels by way of the motor nerves from its site of production in a wound to the nerve cells of the brain and spinal cord. By interfering with synaptic transmission it increases the excitability of motor nerve cells and produces convulsive tonic contractions of voluntary muscles. The spasms may at first be confined to muscles in the proximity of the wound but later become generalized. Spasm of the masseter muscles (trismus or 'lock-jaw') develops early in the disease.

Tetanus is particularly associated with wounds contaminated with soil and foreign bodies, deep puncture wounds and wounds involving extensive tissue destruction. Since patients with severe injuries usually receive antitoxin or other appropriate treatment, trivial injuries caused by splinters, rusty nails and thorn-pricks account for the majority of cases. Tetanus is to a large extent a disease of agricultural communities.

Uterine infection may occur as a result of septic abortion. Tetanus neonatorum due to umbilical infection is extremely rare in the UK but is common in parts of Africa. Tetanus as a complication of surgical operations is rare but very occasionally it follows gall bladder surgery. In other cases it is due to improperly sterilized ligatures, dressings, glove powders, plaster bandages, etc., coming in close contact with the wound; less commonly infection is dust-borne.

Diagnosis

Bacteriological confirmation of the clinical diagnosis is usually impossible because so few *Cl. tetani* are present in the wound. A search is made for 'drumstick' bacilli in films and an attempt is made to isolate the organism by culture and by injection of material from the wound into mice or guinea-pigs.

Treatment

Large doses of tetanus antitoxin are given, but by the time symptoms appear the toxin is largely 'fixed' to the nervous tissues. Intrathecal antitetanus immunoglobulin is of value if given before the onset of spasms. Other important measures include surgical toilet of the wound, sedation, use of muscle relaxants and artificial respiration, and administration of antibiotics to prevent inter-current infection. Tetanus carries a mortality rate of about 50%, but with skilled attention this can be reduced to less than 10%.

Prevention

Tetanus is virtually unknown in individuals who have been properly immunized. All children should be actively immunized with adsorbed tetanus toxoid. One or two booster doses should be given in later years.

Tetanus antitoxin given as soon as possible after a wound has been infected will provide immediate protection for individuals who have not been actively immunized. The safest and most effective antitoxin is human antitetanus immunoglobulin.

If the patient has been immunized there is no need for antitoxin. A single booster dose of adsorbed tetanus toxoid is sufficient.

In the non-immune patient, if thorough wound toilet can be carried out without delay, say within 3 hours, it is justifiable to rely on wound toilet, an antibiotic and an injection of adsorbed tetanus toxoid. The antibiotic of choice is an injection of combined long-acting and short-acting penicillins. A course of tetracycline can be given to patients hypersensitive to penicillin. Treatment must be continued until the wound has healed. The course of active immunization with toxoid should be completed at a later date.

If there is delay in treatment, particularly when this is many hours, or if surgical toilet cannot be completed and there is a possibility of foreign bodies being left in the wound, the patient should be given adsorbed tetanus toxoid in one arm and human antitetanus immunoglobulin in the other. Active immunization with toxoid should be completed later. This regimen is most applicable to countries where the incidence of tetanus is high.

Clostridium perfringens (Cl. welchi)

Morphology

Cl. perfringens is a gram-positive, non-motile bacillus. Capsules are formed in the tissues but are not usually seen in culture. Spores are never found in the tissues and are only rarely seen in culture. When they do occur they are large, oval and either central or subterminal (Fig. 36B, p. 248).

Cultural properties

On blood agar under anaerobic conditions it produces round, smooth, translucent domes surrounded by a zone of complete haemolysis and often an outer zone of partial haemolysis ('target haemolysis'). It produces acid and gas in a characteristic range of sugars, a 'stormy clot' in litmus milk and gives a positive Nagler reaction.

Nagler reaction

The α-toxin of *Cl. perfringens* is a lecithinase and is normally identified by an *in vitro* test. When the organism is grown on plates containing human serum or egg yolk (Nagler medium), dense opalescent zones of lipid material are deposited around the colonies. The reaction is inhibited by *Cl. perfringens* antitoxin (Fig. 37).

Subdivisions

The species is divided into 5 types, A—E, on the basis of toxin production. Type A is responsible for human gas gangrene. Certain strains of type A, some of which possess spores with an unusually high degree of heat resistance, are responsible for a common form of food poisoning (p. 198). Type C occasionally causes a severe form of necrotizing enteritis in man. The disease, pigbel, is caused by β-toxin and is common in children in Papua New Guinea. Types B, C, D and E cause intestinal diseases in animals.

Toxins

Cl. perfringens produces eight lethal toxins as well as a number of extracellular enzymes. Not all these substances are produced by every strain and classification largely depends on different patterns of toxin-production. The most important substance produced by type A strains is the α-toxin. It is the principal lethal toxin and it has marked necrotizing and haemolytic activity. The same α-toxin is produced by other types of *Cl. perfringens* but usually in lesser amounts. Other substances produced by type A strains

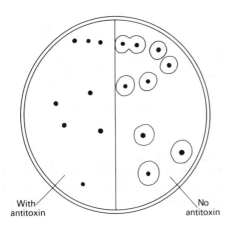

With antitoxin   No antitoxin   **Fig. 37** Nagler reaction.

are an oxygen-labile haemolysin, collagenase, hyaluronidase and deoxyribonuclease.

Other gas gangrene organisms

Cl. novyi (*Cl. oedematiens*) can be differentiated into four types, A—D. Type A is responsible for nearly all human infections. It produces an α-toxin, which is lethal and necrotizing and causes gelatinous oedema at the site of inoculation, a lecithinase which is necrotizing and haemolytic, a haemolysin and a lipase. Types B, C and D cause diseases in animals. Type D is one of the strictest of all anaerobes.

Cl. septicum produces an α-toxin which is lethal, necrotizing and haemolytic, a deoxyribonuclease and a haemolysin.

Cl. histolyticum produces a lethal and necrotizing toxin, a collagenase, a proteinase and an elastase. It is so strongly proteolytic that it can digest living tissues. It grows feebly under aerobic conditions.

Cl. sporogenes (Fig. 36C, p. 248) is one of the most commonly encountered species. It is strongly proteolytic but by itself is of low pathogenicity.

Cl. bifermentans produces a lecithinase antigenically related to the α-toxin of *Cl. perfringens*. Some strains which are often assigned to the species *Cl. sordelli* produce a lethal toxin and are pathogenic.

Cl. fallax resembles *Cl. perfringens* in some respects and is sometimes 'fallaciously' mistaken for it. It produces a toxin and freshly isolated strains are pathogenic.

Cl. bovifaecalis (BS bacillus) is utterly fallacious.

Gas gangrene

Gas gangrene is only likely to occur when there has been extensive damage to the tissues, interruption of the blood supply and contamination of the wound with soil and other foreign matter. Such conditions are particularly associated with war wounds, severe compound fractures (road accidents) and industrial injuries. Uterine infections not infrequently follow septic abortion but are rare after normal childbirth. In the pre-Listerian era gas gangrene was a common complication of surgery.

Three types of wound infection are distinguished:

1 *Simple contamination of wounds.* Small numbers of clostridia can be isolated from 30—40% of septic wounds. This is not surprising since they are very common organisms, e.g. *Cl. perfringens* is invariably present in normal human faeces. In

the vast majority of cases the presence of these organisms in wounds has no significance.

2 *Clostridial cellulitis.* This is an acute, spreading infection of the connective tissue with gas production but little toxaemia. The condition tends to be self-limiting.

3 *Clostridial myositis or true gas gangrene.* The organisms colonize injured muscles and may invade and destroy neighbouring healthy muscles. Toxaemia is severe and there may be haemolytic anaemia and jaundice. Invasion of the blood is common and soon results in death. Gas-containing abscesses may be found after death in the liver and other tissues.

Cl. perfringens is the most important cause of gas gangrene and in most surveys has been isolated in 60—85% of cases. Next in importance are *Cl. novyi* (30—40%) and *Cl. septicum* (10—20%). Other less pathogenic species are frequently isolated but seldom cause gas gangrene by themselves. More than one species is present in about half the cases of gas gangrene. Organisms of other genera, aerobes as well as anaerobes, are frequently present as well.

Diagnosis

Gas gangrene is diagnosed on clinical grounds. Large numbers of gram-positive bacilli are usually seen in direct films, and cultures yield a heavy growth of clostridia. In films from the uterus the presence of capsulated bacilli, damaged leucocytes and the absence of phagocytosis invariably indicate *Cl. perfringens* infection. The presence of non-capsulated bacilli and healthy leucocytes is of no significance.

Treatment

Surgical removal of necrotic tissue and massive doses of penicillin are the basis of treatment. Large intravenous doses of polyvalent horse antitoxin against the three main organisms are of doubtful value and carry the risk of anaphylactic shock. Exposure of the patient to pure oxygen in a pressure chamber has proved very effective.

Other diseases caused by clostridia

Pseudomembranous colitis. Cl. difficile produces a toxin which causes necrosis of the intestinal epithelium and is the cause of most cases of antibiotic-associated pseudomembranous colitis. In its severe form this is a life-threatening illness. The disease has been seen most frequently in patients who have been treated with lincomycin or clindamycin but most antibiotics, including ampicillin, have at times been incriminated. Diagnosis is best made by biopsy. Large amounts of *Cl. difficile* toxin can be demonstrated in the faeces by production of cytotoxic effects on cells in tissue culture and neutralization of these effects by specific antiserum. *Cl. difficile* itself can be isolated by anaerobic culture. *Cl. difficile* toxin is also responsible for many less serious cases of antibiotic-associated diarrhoea without pseudomembrane formation and occasionally contributes to exacerbations, unrelated to antibiotic therapy, in ulcerative colitis and other chronic inflammatory bowel diseases. Pseudomembranous colitis should be treated on clinical suspicion without waiting for laboratory confirmation. Oral vancomycin or metronidazole is usually effective.

Neutropenic enterocolitis. Cl. septicum occasionally causes a fulminating and necrotizing infection of the caecum and adjacent ileum and colon in patients with neutropenia, e.g. following cytotoxic drug therapy for leukaemia.

Neonatal necrotizing enterocolitis. This disease is an important cause of death among premature babies in special-care units. The aetiology is obscure but cases sometimes occur in clusters suggesting that the condition may be caused by an infective agent. Many types of bacteria have been isolated including various species of clostridia. The pathological changes resemble those found in necrotizing enteritis caused by *Cl. perfringens*.

Corynebacterium

This genus consists of gram-positive, non-sporing, non-capsulated, typically non-motile aerobic rods. It includes *C. diphtheriae*, the cause of diphtheria, a number of commensal 'diphtheroid bacilli' and various species which produce disease in animals.

Corynebacterium diphtheriae

Morphology

Certain features taken together give the organism a distinctive appearance:

1 Fission is at first incomplete so that two or more cells remain attached at an angle to give V and Z forms.
2 The cells are often irregular, swollen and club-shaped.
3 Staining is uneven, giving the organism a cross-banded appearance.

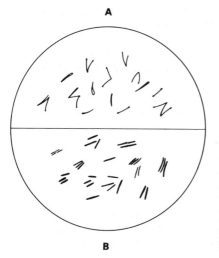

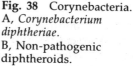

Fig. 38 Corynebacteria.
A, *Corynebacterium diphtheriae.*
B, Non-pathogenic diphtheroids.

4 Metachromatic granules, i.e. granules which stain a different colour from the rest of the cell, are present, particularly at the poles. They can be seen in gram films but are best demonstrated by special stains, e.g. Neisser's or Albert's methods.

The appearance of stained films is said to resemble 'Chinese writing'. Typical morphology is best seen when the organisms are grown on Loeffler serum medium. The appearance is not characteristic on tellurite medium.

Cultural properties

Growth occurs on ordinary media but is better in the presence of blood or serum. From the appearance of the colonies on blood-tellurite agar experts can differentiate three epidemiological types, *gravis, intermedius* and *mitis,* which correspond to the severity of the disease they most frequently produce. The three types differ in other properties. Biochemical reactions are valuable in distinguishing *C. diphtheriae* from diphtheroids which closely resemble it.

Toxin

C. diphtheriae produces a powerful exotoxin which interferes with protein synthesis. This toxin is only formed when the concentration of iron in the medium is very low and may be the protein part of a bacterial cytochrome. It has been suggested that in the absence of iron the organism cannot complete the synthesis of cytochrome, with the result that the protein part of the molecule is excreted into the medium.

Gravis, intermedius and *mitis* strains produce the same toxin. Some strains are non-toxigenic. In recent years *C. diphtheriae* has rarely been isolated in the UK and many of the organisms have been non-toxigenic strains. The capacity to produce toxin depends on infection of the organisms with a temperate phage.

Demonstration that the organism produces the specific toxin is the most certain way of identifying *C. diphtheriae*. This can be done by gel-diffusion precipitin tests or by virulence tests in guinea-pigs.

Diphtheria

There is no animal reservoir of infection and man acquires the disease from a patient with diphtheria or from a healthy person who carries the organism in the nose or throat. The disease begins as an acute inflammatory and ulcerative condition of the mucous membrane of the upper respiratory tract. The process usually starts in the region of the tonsils, but may start in the nose, posterior pharynx or larynx. A tough, whitish 'false membrane' of necrosed tissue, fibrin, polymorphs and bacteria forms over the affected area.

Diphtheria occasionally originates in the ear, conjunctiva or vagina. Skin diphtheria is almost unknown in temperate climates, but in the tropics it is a well-recognized complication of cuts, abrasions and insect bites.

When diphtheritic membrane involves the larynx and trachea the local lesion may cause respiratory obstruction and death. In the great majority of cases the local lesion is of little significance except as a site of toxin-production. The bacilli themselves never invade the blood and the serious and lethal complications of diphtheria can be attributed to the effects of circulating toxin on heart muscles, nerves, kidneys and adrenals.

One attack usually provides lifelong immunity. Immunity may also result from subclinical infection, but in many countries widespread immunization in infancy has greatly reduced the prevalence of diphtheria bacilli and therefore lessened the chances of acquiring immunity in this way. One of the results has been to increase the susceptibility of the adult population. The presence of circulating antitoxin upon which immunity depends can be detected by cell culture methods, indirect haemagglutination and by the Schick test.

Diagnosis

Although diphtheria is now rare. *C. diphtheriae* should always be considered in the routine investigation of sore throats.

Treatment

Antitoxin must be given at the earliest possible moment, i.e. it should be given on clinical suspicion without waiting for bacteriological confirmation. The dose required is large, e.g. 10 000 units for a mild case; up to 100 000 units for severe cases or cases seen at a late stage. Penicillin may be used as an adjunct to antitoxin treatment but never as a substitute.

Prevention

Active immunization with diphtheria toxoid is the most important measure.

Other corynebacteria

C. ulcerans sometimes causes a diphtheria-like illness in man. It produces two toxins, one of which is identical with diphtheria toxin. The organism can be distinguished from *C. diphtheriae* by biochemical tests.

So-called '*C. haemolyticum*' (*Arcanobacterium haemolyticum*) is an occasional cause of sore throat and a maculopapular rash, particularly in young adults. After 48 hours the colonies show an opaque central dot and are surrounded by a zone of β-haemolysis.

'Non-pathogenic' corynebacteria (diphtheroid bacilli) are common commensals of the throat, nose, ear, conjunctiva and skin and are frequently isolated from clinical specimens (Fig. 38B, p. 257). *C. xerosis* produces metachromatic granules and many strains are morphologically indistinguishable from *C. diphtheriae*. It can be distinguished by its fermentation reactions and lack of pathogenicity for animals. It is a common conjunctival commensal. 'Non-pathogenic' diphtheroids occasionally cause serious infections after cardiac surgery and in patients with indwelling plastic devices or undergoing immunosuppressive therapy. Multi-resistant JK strains are particularly dangerous. Anaerobic diphtheroids (*Propionibacterium acnes*) are frequently present on the skin. By liberating fatty acids from skin lipids they contribute to the pathogenesis of adolescent acne.

Mycobacterium

This genus consists of *acid-fast*, non-motile, non-sporing, strictly aerobic rods. They possess complex fatty substances which make them difficult to stain by normal methods. When they can be persuaded to take the stain at all they are gram-positive. They are normally stained by the Ziehl-Neelsen (ZN) method or its fluorescent (auramine) modification. Acid-fastness is a distinguishing feature of the genus and is not found in any other bacteria of medical importance with the exception of a few rarely encountered members of the genera *Nocardia* and *Legionella*. Bacterial and fungal spores and the oocysts of *Cryptosporidium* are also acid-fast.

Mycobacterium tuberculosis and M. bovis

Five types of tubercle bacilli are recognized, each adapted to a different range of animal hosts: human, bovine, murine, avian and cold-blooded. Only the human type (*M. tuberculosis*) and the bovine type (*M. bovis*) play an important part in human pathology.

Morphology

The bacilli are typically very slender. They may occur singly, in pairs joined together at an angle, or in clumps with the individual organisms more or less parallel. Virulent strains characteristically form 'serpentine cords' when growing in culture (Fig. 39B). In stained preparations the organisms often have an irregular beaded appearance. Stained by the ZN or auramine methods they are acid-fast.

Cultural properties

M. tuberculosis and *M. bovis* grow poorly or not at all on ordinary laboratory media. They are usually cultured on coagulated egg medium, e.g. Löwenstein-Jensen medium. Colonies take 2–3 weeks to develop and it may be 6–8 weeks before growth is

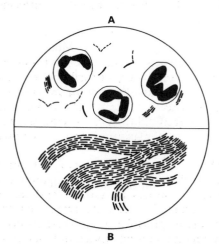

Fig. 39 *Mycobacterium tuberculosis.*
A, Film of sputum.
B, 'Serpentine cords' in culture.

abundant. Dubos medium is a satisfactory liquid culture: it contains a surface-active agent which has a dispersive effect on the organisms and prevents them growing in clumps.

Differentiation of human and bovine types

Typing is of no direct clinical importance but may be required to trace the source of infection.

On glycerol-egg media the human type grows more rapidly and profusely and is described as *eugonic*. The colonies are dry, granular, heaped up, warty, buff or yellowish and not easily broken up. The bovine type grows slowly and less profusely and is described as *dysgonic*. The colonies are moist, smooth, flat, whitish and easily broken up.

Pathogenicity tests are more reliable. The two types are of about the same virulence for guinea-pigs, but the bovine type is highly virulent for rabbits whereas the human type usually causes minimal lesions only.

Strains with intermediate properties ('*M. africanum*', Asian type, etc.) are common. Thus many strains isolated in India and from Asian immigrants in the UK are of low virulence for guinea-pigs, differ from typical *M. tuberculosis* in various cultural and biochemical properties and belong to a distinctive phage type.

Antigenic properties

Various protein and polysaccharide antigens are recognized but are not used in identification. There are no satisfactory serological methods for the diagnosis of tuberculosis, but delayed hypersensitivity to protein components of the organism (tuberculin tests) indicates that the individual has at some time been infected.

Tuberculosis

The human type of bacillus is responsible for the great majority of cases of human tuberculosis, including virtually all cases of pulmonary tuberculosis. During the last century the incidence of the disease has declined dramatically. In the UK about one third of new cases now occur in immigrants. Infection is acquired from another human being, usually by inhalation of droplets or dust, and takes two main forms.

In the primary (or childhood) form there is a single focus of infection in the lung with involvement of the hilar glands (the primary complex). The infection shows a marked tendency to undergo spontaneous cure and usually causes no symptoms. In a few cases the infection spreads to produce progressive forms of the disease such as acute tuberculous bronchopneumonia, miliary tuberculosis, tuberculous meningitis, or isolated foci of infection in bones, joints or kidneys. At one time over 90% of children living in towns acquired a primary infection by the time they reached adult life. This still occurs in some underdeveloped countries, but in the UK childhood infections are infrequent and primary infections are more often encountered in adult life.

The post-primary (secondary or adult) form probably represents reinfection by bacilli acquired from without, but in some cases may be caused by bacilli present in the primary lesions. The usual result is a disease (pulmonary tuberculosis) characterized by one or more lesions near the apex of a lung but without obvious involvement of the regional lymph nodes. The lesions may progress to caseation, cavitation, fibrosis and destruction of lung tissue. The infection shows little tendency to undergo spontaneous cure.

The differences between the primary and post-primary forms of infection mainly depend on immunity and allergy resulting from the primary infection. Age is itself of some importance and primary infection of adults not infrequently produces a progressive form of disease indistinguishable from post-primary infections.

The bovine type of bacillus is rarely conveyed to man by the carcasses and meat of infected animals (pigs and sheep as well as cattle) and the only important source of infection is cow's milk. Cows suffering from tuberculous mastitis may excrete large numbers of the organisms in their milk; the organisms may also find their way into milk from other sources, e.g. faeces of cows with tuberculous enteritis. Human infection is largely confined to children. It is likely to involve the cervical glands, infected via the pharynx, and the abdominal glands, infected from the intestines. Pasteurization of milk and progress in eradicating bovine tuberculosis have made infection by this organism rare.

Tubercle bacilli occasionally cause primary infection of the skin, e.g. self-inoculation by butchers and pathologists. In lupus vulgaris, another type of skin tuberculosis, the mode of infection is obscure: human and bovine strains are about equally represented and the organisms are often peculiar in being avirulent for animals.

Diagnosis

Tubercle bacilli can be demonstrated by microscopy, culture and animal inoculation.

Microscopy. Films of sputum, pus, etc., are stained by the ZN or auramine methods and examined for slender, beaded, acid-fast bacilli. Saprophytic acid-fast bacilli morphologically resembling

M. tuberculosis are occasionally present in dust and may contaminate reagents and equipment. Some species grow in dripping taps. Care must also be taken to avoid confusion caused by dead tubercle bacilli from previous positive specimens and cultures. Specimens should be collected in scrupulously clean containers, slides should be new, and stains should be made up in distilled water. The presence of acid-fast bacilli in sputum nearly always indicates tuberculosis. The number seen in stained films is often very small, but it is justifiable to make a presumptive diagnosis on the presence of only one or two typical bacilli. Positive films from pleural fluid, cerebrospinal fluid (CSF) and pus from closed abscesses also indicate tuberculosis. In specimens of urine saprophytic acid-fast bacilli, particularly *M. smegmatis*, are fairly frequent contaminants and positive films should be interpreted with caution. Specimens of faeces so frequently contain acid-fast organisms and misleading debris that microscopic examination is almost valueless.

Culture. In attempting to culture *M. tuberculosis* from specimens containing other organisms, advantage is taken of the relatively high resistance of *M. tuberculosis* to various chemical agents. Thus incubation of sputum with 4% NaOH, followed by neutralization with HCl, kills off contaminants and enables the specimen to be concentrated in a small volume. Cultures should not be discarded as negative for 8 weeks.

Guinea-pig inoculation. The specimen, if necessary after special treatment and concentration, is injected intramuscularly into the thigh of a guinea-pig. The animal is killed after 6−8 weeks. Postmortem examination shows tuberculosis of the local lymph nodes and usually lesions in other lymph nodes, spleen, liver and lungs. Stained films are prepared to confirm the presence of acid-fast bacilli. Modern methods of culture give about the same proportion of positive results as guinea-pig inoculation and tests using guinea-pigs are now seldom justified.

Prevention

Mass radiography, segregation and treatment of known cases, and supervision of close contacts and those at special risk form the basis of prevention. Immunization with BCG is a valuable supplementary measure. Human infection caused by the bovine bacillus can be virtually eliminated by pasteurization of milk.

Other types of tubercle bacilli

The murine type (*M. microti*, the vole bacillus) causes tuberculosis in voles but is non-pathogenic for man. It has been used as an alternative to BCG for immunization of human beings.

The avian type (*M. avium*) causes tuberculosis in birds and, very rarely, in man. It has an optimum growth temperature of 40–43°C.

The cold-blooded type causes tuberculosis in fishes and other cold-blooded animals. It grows profusely and has an optimum growth temperature of 25°C. It is harmless to man.

Mycobacterium leprae

M. leprae is an exclusively human parasite. It is the cause of leprosy, a chronic granulomatous infection associated with poverty, overcrowding and low standards of hygiene. In the Middle Ages leprosy was relatively common in Europe, but it is now largely confined to tropical countries. In *tuberculoid* leprosy there is infiltration of peripheral nerves leading to anaesthesia and secondary trophic changes. Cell-mediated immunity is active and the lepromin test (a delayed hypersensitivity reaction to intracutaneous injection of extracts of lepromatous tissue) is strongly positive. Few bacilli are present in the lesions. The disease is relatively benign and spontaneous healing may occur. In *lepromatous* leprosy there is progressive formation of chronic inflammatory tissue mainly involving the skin and mucous membranes and frequently leading to ulceration. Cell-mediated immunity is defective and the lepromin test is negative. Large numbers of bacilli are present in the lesions. The prognosis is poor. Intermediate *borderline* forms of leprosy are common. In all forms of leprosy the organisms are usually present in the nasal mucous membranes at some stage. Leprosy is generally contracted only after prolonged and intimate contact with a case of the disease. It is not clear whether this is due to low infectivity of the organisms or because most infections are subclinical and heal spontaneously. Infected nasal secretions are probably the main source of infection.

M. leprae cannot be cultivated on bacteriological media but will produce a localized infection when injected into the foot-pads of mice, rats or hamsters. This provides a means of testing anti-leprosy drugs. Generalized infections may occur in mice whose resistance has been lowered by thymectomy and irradiation. Armadillos are susceptible to *M. leprae* and have been used for the study of leprosy. Sooty mangabey monkeys are also susceptible and may prove to be ideal test animals. The mean generation time of *M. leprae* is about 12 days.

Diagnosis of leprosy depends on finding acid-fast bacilli in smears, scrapings and biopsies from the nasal mucous membrane and from skin nodules. The organisms resemble *M. tuberculosis* and are usually seen in large numbers, especially inside mononuclear cells (lepra cells).

Opportunist (tuberculoid) acid-fast bacilli

Slow-growing acid-fast bacilli which cannot be identified as either human or bovine tubercle bacilli are sometimes isolated from clinical sources. The presence of these organisms often seems to be of little significance, but in some individuals they produce a disease clinically indistinguishable from tuberculosis. The tuberculin reaction may be weakly positive. Case-to-case infection is almost unknown.

These opportunist mycobacteria are a heterogeneous group. They are often highly resistant to the drugs commonly used to treat tuberculosis. They are non-pathogenic for guinea-pigs, but some strains produce an abscess at the site of injection. The following are some of the species at present recognized:

M. ulcerans resembles the tubercle bacillus in many respects but can be distinguished by its ability to grow at temperatures of 25–35°C with an optimum of about 30°C. It fails to grow at 37°C. If the organism is injected into rats or mice progressive lesions develop in the cooler parts of the body, i.e. ends of the limbs, tip of the nose, the tail and the testes. In man the organism colonizes abrasions and causes a chronic ulcerative condition of the skin, particularly of the arms and legs. Human infection is common in some tropical and subtropical countries.

M. marinum is a photochromogen, i.e. it produces a yellow-orange pigment when growing in the light. The organism has an optimum growth temperature of 25–30°C. It produces skin lesions similar to those produced by *M. ulcerans*. In some cases infection has been traced to swimming baths. It may also occur in people who keep tropical fish.

M. kansasi is a photochromogen and is the most important opportunist mycobacterium in the UK. It can produce pulmonary lesions clinically indistinguishable from those of chronic pulmonary tuberculosis.

M. scrofulaceum is a scotochromogen, i.e. it produces pigment in the dark. It is a rare cause of cervical adenitis in children.

M. intracellulare is best regarded as a variant of *M. avium*. It is a non-chromogenic opportunist common in parts of Australia and the USA. It causes infections of the lungs and lymph nodes.

M. xenopi is a non-chromogen that grows best at 42°C. It occasionally causes lung disease. Disseminated infection may occur in immunosuppressed patients.

M. fortuitum is a widely distributed 'rapid grower'. On rare occasions it causes infections of the skin, lymph nodes and lungs.

M. chelonei is another rapid grower which occasionally causes wound infections and abscesses.

Saprophytic acid-fast bacilli

The most important species in this group is *M. smegmatis*, a normal commensal present in smegma on the genital mucous membranes of both sexes and a frequent contaminant of urine. Free-living species are widely distributed in nature.

Morphologically the saprophytic acid-fast bacilli may be indistinguishable from *M. tuberculosis*. Culturally they can be distinguished by the rapidity of their growth and their ability to grow on ordinary media at room temperature, e.g. there may be good growth on nutrient agar after 2 days at 22 or 37°C. Many strains are markedly pigmented. They are non-pathogenic for animals.

Actinomyces

The genus *Actinomyces* consists of microaerophilic gram-positive bacteria which grow in the form of branching filaments and live as parasites of man and animals. Together with the genus *Nocardia* and certain other ill-defined genera of filamentous organisms they are known as the actinomycetes.

Actinomyces israeli

A. israeli is the cause of human actinomycosis, an uncommon, chronic suppurative and granulomatous infection which characteristically occurs in one of four sites: the jaw and surrounding tissues, the lacrimal canaliculi, the lungs, and the ileocaecal region. Growth of actinomyces (*A. israeli* and *A. odontolyticus*) is frequently associated with the long-term use of plastic (non-copper-containing) intrauterine contraceptive devices, but clinical pelvic actinomycosis is extremely rare. Actinomycosis probably represents an endogenous infection by strains which are normally present as harmless commensals around the teeth and in the tonsillar crypts.

Morphology

In the tissues *A. israeli* develops in the form of colonies. These are discharged in the pus as yellow 'sulphur granules', about the size of a pin-head and often gritty from calcification. They are usually scanty and may not be seen unless the pus is spread out and

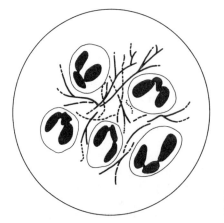

Fig. 40 *Actinomyces israeli* in pus.

examined in a thin layer. When crushed and stained the granules are seen to consist of a tangled mass of very slender, gram-positive, branching filaments. The filaments stain irregularly and often appear to be fragmented into bacillary and coccal forms and rows of small dots. In tissue sections the filaments radiate from the central mass of mycelium and may terminate in club-like swellings. The clubs are gram-negative and may be weakly acid-fast. They are not part of the organism but are formed by deposition of material by the tissue.

In culture *A. israeli* grows in short bacillary forms and may be mistaken for a diphtheroid. Careful search usually reveals a few branched filaments.

Cultural properties

Cultures are usually unsuccessful unless a sulphur granule is obtained. The granule should be washed in saline and crushed. Growth is slow and does not occur under ordinary atmospheric conditions. On blood agar incubated anaerobically for 4–7 days the organisms develop in the form of small, white, irregular colonies which look like breadcrumbs. They are firmly adherent to the medium. Slight growth may occur in air with 5–10% CO_2. In cooked meat medium the organisms grow as compact, white, mulberry-like masses. In shake cultures there is no surface growth and the organisms grow best several millimetres below the surface (Fig. 16, p. 51).

Filamentous organisms which resemble *A. israeli* but which grow aerobically are often isolated from clinical specimens. In the vast majority of cases these aerobic organisms are harmless.

Actinomyces bovis

A. bovis is the cause of actinomycosis ('lumpy jaw') in cattle. Minor cultural and antigenic differences between *A. bovis* and *A. israeli* have been described, but some workers consider that they are variants of the same species. There is no reason to suppose that human infections are derived from cattle.

Nocardia

The genus *Nocardia* consists of aerobic gram-positive bacteria which grow in the form of branching filaments. They normally live as saprophytes in the soil, but three species, *N. asteroides*, *N. brasiliensis* and *N. madurae*, are occasionally pathogenic for man.

Nocardia asteroides

N. asteroides is occasionally responsible for a granulomatous infection of the lungs. The organisms may spread by the blood to involve the subcutaneous tissues and the brain. The disease is of world-wide distribution but is rare. Small outbreaks of *N. asteroides* infection have occurred among patients undergoing immuno-suppressive therapy. The organism is aerobic, acid-fast and produces a generalized infection when injected into rabbits.

Nocardia brasiliensis

N. brasiliensis is generally associated with infections of the skin and soft tissues. Pulmonary and disseminated infections may occur. The organism closely resembles *N. asteroides*.

Nocardia madurae

N. madurae is one of the causes of mycetoma or 'Madura foot', a chronic granulomatous infection occurring in tropical countries. The organism is aerobic, non-acid-fast and non-pathogenic for animals.

Micropolyspora

M. faeni, a saprophytic thermophilic actinomycete, is the main cause of 'farmer's lung', an allergic pulmonary disease due to inhalation of the dust of mouldy hay or other vegetable produce. In typical cases cough and difficulty in breathing begin 5—6 hours after exposure. In the chronic disease granulomatous infiltration occurs in the peripheral parts of the lungs. Antibodies against *M. faeni* are found in the serum of 90% of cases.

Thermoactinomyces vulgaris resembles *M. faeni* and is also a common cause of farmer's lung.

Streptomyces

The genus *Streptomyces* consists of a large group of saprophytic filamentous organisms which grow in the soil. They do not cause disease in man, but are of medical importance as they are the main source of antibiotics.

Lactobacillus

Lactobacilli are long, slender, non-motile gram-positive rods which tend to grow in chains. They tolerate extremely acid conditions and will grow at a pH of 3–4. Many species are microaerophilic, particularly when first isolated, and some are strict anaerobes. The colonies are often minute.

L. acidophilus (Döderlein's bacillus) is a normal inhabitant of the human vagina during the child-bearing years. By converting glycogen into lactic acid it creates a highly acid environment which inhibits the growth of other organisms.

Various species of lactobacilli are normal inhabitants of the mouth. In conjunction with oral streptococci (p. 237) they play an important part in the production of dental caries, i.e. the acids they produce from carbohydrates present in food may decalcify the enamel and dentine.

Lactobacilli are normally present in the intestinal tract and are often the predominant organism in the faeces of breast-fed infants. Lactobacilli in unpasteurized milk are one of the main causes of souring. The production of yoghurt and 'lactic' cheese depends on the action of these organisms.

Erysipelothrix

Erysipelothrix rhusiopathiae

This organism is a slender, non-motile gram-positive bacillus which tends to produce filamentous forms in culture. It is the cause of swine erysipelas. It also infects a wide variety of other animals and birds and is found as a commensal on the scales of fishes.

Human infection mainly occurs among abattoir workers,

butchers, fishmongers, etc. The organism gains access through an abrasion, often caused by a prick from a bone, and produces a characteristic, localized, dusky, inflammatory lesion known as erysipeloid of Rosenbach. On rare occasions it produces a septicaemic condition. Isolation of the organism is difficult.

Listeria

Listeria monocytogenes

This organism is a motile gram-positive bacillus which tends to produce filamentous forms in culture. It is a common inhabitant of soil and a pathogen of a wide variety of animals. It closely resembles *Erysipelothrix rhusiopathiae* in cultural characteristics and pathogenicity but differs in certain biochemical and antigenic properties.

Human infections take three main forms: meningitis, septicaemia and infection of the fetus *in utero*. Fetal infection may cause fetal death and abortion, or the infant may be born alive and shortly afterwards succumb to a generalized infection characterized by focal necrosis in the liver and spleen. The mother usually shows no symptoms. Listeriosis is relatively common in patients undergoing immunosuppressive therapy. Contaminated food is probably the main source of human infection. Small outbreaks have been associated with consumption of coleslaw, unpasteurized milk and cheese. Infection of man and small animals is often associated with monocytosis.

L. monocytogenes grows on ordinary media, but unless it is isolated in pure culture from the CSF or the blood it is liable to be dismissed as a 'diphtheroid' of no significance. Identification is assisted by the appearance of a zone of haemolysis around the colonies on blood agar after incubation for 48 hours.

Gram-negative Bacilli

A dreadful plague in London was
In the year sixty-five,
Which swept an hundred thousand souls
Away; yet I alive!
[Yersinia pestis]

Daniel Defoe, 1722

From the practical point of view gram-negative bacilli can be divided into two broad groups:

1 Coliforms or intestinal bacilli (enterobacteria). These grow profusely on simple media such as peptone water and plain nutrient agar and form colonies on MacConkey medium, e.g. *Escherichia, Klebsiella, Salmonella, Shigella, Proteus* and miscellaneous coliform organisms. It is also convenient to consider the genera *Pseudomonas, Vibrio* and *Yersinia* in this group.
2 Small, nutritionally exacting bacilli, often referred to as parvobacteria. These grow comparatively poorly even on enriched media such as blood agar and usually not at all on MacConkey medium, e.g. *Haemophilus, Bordetella, Brucella, Pasteurella* and various other delicate bacilli.

Intestinal bacilli (coliforms)

Morphology

Most species are morphologically indistinguishable. They resemble *Escherichia coli* and can be described as 'coliform'. They are usually straight rods 2–3 μm long and about 0.6 μm wide, but much variation occurs. *Proteus* is more pleomorphic than other species. *Klebsiella* has a capsule.

Motility

Shigellae and klebsiellae are non-motile. Nearly all the other intestinal organisms are motile, but non-motile variants are sometimes encountered.

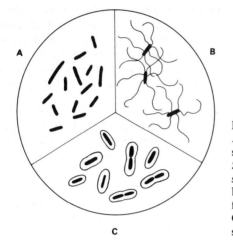

Fig. 41   Intestinal bacilli.
A, Typical intestinal bacilli
such as *Escherichia coli*,
Salmonella typhi or *Shigella
sonnei*.
B, *E. coli* stained to show
flagella.
C, *Klebsiella pneumoniae*
stained to show capsules.

Cultural properties

The colonies of most species look alike. After 24 hours they are
typically large, 2–3 mm, round, smooth, glistening domes. There
are three exceptions: *Pseudomonas aeruginosa* produces colonies
with a metallic sheen, a green discoloration of the medium and a
distinctive smell; *Proteus* (most strains) 'swarms' over the medium
and smells of ammonia; *Klebsiella* produces large, mucoid colonies.

Biochemical reactions

1   Fermentation of lactose is the most important differential
    feature. *E. coli* and closely related species, including *Klebsiella*,
    produce acid and gas from lactose. Other species are non-
    lactose fermenters, with the important exception that *Shigella
    sonnei* is a late-lactose fermenter; fermentation is not apparent
    at 24 hours and is usually delayed for several days.
2   Salmonellae typically produce acid and gas from glucose,
    mannitol and dulcitol but do not ferment lactose, sucrose or
    salicin. *S. typhi* is distinguished from other salmonellae by its
    failure to produce gas from any carbohydrate and failure to
    ferment dulcitol.
3   Shigellae do not produce gas from carbohydrates. *Sh. flexneri*,
    Sh. boydi and *Sh. sonnei* produce acid from glucose and mannitol
    but do not ferment lactose, sucrose and salicin; *Sh. sonnei* is,
    however, a late fermenter of lactose and sucrose. *Sh. dysenteriae*
    is distinguished from the other species by its failure to ferment
    mannitol. Rarely encountered varieties of *Sh. flexneri*, e.g.
    Newcastle variety, produce a small bubble of gas and fail to
    ferment mannitol.

4 Production of indole from tryptophan excludes salmonellae. *Sh. sonnei* does not produce indole, but some types of the other shigellae do. Indole is produced by *E. coli*, some strains of *Proteus* and various unimportant coliform organisms.

5 Liquefaction of gelatin excludes salmonellae and shigellae. It is characteristic of *Proteus, Pseudomonas* and a few unimportant coliforms.

6 Rapid splitting of urea excludes salmonellae and shigellae. It is characteristic of *Proteus*. Other coliforms split urea slowly.

Note. There are rare exceptions to all the above features. They are mainly of interest experts working in reference laboratories.

Serological reactions

Final identification of the more important species depends on detection of specific antigens by agglutination reactions.

Escherichia

The genus *Escherichia* consists of lactose-fermenting, gram-negative bacilli and includes the important species, *E. coli*.

Escherichia coli

E. coli is the typical coliform of the intestinal tract. It is of importance (1) as a normal commensal which must be distinguished from the intestinal pathogens, salmonellae and shigellae; (2) as a pathogen particularly of the urinary tract and also in appendicitis, peritonitis, cholecystitis, wound infection, neonatal meningitis and gastroenteritis in infancy; (3) in providing evidence of faecal contamination of water supplies.

Cultural properties

It grows well on all ordinary media but the colonies are not distinctive. About 10% of strains are late-lactose fermenters. Some strains produce haemolysis on blood agar.

Subdivisions

Many varieties of *E. coli* can be distinguished by a battery of biochemical tests. Serological classification is more precise. Strains can be classified into at least 170 groups on the basis of their O antigens and further subdivided on the basis of H and K (envelope) antigens.

E. coli gastroenteritis

E. coli is an important cause of gastroenteritis. In particular the organism is responsible for outbreaks of gastroenteritis among infants and young children in nurseries and children's wards. The disease mainly affects babies under 18 months of age. Diarrhoea and vomiting lead to severe dehydration. The mortality may be high in very young babies.

The strains of *E. coli* responsible for gastroenteritis (*enteropathogenic strains*) are of at least two kinds:

Enterotoxigenic strains produce one or both of two enterotoxins, one heat-labile the other heat-stable. The heat-labile toxin closely resembles the enterotoxin of *Vibrio cholerae*. Ability to produce enterotoxins depends on the possession of particular plasmids. The organisms cause outbreaks of gastroenteritis in infants and often affect adults as well. Many cases of traveller's diarrhoea are caused by these organisms. Unlike the residents, newcomers do not possess antibodies to the prevailing strains of *E. coli*.

Enteroinvasive strains invade the epithelial cells of the large gut. The organisms are particularly liable to cause illness in older children and adults. Large outbreaks among adults have been described.

Various other properties seem to be necessary for the expression of enteropathogenicity, e.g. the ability to adhere to the intestinal mucosa, but the role of certain O antigens, which at one time were thought to be associated with epidemics of infantile gastro-enteritis, is obscure. Some strains of *E. coli* produce a toxin (Vero toxin) which has a cytotoxic effect on Vero cells and closely resembles the Shiga toxin produced by *Shigella dysenteriae* type 1. Certain of these strains have caused outbreaks of haemorrhagic colitis and have been associated with haemolytic uraemic syndrome.

Serotyping of *E. coli* is sometimes of value in investigating outbreaks of the disease (p. 170). Control of outbreaks is considered elsewhere (p. 197).

Gram-negative bacteraemia

This condition, also known as bacteraemic or endotoxic shock, is caused by the entry into the blood stream of large numbers of coliforms. The bacteria commonly gain access from the urethra following such procedures as catheterization and cystoscopy. They may also arise from abdominal and pelvic sepsis, wounds and burns, particularly after surgical intervention. Transfusion of infected blood is a rare cause.

Typically, the symptoms are a sudden onset of rigor and high fever and a profound drop in blood pressure. Sometimes the patient develops shock with little fever. The symptoms are caused by the endotoxins of the organisms (p. 76). Later the organisms may multiply in the tissues. Apart from general measures to treat shock, the patient should be given an antibiotic active against a wide range of gram-negative bacilli, e.g. gentamicin. This should be done without waiting for the results of blood culture. Chemotherapy, especially with agents such as β-lactam antibiotics which act by damaging the bacterial cell wall, sometimes exacerbates endotoxic shock. The high mortality of gram-negative bacteraemia can be reduced by giving antibody against endotoxin.

Faecal contamination of water supplies

A direct search for faecal pathogens such as salmonellae is seldom worth while, but the presence of even a few *E. coli* suggests recent faecal contamination. The investigation usually entails a quantitative estimation of all coliform bacilli (presumptive coliform count) and differential tests to distinguish 'typical' or 'faecal' (type 1) coliforms such as *E. coli* from 'atypical' (type 2) coliforms such as *Enterobacter* spp. and various intermediate types. Whereas type 1 coliforms are almost exclusively derived from human or animal faeces, type 2 coliforms are mainly saprophytes of soil and crops and their presence in water is of much less significance. Direct enumeration of colonies on the surface of membrane filters is more satisfactory than methods using multiple tubes and probability tables.

Klebsiella

The genus *Klebsiella* consists of non-motile, lactose-fermenting, capsulated, gram-negative bacilli. Klebsiellae can be classified on the basis of their polysaccharide capsular (K) antigens into more than 70 types. There is one important species, *K. pneumoniae.* Several subspecies or biotypes are distinguished by their biochemical reactions. *K. pneumoniae* subsp. *aerogenes* accounts for nearly all human infections. Other subspecies are *pneumoniae*, *rhinoscleromatis* and *ozaenae*. *K. oxytoca* closely resembles *aerogenes* strains but is regarded as a separate species.

Klebsiella pneumoniae

Cultural properties

Typical strains have large capsules (Fig. 41C, p. 272) and produce a characteristic profuse mucoid growth on solid media.

Infections

K. *pneumoniae* is often found in the intestinal tract and is an occasional commensal of the upper respiratory tract. Its main importance is that it frequently causes hospital-acquired infection. Urinary tract infections are particularly common. Surgical wound infection and bacteraemia may occur. Colonization of the respiratory tract is very common, especially in patients being treated with antibiotics. In most cases the organism is probably a secondary invader of little significance but in some cases of pneumonia it appears to be the primary infective agent. Certain strains of K. *pneumoniae* are the cause of a rare type of destructive pneumonia, Friedländer's pneumonia, usually occurring outside hospitals in elderly dehabilitated patients. The *rhinoscleromatis* subspecies is the cause of rhinoscleroma, a granulomatous nasal condition, and *ozaenae* strains have been isolated from cases of ozaena, a form of atrophic rhinitis.

Salmonella

This genus consists of motile, non-lactose-fermenting, gram-negative bacilli which are parasites of the intestinal tract of man and animals, including birds. In their distribution and pathogenicity they fall into two groups:

1 S. *typhi* and S. *paratyphi* A, B and C are human pathogens, though S. *typhi* has been isolated from fruit-eating bats in Madagascar (!) and S. *paratyphi* B has occasionally been isolated from animals. They are highly pathogenic for man. After a long incubation period they typically produce a severe, generalized illness of long duration in which septicaemic symptoms predominate over intestinal symptoms (enteric fever).
2 All other salmonellae are primarily animal pathogens which occasionally cause disease in man. They are less pathogenic for man. After a short incubation period they typically produce a more benign and less invasive illness of short duration in which intestinal symptoms predominate (salmonella food poisoning; salmonellosis).

Subdivisions

Biochemical reactions serve to define the group as a whole and aid in the differentiation of a few species which have special peculiarities. Classification mainly depends on antigenic composition. In the Kauffmann-White scheme the salmonellae are divided into groups on the basis of their O or somatic antigens;

within each group 'species' are differentiated on the basis of their H or flagellar antigens. About 2000 'species', i.e. different serotypes, can be recognized in this way. Some species possess additional Vi or virulence antigens.

O antigens. These are protein-polysaccharide-lipid complexes. About 45 distinct O antigens are recognized. Most species possess several O antigens which they share with a number of other species. Salmonellae are divided into nine main groups (A, B, C etc.) each characterized by an O antigen which is not found in the other groups.

H antigens. These are protein in nature. Over 70 distinct H antigens are recognized. Many species such as *S. paratyphi* B and C and *S. typhimurium* are diphasic, i.e. they possess two alternative sets of H antigens, either of which may predominate in a particular culture. Antigens of phase 1 (specific phase) are shared by only a few species or may be entirely specific. Antigens of phase 2 (non-specific or group phase) are usually shared by a large number of species. Other species such as *S. typhi, S. paratyphi* A, and *S. enteritidis* are monophasic, i.e. their H antigens can exist in only one phase, usually phase 1. Each species may possess more than one H antigen in phase 1 or phase 2. Rare species are permanently non-motile and do not possess H antigens.

Vi antigens. These are superficial (envelope) antigens found in freshly isolated, virulent strains of *S. typhi* and rarely in some other species.

Antigenic variation

In addition to diphasic flagellar variation (see above) strains may show other types of variation in their antigenic components:

1 Motile strains may lose their flagella and become non-motile (H → O variation). Non-motile cultures usually contain small numbers of motile organisms which can be recovered by special means, e.g. allowing the culture to grow through a tube containing semi-solid medium. A few strains are permanently non-motile.
2 Organisms may lose their Vi antigen partially or completely.
3 Organisms may lose some or all of their O antigens. This is associated with change of colonial appearance from smooth to rough (S → R variation), loss of virulence and exposure of non-specific R antigens which are common to the salmonella group as a whole and are sometimes found in rough variants belonging to other genera of intestinal bacilli.

Phage-typing

Strains of *S. typhi* possessing Vi antigen can be assigned to one of a large number of Vi types on the basis of their susceptibility to bacteriophages (Vi phages). The method is of great value in investigating outbreaks of typhoid fever, e.g. correlating strains isolated from cases, carriers and other sources. Phage-typing is also applicable to *S. paratyphi* B, *S. typhimurium* and certain other species.

Enteric fever

The classical example is typhoid fever caused by *S. typhi*. In the UK *S. paratyphi* B is a more common cause of paratyphoid fever than *S. paratyphi* A; *S. paratyphi* C is almost unknown. Most cases of enteric fever encountered in the UK are contracted abroad. On rare occasions other salmonellae such as *S. typhimurium* and *S. enteritidis* produce the clinical picture of enteric fever. Typhoid fever tends to be more severe than the paratyphoid fevers, but all of them sometimes appear in a mild, 'ambulant' form in which the disease is unrecognized.

Source

The source of infection is a human case or carrier who excretes the organisms in the faeces or less commonly in urine. The infective dose of organisms is very small. Contaminated drinking water and milk offer the greatest possibilities for large-scale epidemics, but public health measures have greatly reduced the dangers from these sources. The disease is now mainly transmitted by food which has been handled by carriers. Other channels of infection are oysters and other shellfish from infected estuaries, and watercress from infected streams. The 1964 Aberdeen epidemic of typhoid fever involved over 500 cases and probably originated from a single can of infected corned beef. Flies and dust are important in countries with a low standard of hygiene. Person-to-person transmission by use of a contaminated duo-denal tube and fibreoptic gastroscope has been reported.

Pathogenesis

The organisms enter the body by the mouth and multiply in the lymph follicles of the intestinal tract and in the mesenteric lymph nodes. Some gain access to the blood and are taken up by the reticuloendothelial cells of the liver, spleen and bone marrow. The organisms multiply intracellularly. Headache, prostration, nose-bleeds, bronchitis, constipation, abdominal tenderness and high fever are common. Diarrhoea is unusual at this stage. The cellular reaction is mononuclear in type and the peripheral blood shows a leucopenia. After a few days 'rose spots' appear in the skin and the spleen is enlarged. Ulcerative inflammation of Peyer's patches and the solitary lymph follicles of the small intestine may lead to diarrhoea and later to the two most serious complications, intestinal haemorrhage and perforation. The gall-bladder is invariably infected and is probably the main source of salmonellae in the faeces, particularly in the later stages of the disease. Abscesses sometimes form in bones and other organs. Relapses are common.

Carriers

After an attack of typhoid fever a few individuals continue to harbour *S. typhi* in their gall-bladders and intermittently excrete the organisms in their faeces. After a year 2–5% of cases are still excreting the organisms and some of these individuals continue to do so indefinitely (Fig. 19, p. 59). Nearly all permanent faecal excreters are women. The most notorious carrier of all times was 'Typhoid Mary' who, in her career as a cook to many households and institutions from 1901 onwards, left a trail of typhoid victims in the USA and Canada. Persistent urinary excretion may occur but is rare unless there is an abnormality of the urinary tract, e.g. urinary excreters are common in countries where schistosomiasis is rife. The incidence of urinary excretion is the same in the two sexes.

Patients who excrete *S. typhi* (or any other salmonellae) for less than a year are known as *temporary excreters*. They are of two sorts: *convalescent excreters* who have recently had the disease, and *symptomless excreters* who have had no apparent illness. Patients who excrete the organisms for more than a year are known as *chronic carriers*. The carrier state following infection with *S. paratyphi* B is usually less prolonged than that found with *S. typhi*, but some individuals become chronic carriers.

Diagnosis

This depends on isolation of the organisms from the blood, faeces or urine and detection of specific antibodies in the patient's serum (Widal reaction).

Isolation of the organism. Blood cultures are usually positive in the early stages of the illness. About 80% of cases give positive results in the first week; thereafter the chances of success progressively diminish. Stool cultures are often positive in the first week, but are more likely to be positive (70–80%) in the second

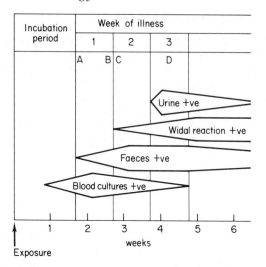

Fig. 42 Diagnosis of typhoid fever, showing time-scale of positive laboratory findings. A, Insidious onset (headaches, constipation). B, Severe illness (high fever, diarrhoea, enlarged spleen). C, Rose spots. D, Complications (intestinal haemorrhage and perforations); relapses with positive blood cultures may occur at this stage.

and third weeks. Urine cultures are positive in about 20% of cases, but usually not before the third week. Whatever the stage of the disease, repeated blood and stool cultures should be made until the organisms have been isolated. Culture of urine, bile (duodenal juice) and bone marrow may sometimes succeed when other methods fail.

Widal reaction. This is an agglutination test for antibodies which appear in the course of enteric fever and other salmonella infections. In the UK a suitable range of suspensions for routine use consists of *S. typhi* (H, O and Vi), *S. paratyphi* A (H), *S. paratyphi* B (H and O) and a 'non-specific salmonella' suspension containing several H phase 2 antigens; the most useful additional suspension is *S. typhimurium* (H phase 1). In other parts of the world or when patients come from abroad it is usual to add *S. paratyphi* A (O) and *S. paratyphi* C (H and O). Further salmonella suspensions can be included when necessary. Suspensions of *Brucella abortus* and *Br. melitensis* are commonly included in the test.

Interpretation is often difficult and factors such as the stage of the illness, previous infection or vaccination and the occurrence of low titres in healthy individuals need to be taken into account.

Identification of carriers

Urine and faeces should be obtained from everyone who is a possible source of infection. Knowledge that the incubation period of typhoid fever is about 12 days may narrow the field of investigation. Swabs placed in sewers and drains may help to trace a carrier to a particular street, block of buildings or an individual home. The Widal reaction is a useful screening procedure, since a high proportion of carriers of *S. typhi* have Vi titres of 10 or more. Excretion by carriers is intermittent and repeated examination of faeces and urine may be necessary.

Control

This involves (1) eliminating the source of infection, particularly by control of carriers; (2) preventing the spread of infection by public health measures, e.g. safe sewage disposal, clean water supplies, pasteurization of milk, hygienic preparation of food; and (3) when sanitary control of the environment is difficult, active immunization with typhoid vaccine.

Salmonella food poisoning (salmonellosis)

This variety of 'food poisoning' should be regarded as a 'food infection' as the organisms multiply in the body and toxins are not responsible. The patient may have diarrhoea, vomiting and fever for several days, but intestinal perforation and haemorrhage are almost unknown and death is rare except at the extremes of life. Relapses are infrequent and chronic carriers are very rare. Temporary convalescent carriers (convalescent excreters) and ambulant subclinical cases (symptomless excreters) are more important as sources of infection. Chemotherapy is seldom necessary and may actually prolong the period during which organisms are excreted.

S. typhimurium is the most common cause of this condition. The prevalence of other species varies from year to year. *S. paratyphi* B not infrequently causes gastroenteritis rather than enteric fever. Diagnosis depends on isolating the organisms from the faeces. Blood cultures are seldom positive and the disease is usually over before the Widal reaction becomes positive. The investigation of salmonella food poisoning is considered elsewhere (p. 198).

Salmonella septicaemia

Salmonella septicaemia is characterized by persistent fever and a tendency for the organisms to cause localized abscesses. Intestinal involvement is usually absent or a minor feature, but salmonella septicaemia sometimes complicates gastroenteritis in children. Salmonellae of both the enteric and food poisoning groups can cause this syndrome. *S. choleraesuis* has often been incriminated. Diagnosis can usually be made by blood culture. At other times the diagnosis is made unexpectedly, e.g. during routine examination of pus from a septic joint or a pelvic abscess.

Shigella

This genus consists of non-motile, non-lactose-fermenting, non-gas-producing, gram-negative bacilli. They are parasites of the human intestinal tract and are the cause of bacillary dysentery.

Subdivisions

Classification is based on a combination of biochemical properties and antigenic analysis. Since shigellae do not possess flagella there are no H antigens to be considered. Four species are recognized:

Sh. dysenteriae consists of ten antigenic types: type 1 is also known as *Sh. shigae* and type 2 as *Sh. schmitzi*.

Sh. flexneri is divided into six types each possessing a specific antigen. Two variants, X and Y, are strains which have lost their specific antigens but retain their group antigens. Type 6 includes biochemical varieties, Newcastle and Manchester, which differ from other shigellae in their ability to produce a tiny bubble of gas in fermentation.

Sh. boydi consists of 15 serological types.

Sh. sonnei consists of only one serological type, but the organisms often undergo S → R variation. The two forms, smooth (phase 1) and rough (phase 2), are antigenically distinct. Colicin-typing can be used to type strains for epidemiological purposes.

Infections

Bacillary dysentery is an acute inflammatory condition of the large bowel associated with the passage of thin stools containing blood, pus and mucus. The infective process is confined to the intestinal tract and there is no bacteraemic phase. In severe cases there may be extensive ulceration and sloughing of the intestinal mucosa.

Sh. dysenteriae type 1 causes the most severe forms of dysentery (Shiga dysentery); the organism is mainly confined to the Indian subcontinent and the Far East. *Sh. flexneri* and *Sh. boydi* tend to produce less severe disease; they are mainly found in tropical and subtropical countries, but may be found in temperate climates. *Sh. sonnei* usually produces a very mild disease; it is the most common cause of dysentery in temperate climates.

Source

Infection is acquired by mouth. The source of the organisms is faeces from a case or carrier. No animal reservoir of infection is known. Individuals with mild or inapparent infections outnumber clinical cases and constitute the main source of infection, particularly in Sonne dysentery. Convalescent patients may continue to excrete the organisms for a few weeks, but chronic carriers are rare.

In tropical countries major epidemics are associated with low standards of hygiene. Flies are an important vector in transferring the organisms from faeces to food.

In the UK over 95% of cases are due to *Sh. sonnei* and the remainder are nearly all due to *Sh. flexneri*. The disease is mainly transmitted by faecal contamination of the hands and environmental objects such as crockery, door handles, lavatory chains and lavatory seats. The organisms may also be conveyed by food infected by a carrier. Flies are probably of minor importance. Sonne dysentery has its greatest incidence in children and is often endemic in nurseries and schools. Widespread community epidemics have occurred. Dysentery is common in hospitals for the mentally handicapped.

Diagnosis

This depends on isolating the organisms from the faeces. Agglutination reactions on the patient's serum are of no value.

Control

Detection and elimination of mild and inapparent cases presents an almost insuperable problem. Prevention mainly depends on hygienic measures (individual and communal) which limit the transference of faeces from one individual to another.

Proteus

The genus *Proteus* consists of motile, non-lactose-fermenting, gram-negative bacilli. It derives its name from the tendency of the organisms to vary from an almost coccal form to very long filaments (Proteus, a Greek god who often changed his shape).

Cultural properties

The chief peculiarity is a tendency to spread rapidly ('swarm') over the surface of moist solid media in a thin, transparent film. Other organisms in the culture become overgrown and are liable to be overlooked. Swarming can be prevented by using MacConkey medium or salt-free media. Some strains of *Proteus* do not swarm. All strains rapidly hydrolyse urea and cultures have a characteristic ammoniacal smell.

Subdivisions

Two species of *Proteus, Pr. mirabilis* and *Pr. vulgaris,* and two closely related urea-splitting organisms, *Morganella morgani (Pr. morgani)* and *Providencia rettgeri (Pr. rettgeri),* can be distinguished by biochemical reactions. *Pr. mirabilis,* the most common species, is usually sensitive to ampicillin.

On the basis of their O and H antigens strains of *Proteus* can be divided into numerous serological types. A similarity between certain *Proteus* O antigens and rickettsial antigens is the basis of the Weil-Felix test for typhus fever.

Infections

Proteus is primarily a free-living organism of soil and water. It is a frequent inhabitant of the intestinal tract. It can cause severe infections of the urinary tract and often colonizes wounds and bed sores. It is resistant to many of the commonly used antibiotics and is liable to cause superinfection during antibiotic therapy.

Other coliform organisms

Other species of coliform bacilli are frequently isolated from clinical specimens, e.g. species of *Enterobacter, Citrobacter, Serratia, Acinetobacter* and *Aeromonas.* In general they have much the same significance as *E. coli.* Some of the infections in hospital patients are severe. Multi-resistant strains are common. For most practical purposes the organisms can be referred to as 'coliforms', but full identification may be necessary when tracing outbreaks of hospital cross-infection.

Serratia marcescens has the unusual property that 10% of strains produce a bright red pigment which can cause red discoloration of food and the appearance of 'blood' in sputum or on babies' nappies.

Pseudomonas

The genus *Pseudomonas* consists of motile, non-lactose-fermenting, gram-negative bacilli. They differ from enterobacteria in their higher G + C content and in being strict aerobes which attack sugars by oxidation.

Pseudomonas aeruginosa (Ps. pyocyanea)

The most striking feature of *Ps. aeruginosa* is its ability to produce green discoloration of the medium. This is due to the production of two pigments: pyocyanin which is blue and fluorescin which is greenish-yellow. Pigment production is most abundant at room temperature. Growth occurs over a wide temperature range and some strains can multiply at 4°C. Cultures have a characteristic smell. On solid media the growth often has an irregularly distributed, iridescent, metallic sheen. Some strains produce highly mucoid colonies. Pyocyanin is a powerful antibiotic and other organisms in the culture tend to be killed.

Infections

Ps. aeruginosa is essentially a free-living species, but it sometimes parasitizes the intestinal tract. It rarely initiates infection, but it is a common cause of infection of burns, wounds and ulcers and may cause severe infections of the urinary tract, particularly following instrumentation. It occasionally causes meningitis. It is an important cause of respiratory tract infection in patients with cystic fibrosis. The pus in *Ps. aeruginosa* infections is often blue-green with a distinctive smell. The incidence of severe and generalized infections has increased markedly in recent years. The organism is a major pathogen in immunosuppressed patients. It is resistant to many antibiotics and is liable to cause super-infection during antibiotic therapy for other conditions. Many strains produce an exotoxin that inhibits protein synthesis and is probably responsible for necrotic lesions of the skin (ecthyma gangrenosum) found in generalized infections. Because of its simple growth requirements, ability to grow at room temperature and resistance to many disinfectants, *Ps. aeruginosa* is liable to survive and multiply in almost any moist situation (p. 194). It may contaminate swimming pools and whirlpools (Jacuzzis) and cause extensive rashes and otitis externa in people who bathe in them. It was quick to move in on the North Sea oil boom. It thrives in the pressurized chambers used as living quarters in saturation diving and has caused incapacitating otitis externa among the divers.

Other pseudomonads

Ps. mallei causes glanders, a disease of horses in Asia, Africa and parts of eastern Europe. It has been eradicated from western Europe and the UK. Human glanders is rare. Infection usually originates in the skin, but granulomatous and suppurative lesions later occur throughout the body. The disease is usually fatal if untreated.

Ps. pseudomallei is the cause of melioidosis, a rare highly lethal glanders-like disease occurring in south-east Asia. The organism lives in soil and water. Man acquires infection by inoculation through the skin, inhalation of dust or immersion in contaminated water. In the Vietnamese wars the organism was a common cause of wound infection. Some ex-servicemen developed melioidosis many years after leaving the endemic areas. Melioidosis occurs in various animals but there is little evidence that these are a source of human infection.

Other species of Pseudomonas. These include some important plant pathogens and various free-living organisms of soil and water. Pseudomonads of this sort are often isolated from clinical material and the hospital environment. They are opportunists of low pathogenicity and sometimes contaminate hospital equipment and medical fluids. *Ps. cepacia* has caused serious sepsis in hospital patients.

Vibrio

The genus *Vibrio* consists of gram-negative, motile, *curved* rods. It includes: (1) *V. cholerae*, the cause of cholera, (2) 'non-cholera vibrios' which sometimes cause disease in man, (3) halophilic vibrios, e.g. *V. parahaemolyticus*, and (4) saprophytic species found in water, soil and sewage.

Vibrio cholerae

The organisms which cause cholera can be classified into 'classical' and El Tor vibrios. The two groups differ in minor properties only. Vibrios can be divided into many serological types on the basis of their main O antigens. Classical and El Tor varieties of *V. cholerae* are characterized by possession of antigen O1.

Morphology

In the stools from cases of cholera and in freshly isolated cultures the organisms are short, curved ('comma-shaped') rods. Sometimes

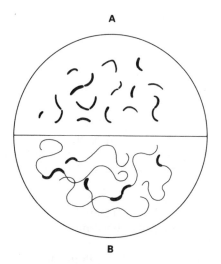

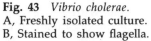

Fig. 43 *Vibrio cholerae.*
A, Freshly isolated culture.
B, Stained to show flagella.

two or three vibrios are attached end-to-end producing S-shaped and spiral forms. In subcultures the characteristic curvature may be largely lost and the organisms become straight rods indistinguishable from coliforms.

Cultural properties

V. cholerae can grow in strongly alkaline media which suppress the growth of many other bacteria. Preliminary incubation of faeces for 5—6 hours in alkaline peptone water and use of special selective media (such as thiosulphate-citrate-bilesalt-sucrose medium) facilitates isolation. Fermentation reactions and biochemical tests are used for provisional identification but many other vibrios show the same range of reactions.

Toxins

The copious outpouring of fluid from the intestinal tract which is characteristic of cholera depends on a potent protein enterotoxin. The toxin, which consists of two subunits, stimulates adenylate cyclase activity in the gut and produces an accumulation of cyclic adenosine monophosphate which causes the intestinal wall to secrete chloride and water into the lumen. *V. cholerae* produces various enzymes including a neuraminidase ('receptor destroying enzyme' or RDE) which breaks down the mucoprotein receptors by which certain viruses attach themselves to cells (p. 41). It has been suggested that motility and their neuraminidase enables

V. cholerae to gain access to the intestinal mucosal surface and initiate infection.

Cholera

Cholera is classically a violent infection of the intestinal tract, especially the small intestine, resulting in the almost incessant passage of thin 'rice-water' stools containing flakes of mucus and desquamated epithelial cells. General invasion of the body does not occur. Dehydration, collapse and toxaemia are marked features, and death may occur within a few hours of the onset of symptoms.

Patients often excrete the organisms for a few days during convalescence, but chronic carriers are rare. Healthy individuals in contact with a case (contact carriers) may become infected and excrete the organisms for some days without developing symptoms. Outside the body the life of the organism is usually short, but it is sometimes able to survive for 1–3 weeks in water.

Human faeces are the only source of *V. cholerae*. Cholera is spread by contaminated water, food, flies and by direct contact. In endemic areas there may be widespread contamination of the environment. The explosive outbreaks which in bygone years occurred in temperate climates were mainly water-borne, e.g. the epidemic of the Broad Street pump (1854) was correctly attributed by John Snow to an agent transmitted by contaminated water: the epidemic ceased when the pump handle was removed.

Cholera is endemic in parts of India, Pakistan, Bangladesh, China and other regions in the Far East. The Ganges delta is a particularly important endemic focus. Classical strains of *V. cholerae* have now become very rare and the El Tor vibrio, which was once a relatively unimportant cause of cholera, has in recent years caused extensive outbreaks with a high mortality. Outbreaks have occurred in the Middle East and in West Africa, a region where hitherto this century cholera had not been known to occur. In 1973 an epidemic in Naples resulted in over 100 confirmed cases with at least 12 deaths. It is unlikely that cholera could gain a widespread footing in western Europe but there are parts of Africa where there is little to stop the disease spreading rapidly.

Diagnosis

Numerous vibrios lying with their long axes parallel 'like fish in a stream' can be seen in films of mucus from a 'rice-water' stool. The organisms are identified by cultural and biochemical reactions and agglutination with *V. cholerae* O1 antiserum.

Agglutination reactions on the patient's serum are of little value since they do not become positive until convalescence.

Prevention

Cholera epidemics can occur only under conditions of poor hygiene. Purification of water supplies, safe disposal of sewage and hygienic handling of food are of prime importance. Active immunity can be provided by means of killed vaccines, but protection is limited and short-lived. Reinoculation is necessary every six months.

Treatment

Oral rehydration therapy (ORT) with a solution of sodium chloride and glucose ('a handful of sugar and pinch of salt') has saved the lives of thousands of victims of cholera and other diarrhoeal diseases. Antibiotics are largely irrelevant.

Other vibrios

Non-cholera vibrios ('non-O1 *V. cholerae*') cause limited outbreaks of diarrhoeal disease in tropical and subtropical countries. Occasionally the symptoms are severe and the illness resembles classical cholera. Over 80 serological types are recognized. Each type tends to have a limited geographical distribution.

V. parahaemolyticus causes food poisoning, particularly in the Far East where raw fish is a major item of diet. It is a marine organism and sea-food is invariably incriminated.

Yersinia

This genus consists of small, delicate, gram-negative rods. They are primarily parasites of animals in which they cause generalized infections. Man is an incidental host. The most important species is *Y. pestis*, the cause of plague.

Yersinia pestis

Morphology and culture

Y. pestis often shows bipolar staining. In material from lesions the organisms are seen as short, fat, ovoid bodies dark at the ends and almost clear in the centre (Fig. 44A, p. 290). The morphology may be less typical in cultures. In liquid cultures chain formation is common. In the tissues a thin capsule is formed, but this is not

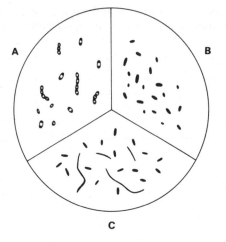

Fig. 44 Parvobacteria.
A, Yersinia pestis,
showing bipolar staining.
B, Brucella abortus.
C, Haemophilus influenzae.

seen in ordinary cultures. The organism grows slowly on most media including MacConkey agar. The colonies are not distinctive.

Antigens and toxins

Y. pestis has superficial envelope or capsular antigens and several somatic antigens. The organism produces a protein endotoxin which causes vascular damage and tissue necrosis.

Plague

Plague is a disease of rats and other rodents. Rats constitute the main reservoir of infection for man. Plague is transmitted from animal to animal by fleas, e.g. the rat flea, *Xenopsylla cheopis*. Just as rats are said to leave a sinking ship so rat fleas will leave a dying rat. If the rat is dying of plague the last feed will consist of rat blood swarming with *Y. pestis*. The organisms multiply inside the flea and are regurgitated and inoculated into a new host when the flea next feeds. Usually the victim will be another rat, but if no rat is available the flea will bite man.

Three clinical types of plague are recognized:

1 *Bubonic plague* is most common. Following the bite of an infected flea there is enlargement of the regional lymph nodes, most frequently the inguinal, to form the characteristic buboes. The blood is invaded and widespread infection results. This form of the disease is not readily transmitted from man to man.

2 *Pneumonic plague*. If in the course of bubonic plague the

organisms set up a focus of infection in the lungs the result is a rapidly spreading haemorrhagic bronchopneumonia. The sputum teems with *Y. pestis* and the patient is highly infectious. Case-to-case transmission of pneumonic plague occurs by droplet infection and rat fleas are not involved.

3 *Septicaemic plague.* There is early invasion of the blood. Involvement of lymph nodes and lungs is not an obvious feature.

Plague is typically a very severe disease with a high mortality, e.g. recovery from pneumonic plague is unusual. A mild ambulatory form of plague is also recognized. Plague occurs in epidemic and sporadic forms. Epidemics are preceded by an outbreak among rodents in one of the permanent endemic centres notably in India and also in parts of Asia, Africa and America. From time to time the disease has appeared in most countries. In England the Black Death of the fourteenth century was a pandemic of pneumonic plague. In countries where plague is endemic in wild rodents other than rats sporadic cases of infection in hunters and other workers in rural areas occur as a result of handling infected animals.

Diagnosis

Characteristic organisms are found in fluid aspirated from the bubo or in sputum from cases of pneumonic plague. They are identified by their cultural and biochemical properties, agglutination with specific antiserum, susceptibility to a specific phage, and inoculation of rats or guinea-pigs. Blood culture is of value in the early septicaemic stages.

Prevention

This depends on measures which reduce contact between rats and man, e.g. improvements in housing, domestic hygiene and refuse disposal; reduction of the rat population by poisons; preventing rats entering and leaving ships by rat-guards placed on hawsers and by fumigation; control of fleas with insecticides when epidemics threaten. Masks and protective clothing should be used when caring for cases of pneumonic plague. Killed or living attenuated vaccines can be used for active immunization.

Other yersiniae

Y. enterocolitica is an animal pathogen which not infrequently infects man causing fever, diarrhoea, abdominal pain, erythema nodosum and arthritis. Fatal cases have occurred. Pets and domestic animals are the usual source of infection but subsequent person-to-person spread may result in small outbreaks. Food-borne transmission has been described. Eating raw pork is particularly hazardous. The disease is diagnosed by isolating the organism from the faeces using selective media containing cefsulodin, novobiocin and triclosan and by detecting antibodies in the patient's serum.

Y. pseudotuberculosis may cause error in the diagnosis of plague in rats and in the diagnosis of tuberculosis in laboratory guinea-pigs. A few cases of human infection have been recorded. Involvement of the mesenteric lymph nodes with production of gastrointestinal symptoms is the most common finding. Severe septicaemic forms of the disease also occur.

Pasteurella

This genus consists of small gram-negative bacilli which closely resemble the yersiniae. They are primarily animal pathogens.

P. multocida consists of a number of varieties each adapted to different animal hosts in which they typically produce haemorrhagic septicaemia. In man localized infections frequently follow cat and dog bites. Infections of the respiratory tract are not uncommon. Severe generalized infections have been described.

P. haemolytica is an animal pathogen serologically distinct from *P. multocida*. It is sometimes responsible for infections of the human respiratory tract.

P. ureae sometimes causes respiratory tract infections.

Cardiobacterium hominis is a small pasteurella-like bacillus which occasionally causes endocarditis in man.

Francisella

F. tularensis is a small gram-negative bacillus. Freshly-isolated virulent strains have a capsule. The organism is the cause of tularaemia, a plague-like disease first observed in wild rodents in Tulare, California, and later recognized in other parts of the USA and in the USSR, Norway and Japan. Infection is transmitted to man by handling infected rabbits, hares, ground squirrels, etc., and by ticks and other blood-sucking insects. The organisms usually enter by the skin and produce a local ulcerative lesion and often a severe generalized infection.

Brucella

This genus consists of very small, very short, non-motile, non-capsulated, gram-negative coccobacilli (Fig. 44B, p. 290). They grow poorly on ordinary media and enriched media are necessary for isolation. Brucellae are primarily animal pathogens and man becomes infected as a result of contact with infected animals or their products. Three species are recognized:

1 *Br. abortus* infects cows and is by far the most common cause of human brucellosis (abortus or undulant fever) in the UK.
2 *Br. melitensis* infects goats and is common in Malta and other Mediterranean countries. It is the cause of Malta fever.
3 *Br. suis* infects pigs and is chiefly found in the USA, South America and Denmark.

All three species can cause natural infections in domestic animals other than those for which they have a special predilection.

Differential features

The three species are very similar and strains with intermediate properties are common. They are differentiated by their CO_2 requirements, H_2S production, oxidation of amino acids and sugars, sensitivity to dyes, phage sensitivity and antigenic properties. Each species is subdivided into varieties or biotypes. There are eight biotypes of *Br. abortus*, three biotypes of *Br. melitensis* and at least four of *Br. suis*. Most strains of *Br. abortus* isolated in the UK belong to biotype 1. The differences in antigenic structure are quantitative. *Br. abortus* contains a large amount of antigen A and a small amount of antigen M. *Br. melitensis* contains a large amount of M and a small amount of A. *Br. suis* is intermediate with a moderate excess of A. Brucellae readily undergo $S \rightarrow R$ variation with loss of A and M antigens and emergence of a common rough antigen. The three species are serologically indistinguishable in this state.

Infections

In cows and goats brucellae are responsible for contagious abortion. The organisms later localize in the mammary glands and are often excreted in the milk for long periods. They are also excreted in the uterine discharges, faeces and urine. In pigs, genital and mammary gland involvement may occur but silent infections are common.

Human brucellosis is mostly found among farmers, veterinary surgeons and others who work with infected animals. The organisms gain access through abrasions in the skin and through the alimentary tract, but mainly through the respiratory tract. In the general population infection is usually due to close contact with infected animals and rarely to consumption of raw milk, i.e. unpasteurized cow's milk in rural areas of the UK and goat's milk in Mediterranean countries. Veterinary surgeons are often infected with the S19 vaccine strain. Infection from laboratory cultures is not uncommon.

In its most characteristic form human brucellosis is a long-continued bacteraemic state with a remittent 'undulant' fever. The organisms multiply inside the cells of the reticuloendothelial system producing a granulomatous reaction. The liver, spleen and lymph nodes are frequently enlarged. The relative inaccessibility of the organisms probably explains why the disease often persists for many months despite high levels of antibodies, why chemotherapy is often ineffective and why relapses are common. Subclinical infections and chronic low-grade infections with minimal symptoms are common.

Diagnosis

Repeated attempts should be made to isolate the organisms by blood culture. The results are often negative. Brucellae can sometimes be grown from bone marrow or lymph nodes when blood cultures are negative. The organisms are intermittently excreted in the urine and urine culture should not be omitted. All cultures should be incubated in an atmosphere of $5-10\%$ CO_2 as this is essential for primary isolation of *Br. abortus*.

In acute brucellosis antibodies can usually be detected by agglutination, complement fixation and antiglobulin tests. The standard test is the agglutination reaction using suspensions of *Br. abortus* and *Br. melitensis*. Interpretation is difficult when the titres are low, e.g. 80 or less. Inhibition of agglutination at high serum concentrations (prozone phenomenon) is common (Fig. 25, p. 116). IgM antibodies are mainly responsible for agglutination.

In chronic brucellosis little or no IgM is produced and the agglutination reaction is often negative. The diagnosis can usually be made by means of the complement fixation and antiglobulin tests. These two tests detect IgG and IgA antibodies which are relatively ineffective in causing agglutination.

In some cases of acute or chronic brucellosis all the conventional tests are negative. In such cases antibodies can be measured by radioimmunoassay of IgM, IgG and IgA. If radioimmunoassay tests are negative the diagnosis of brucellosis can be excluded.

Prevention

Brucellosis can be eradicated from animals by testing them and slaughtering positive reactors. Immunization of animals with a living attenuated vaccine (S19) has also been of value. Most herds of cattle in the UK are now free from infection, but *all* milk should be pasteurized.

Haemophilus

This genus consists of tiny, non-motile, aerobic, gram-negative coccobacilli which require one or both of two accessory growth substances which can be provided by blood:

X factor is haematin. It is provided by blood agar but not by nutrient agar.

V factor is nicotinamide adenine dinucleotide. It is provided in small quantities by blood agar but not by ordinary nutrient agar. It is present in yeast and vegetable extracts and is produced by most bacteria. Some bacteria such as *Staphylococcus aureus* excrete relatively large amounts into the medium.

Haemophilus influenzae

This organism is a commensal in the throat of most healthy people. It is associated with infections of the respiratory tract and has been particularly incriminated as the cause of acute exacerbations in chronic bronchitis. It is not the cause of influenza but is sometimes a secondary invader in this disease which is due to a virus. It can cause sinusitis, otitis media and, mainly in young children, acute epiglottitis which may produce respiratory obstruction. It is an important cause of meningitis in young children. Sometimes it causes septic arthritis. Rarely it may cause infective endocarditis.

Morphology

Coccobacilli predominate but characteristically a few long bacilli and filamentous forms are present (Fig. 44C, p. 290). Filaments are particularly common in strains causing meningitis. Virulent strains isolated from the cerebrospinal fluid possess capsules.

Cultural properties

It requires X and V factors and will not grow on nutrient agar. On blood agar after incubation for 24 hours the colonies are usually minute clear domes barely visible to the naked eye. Growth is better on heated blood ('chocolate') agar and on media containing a peptic digest of blood. Virulent capsulated strains produce smooth mucoid colonies with a characteristic iridescence. Noncapsulated strains, such as those commonly isolated from the throat, produce small rough colonies which are not iridescent.

In mixed cultures *H. influenzae* can often be detected by the fact that the colonies are bigger, or only appear at all, in the immediate neighbourhood of colonies of *Staph. aureus*. This phenomenon is known as *satellitism* (Fig. 45) and is due to production of V factor by the staphylococci. It is a valuable method of identification. *Staph. aureus* can be streaked across routine blood agar culture plates before incubation when it is thought that *H. influenzae* may be present.

Subdivisions

Smooth, capsulated strains can be differentiated into six types (a—f) on the basis of differences in their capsular polysaccharides as determined by agglutination or capsule-swelling reactions. Type b is responsible for nearly all cases of meningitis. It also causes acute obstructive laryngotracheitis and epiglottitis. Type b is not often found in the respiratory tract of healthy individuals, but a high carrier rate is common in families of patients with meningitis. Most strains from healthy subjects and patients with chronic bronchitis are rough, non-capsulated and non-typable.

Toxic products

H. influenzae produces several toxic substances which may aid colonization of the respiratory tract, including histamine, an IgA1 protease and a factor which causes slowing and incoordination of ciliary beating.

Haemophilus ducreyi

H. ducreyi is the cause of chancroid (soft sore or soft chancre), a sexually transmitted disease which may be confused with syphilis. The organism is found in exudate from the genital sore and in pus from infected inguinal lymph nodes (buboes). It is also

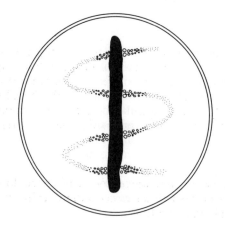

Fig. 45 Satellitism. The vertical streak is *Staphylococcus aureus* and the zig-zag streak *Haemophilus influenzae*.

sometimes found as a secondary invader in other types of genital ulceration, e.g. genital herpes. In stained films the bacteria are characteristically arranged in parallel rows. The organism can be grown on special supplemented 'chocolate' agar incubated in air with $5-10\%$ CO_2. It requires X factor but not V factor. Intact colonies can be pushed around on the surface of solid media. Agglutination with a specific serum is used in identification.

Other species of Haemophilus

H. aegyptius (Koch-Weeks bacillus) is a cause of acute contagious conjunctivitis. It is probably identical with *H. influenzae*.

H. parainfluenzae closely resembles *H. influenzae* but does not require X factor. It is a common respiratory tract commensal and has been isolated occasionally in infective endocarditis.

H. haemolyticus requires X and V factor and *H. parahaemolyticus* requires V factor only. They are frequently found in the respiratory tract. The colonies on blood agar are haemolytic and may be confused with those of β-haemolytic streptococci.

H. aphrophilus (requires X factor) and *H. paraphrophilus* (requires V factor) are respiratory tract commensals and rare causes of endocarditis.

Bordetella

The genus *Bordetella* consists of tiny gram-negative coccobacilli. It differs from *Haemophilus* in that the organisms do not require X or V factors.

Bordetella pertussis

B. pertussis is the causative organism of whooping cough. It is found in the exudates of the upper respiratory tract in whooping cough and later in the lung lesions which often complicate this disease. In contrast to *H. influenzae* it is not found in the healthy throat. An illness clinically indistinguishable from whooping cough is sometimes caused by viruses, particularly adenoviruses.

Morphology

It closely resembles *H. influenzae*, but filamentous forms are seldom seen in young cultures. Freshly isolated strains possess thin capsules which are readily lost on subculture.

Culture

An enriched medium containing blood is needed for primary isolation. The blood is believed to neutralize toxic substances in the medium and is not primarily important as a source of nutrient factors. Charcoal blood agar with added cephalexin or the blood-potato-glycerol agar of Bordet and Gengou are very satisfactory. After incubation for 3 or 4 days the colonies are small, about 0.5 mm diameter, have a characteristic sheen and stand up from the medium like half pearls or droplets of mercury. Areas of confluent growth resemble streaks of aluminium paint.

Antigenic properties

Freshly isolated virulent smooth (phase 1) strains share a common antigen and are all agglutinated by the same antiserum. Other antigens are variable and several serotypes of the organism are distinguished. Subculture results in progressive loss of antigens. These rough variants are no longer agglutinated by specific antiserum and are of low virulence and low toxicity. Of particular importance, they lack the antigens necessary for production of effective vaccines.

Diagnosis

Organisms for culture are best obtained by means of a *pernasal swab* consisting of a small pledget of cotton-wool on a flexible wire. The swab is passed along the floor of the nasal passages to sample the nasopharynx and is plated out immediately on charcoal blood agar or Bordet-Gengou medium. If delay is inevitable the swab should be sent to the laboratory in special pertussis transport medium. The *cough plate* method in which a culture plate is exposed directly in front of the child's mouth during a paroxysm of coughing is less reliable but does not distress the patient.

Fluorescent antibody staining has been used for rapid identification of B. pertussis in smears of secretions.

Prevention

Vaccines prepared from killed virulent phase 1 organisms give a high degree of protection.

Bordetella parapertussis

B. parapertussis is responsible for a mild form of whooping cough. It closely resembles B. pertussis but is less fastidious in its growth requirements. The two species have some antigens in common, but B. parapertussis possesses specific surface antigens.

Moraxella

M. lacunata (Morax-Axenfeld bacillus) is the cause of angular conjunctivitis. It is a small gram-negative bacillus which tends to grow end-to-end in pairs. Growth is best on serum media: characteristically the colonies are surrounded by small pits, *lacunae,* due to liquefaction of the serum. It grows poorly on blood agar and not at all on simple nutrient agar.

Bartonella

The genus *Bartonella* consists of minute, motile, gram-negative bacilli which are parasites *inside* the red blood cells and reticulo-endothelial cells of various animal species.

B. *bacilliformis* is a human pathogen peculiar to mountainous regions of Peru and neighbouring countries. It is the cause of Oroya fever, a severe and often fatal form of acute, febrile, haemolytic anaemia, and of verruga peruviana, a relatively benign nodular skin eruption occurring in individuals who have developed some immunity. Infection is transmitted by night-feeding sand-flies and insecticides are effective in prevention. No other bacterium is ever found inside human red cells and the appearance of blood films is diagnostic (Fig. 46A). It can be cultivated from the blood using special semi-solid media.

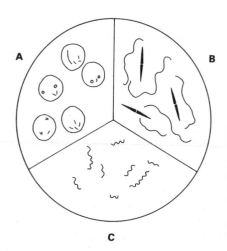

Fig. 46 Miscellaneous gram-negative bacilli.
A, *Bartonella bacilliformis* inside red blood cells.
B, *Leptotrichia buccalis* and spirochaetes (*Borrelia vincenti*) in a film from a case of Vincent's angina.
C, *Spirillum minus.*

Bacteroides group

This group consists of a large and heterogeneous collection of *anaerobic*, non-sporing, gram-negative bacilli. They are parasites of the intestinal tract and other mucous membranes of man and animals. They are very pleomorphic, and organisms which are fusiform (spindle-shaped) in direct films may be filamentous or coliform in culture. On blood agar the colonies are usually very small and may not appear for several days. Classification is mainly based on biochemical properties. Three genera are distinguished: *Bacteroides* in which the bacilli usually have rounded ends and *Fusobacterium* and *Leptotrichia* in which the bacilli are usually fusiform with pointed ends.

Bacteroides

Organisms of this genus are the predominant bacteria in the lower part of the intestinal tract where strict anaerobes, mainly *Bacteroides*, outnumber aerobes and facultative anaerobes, such as *E. coli*, by as much as 1000 to one. *Bacteroides* are found in smaller numbers in the mouth and vagina. They are frequently isolated, usually in association with other organisms, from cases of acute appendicitis, pelvic inflammatory disease and puerperal sepsis and from suppurative, necrotic and gangrenous lesions elsewhere in the body. In severe infections they can often be recovered from the blood. *Bacteroides* are by far the commonest cause of anaerobic infections in man, though by themselves the organisms are usually of low pathogenicity. Many species have been described of which *B. fragilis* is the most commonly encountered. Anaerobic infections are typically associated with the presence of foul-smelling pus. Gas-liquid chromatography will identify volatile products and can be used for the immediate detection of anaerobes in pus and for identification of organisms recovered in culture.

Fusobacterium

This genus consists of a miscellaneous collection of fusiform bacilli which are normal inhabitants of the upper respiratory and intestinal tracts. *F. necrophorum* is one of the more pathogenic species. It is often isolated from necrotic lesions.

Leptotrichia

L. buccalis (*Fusobacterium fusiforme*) is a long, slender fusiform bacillus pointed at both ends (Fig. 46B, p. 299). It differs from fusobacteria in its metabolic properties. It is a normal commensal of the mouth and intestinal tract. Together with the spirochaete *Borrelia vincenti* it is found in the lesions of Vincent's angina and in ulcerative and necrotic processes in other parts of the body.

Capnocytophaga

C. ochracea belongs to a genus of motile gram-negative 'gliding bacteria'. On solid media they show gliding movements associated with rapid flexing of the cells. Added carbon dioxide is essential for growth and isolation. *C. ochracea* is a normal inhabitant of the gum margins. It has been isolated in large numbers from the lesions of ulcerative gingivitis. Septicaemic states may occur in patients with neutropenia.

Streptobacillus

S. moniliformis is a commensal of the respiratory tract of rats. It causes one variety of rat-bite fever (the other is caused by *Spirillum minus*, see below). The illness is characterized by fever, rashes and polyarthritis. On rare occasions outbreaks have been caused by ingestion of contaminated milk or food (Haverhill fever: Haverhill, Mass., USA). The organism can be isolated from the blood. It is aerobic, slow-growing and requires blood or serum. It is highly pleomorphic and may appear in the form of bacilli, long filaments, chains of bacilli or cocci, large oval or round bodies resembling yeasts, and minute L-forms. The L-forms are found in minute colonies distinct from the normal colonies.

Spirillum

This is a genus of highly motile, spiral gram-negative rods. They resemble spirochaetes but are in fact closely related to the vibrios. Unlike spirochaetes the organisms are rigid and owe their motility to terminal flagella. Most species are free-living in soil and water. One species, *S. minus*, is a parasite of the respiratory tract of rats and causes one variety of rat-bite fever (another variety is caused by *Streptobacillus moniliformis*, see above). *S. minus* is 2–5 μm long and usually shows 2 or 3 spirals (Fig. 46C, p. 299). It cannot be cultured. It can sometimes be demonstrated in the local lesions by dark-ground illumination or by ordinary stains, but diagnosis is more readily achieved by inoculating blood into a guinea-pig or mouse and detecting the spirilla in their blood after 1–2 weeks.

Campylobacter

This genus consists of highly motile, gram-negative, *curved* rods. Spiral, S-shaped and seagull-like forms are common (Fig. 47A). The organisms are microaerophilic, i.e. grow best at reduced oxygen tensions.

C. *jejuni*, C. *coli* and other 'thermophilic' campylobacters are a common cause of gastroenteritis in man. Family outbreaks may occur and children are especially liable to be affected. Infection is occasionally associated with urticarial rashes. In most outbreaks the source of infection is unknown. Large milk-borne outbreaks have been associated with inefficient pasteurization. Water-borne outbreaks have occurred. A hospital outbreak of campylobacter meningitis in newborn babies has been described. Campylobacters have been isolated from a wide variety of animals and birds, both wild and domestic. Human infection is sometimes acquired from dogs. Poultry frequently excrete campylobacters and are an important reservoir of infection. Campylobacters can be isolated from the faeces by using selective media containing vancomycin, polymyxin and trimethoprim and by incubating at 43°C in an atmosphere containing 5% oxygen and added carbon dioxide. Some strains of C. *jejuni* produce a heat-labile enterotoxin which resembles the enterotoxin of *Vibrio cholerae*.

C. *fetus* causes abortion in sheep and cattle. Human infection is rare and usually presents as a pyrexial illness. The diagnosis is most often made by finding the organism in blood cultures. Occasionally infection localizes in the meninges, joints or the developing fetus.

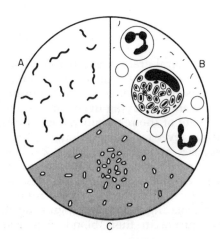

Fig. 47 Miscellaneous gram-negative bacilli. A, *Campylobacter jejuni*. B, *Calymmatobacterium granulomatis* ('Donovan bodies') inside macrophage. C, *Legionella pneumophila* stained with fluorescent antibody.

C. pylori ('campylobacter-like organisms') are found in large numbers on the gastric epithelium in patients with gastritis. They may contribute to the pathogenesis of duodenal ulcers.

Calymmatobacterium

C. granulomatis (*Donovania granulomatis*) is responsible for granuloma inguinale (not to be confused with lymphogranuloma venereum), a sexually transmitted disease prevalent in tropical and subtropical countries. It causes a chronic ulcerative condition involving the genitalia, perineum and groins. Films from the lesions show short, capsulated gram-negative bacilli (*Donovan bodies*) within mononuclear cells (Fig. 47B). The organisms fail to grow on ordinary media, but growth can be obtained in the yolk sac of the chick embryo.

Legionella

L. pneumophila is the cause of legionnaires' disease, a severe respiratory illness first recognized in 1976 when there was an outbreak among those attending a convention of the American Legion in Philadelphia. The organism is a tiny motile gram-negative coccobacillus (Fig. 47C). It fails to grow on ordinary media but it can be isolated on special media supplemented with iron and cysteine. The colonies take several days to develop. It can also be isolated by inoculation of guinea-pigs. *L. pneumophila* can be identified by immunofluorescent tests. At least ten serogroups of the organism are recognized. Gas-liquid chromatography of fatty acids extracted from the organism gives a characteristic profile rich in branched-chain acids.

L. pneumophila normally lives in soil and water. Human infection is acquired by inhalation of contaminated aerosols from such sources as the water of air-conditioning systems and shower units. A few outbreaks have been associated with whirlpools (Jacuzzis). *L. pneumophila* is found in up to 75% of water cooling systems. Patients who have had major surgery for head and neck cancer have a high incidence of legionella pneumonia, presumably from aspiration of contaminated water. The organism has been isolated from water from dental equipment such as high speed drills and mouth sprays but there is no evidence that these sources have caused infection. Stagnation and temperatures between 20 and 45°C favour colonization. Free-living amoebae readily ingest legionellae and may be important in ensuring the survival of legionellae in water and their subsequent transmission to man. Many outbreaks have originated in hospitals and hotels. A large outbreak at Stafford District General Hospital in 1985 caused 28 deaths. It was probably due to contamination caused by a fault in the design of the ventilation system in the out-patients department. Case-to-case spread of infection does not occur. Legionnaires' disease usually takes the form of severe pneumonia but patients may present with diarrhoea or mental confusion. In the early stages of the disease it is usually possible to demonstrate the organism in respiratory secretions by staining with fluorescent antibodies or by culture. Blood cultures are often positive if suitable media are used. Confirmatory diagnosis is made by means of an indirect fluorescent antibody test on the patient's serum. Non-pneumonic legionellosis (Pontiac fever) may present as a mild respiratory illness. Endocarditis has been described. Subclinical legionellosis is common.

Organisms which are distinct from *L. pneumophila* but resemble it closely ('atypical legionella-like organisms') are also associated with the production of pneumonia in man. Most of them have at some time been isolated from water. They include other species of *Legionella* such as *L. micdadei* ('Pittsburgh pneumonia agent'), a weakly acid-fast bacillus which has caused pneumonia in patients undergoing immunosuppressive therapy.

Spirochaetes

A shepherd once (distrust not ancient Fame)
Possest these Downs and Syphilus *his Name.*

. . . .

And first th'offending Syphilus *was griev'd*
Who rais'd forbidden Altars on the Hill. . .
                                    Fracastorius, 1530

Spirochaetes are thin, spiral, motile, flexible bacteria. Their motility is due to a combination of corkscrew-like and bending movements. They are structurally more complex than ordinary bacteria. Electron microscopy has shown that most of them possess a number of fine filaments anchored to the two poles of the organism and twisted round the cytoplasm in a helical fashion between the cytoplasmic membrane and the outer cell wall. Spirochaetes are thinner than other bacteria and stain poorly with ordinary dyes. If they can be persuaded to take the stains at all they are gram-negative. They can usually be stained by Giemsa or Leishman stains. Silver impregnation methods can be used to demonstrate them in tissue sections. For most purposes spirochaetes are best seen in wet preparations examined under dark-ground illumination. The pathogenic spirochaetes are assigned to three genera, *Borrelia, Leptospira* and *Treponema*.

Borrelia

Borreliae tend to be relatively large and thick and can usually be stained by Gram's method. Their spirals are looser, wider and more irregular than those found in the genus *Treponema*. The wavelength of the spirals is usually 2–3 μm. Borreliae are extremely difficult to culture on artifical media.

Borrelia vincenti

B. vincenti (Treponema vincenti) is 5–10 μm long with 2–5 loose, irregular spirals. It is often accompanied by a fusiform bacillus,

Leptotrichia buccalis. The two organisms are present in small numbers around the gum margins of most normal individuals. They are found in large numbers in the lesions of Vincent's angina, an ulcerative condition of the mouth and throat, in acute gingivitis, in necrotic lesions of the throat such as occur in infectious mononucleosis, and sometimes in gangrene of the lung and ulcerative and gangrenous lesions of the skin. Diagnosis of Vincent's infection (fusospirochaetal disease) depends on finding large numbers of the two organisms in stained films (Fig. 46B, p. 299).

Borrelia recurrentis

B. recurrentis is a human parasite and is the cause of European louse-borne relapsing fever. It is 10–20 μm long with 5–10 loose, irregular spirals (Fig. 48A). The disease is transmitted by the human body louse, *Pediculus humanus*. The louse becomes infected when it feeds on the blood of a human host. At first it cannot transmit infection, but after a few days spirochaetes appear in the body cavity and can be transmitted to a new host if the louse is crushed near a bite or an abrasion. There is no known animal reservoir of infection. Epidemics are associated with cold, over-crowding, famine and war, i.e. conditions which favour human lousiness. Louse-borne typhus fever may occur concomitantly.

Relapsing fever is characterized by bouts of fever lasting 2–6 days, separated by afebrile intervals of a week or so. Each relapse represents the emergence of a new antigenic type of organism. There may be as many as ten relapses before the repertoire of the spirochaete is exhausted.

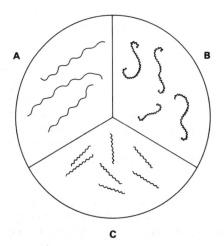

Fig. 48   Spirochaetes.
A, *Borrelia recurrentis*.
B, *Leptospira interrogans*.
C, *Treponema pallidum*.

Diagnosis is made during the febrile period by demonstrating the spirochaetes in blood films stained by Giemsa or Leishman stains, by examining fresh preparations by dark-ground illumination, or by inoculating mice and rats and detecting the organisms in their blood after 48 hours.

Borrelia duttoni

This spirochaete is the cause of African tick-borne relapsing fever. It closely resembles *B. recurrentis*. It is found in various species of ticks. The spirochaetes are transmitted from one generation of ticks to the next. Wild rodents probably constitute an additional reservoir of infection. The tick transmits infection to man by biting or by contamination of the bite wound with infected secretions. Tick-borne relapsing fever is mainly a sporadic disease.

Other borreliae

Borreliae not clearly distinguishable from *B. recurrentis* and *B. duttoni* cause relapsing fever in various parts of the world. Other species occur as human commensals in the mouth and on the genital mucous membranes.

Lyme disease (Lyme: a small community, Conn., USA) is a tick-borne spirochaetal illness with fever, a characteristic rash (erythema chronicum migrans), chronic meningitis and recurrent arthritis. The disease is not uncommon in the UK. Spirochaetes (*B. burgdorferi*) can be isolated from skin lesions, blood and cerebrospinal fluid (CSF) and from the ticks. Deer are an important reservoir of infection. Antibodies against *B. burgdorferi* can be detected by an immunofluorescent test.

Leptospira

Spirochaetes of the genus *Leptospira* are 5–20 μm long, 0.1–0.2 μm wide and have a large number of spirals with a wavelength of about 0.5 μm. The spirals are so tightly coiled that at first sight the organism looks like a chain of granules. Characteristically one or both ends of the organism are bent in the form of a hook (Fig. 48B). Leptospirae, unlike borreliae and the pathogenic treponemas, can be cultured fairly readily on media containing serum. Suspensions can therefore be obtained for serological investigation.

The genus can be subdivided into two species: *L. biflexa* consists of saprophytic and non-pathogenic strains and *L. interrogans* consists of parasitic and pathogenic strains. *L. interrogans* strains can be classified into over 160 serotypes (serovars), many of which show antigenic overlap. Serotypes with important antigens in common are grouped together in 16 serogroups.

Leptospirae are parasites of cattle, pigs, dogs and a wide variety of wild animals, particularly rodents. Man is an occasional host. Human leptospirosis takes many clinical forms including Weil's disease, a syndrome that can be caused by various serotypes.

Leptospirosis

Leptospirae belonging to the Icterohaemorrhagiae serogroup (serotypes *copenhageni, icterohaemorrhagiae*, etc.) are of worldwide distribution and are responsible for most of the more serious infections in the UK. A high proportion of wild rats harbour the organisms in their kidneys and are the main reservoirs of infection. The animals usually suffer little harm and excrete the organisms in their urine for life. Dogs are occasionally infected. The spirochaetes can survive for several weeks in water and damp soil. Leptospirosis is an occupational disease of farm-workers, sewer-workers, miners, fish-cleaners, workers on fish farms and others who come into close contact with rats. Infection can also be acquired by watersport enthusiasts from immersion in infected canals, rivers and lakes. The organisms probably enter through abrasions of the skin and through the conjunctiva and mucous membranes of the nose and mouth.

The Hebdomadis serogroup (serotypes *hardjo, sejroe*, etc.) is also an important cause of leptospirosis in the UK. The organisms tend to cause a less serious illness than the Icterohaemorrhagiae serogroup. Infection is usually acquired from cattle. Serotype *hardjo* has become the commonest serotype infecting farmers.

The Canicola serogroup (serotype *canicola*, etc.) is the cause of most other cases of leptospirosis in the UK. The organisms are particularly liable to cause meningitis. Infection is acquired from dogs.

Other serotypes characterized by their antigenic properties, host range and limited geographical distribution cause human leptospirosis in various parts of the world, e.g. *grippotyphosa* in central Europe, *sejroe* in Denmark, *hebdomadis* in Japan and *pomona* in Australia.

Weil's disease classically takes the form of an acute illness with fever, conjunctivitis, albuminuria, haemorrhages and jaundice. Renal failure often occurs. Some patients develop meningitis. However, cases of leptospirosis with no jaundice and mild symptoms are common, e.g. patients may present with an influenza-like illness or a pyrexia of obscure origin. Many cases can be recognized only by serological means.

Diagnosis

In the first week the organisms can occasionally be demonstrated in the blood by dark-ground microscopy, but diagnosis is more readily achieved by culture on special media or by intraperitoneal inoculation of a guinea-pig. The animal becomes jaundiced and usually dies within 14 days. The organisms can be demonstrated in the peritoneal fluid, blood, liver or spleen.

In the second week the organisms can often be demonstrated in the urine by dark-ground microscopy or guinea-pig inoculation. It is important to render the urine alkaline as the spirochaetes rapidly disintegrate in acid urine.

Serological tests are of great value. Antibodies appear towards the end of the second week and can be detected by a genus-specific complement fixation test using antigens from a *L. biflexa* strain and various pathogenic serotypes. Identification of the serotype causing infection is made by agglutination reactions using suspensions of spirochaetes. The titre is highest against the infecting organism.

Treponema

The important spirochaetes of the genus *Treponema* are extremely slender and have small, sharp, *regular* spirals with a wavelength of about 1 μm. The genus includes the human pathogens *Tr. pallidum*, *Tr. pertenue* and *Tr. carateum*, none of which can be cultured on laboratory media, and non-pathogenic species present in the mouth and around the genitalia, most of which can be cultured.

Treponema pallidum

Tr. pallidum is an exclusively human pathogen and is the causative agent of syphilis.

Morphology

It is a thin, spiral organism, 6−12 μm long and less than 0.2 μm wide, with 6−12 regular spirals (Fig. 48C, p. 306). In wet preparations examined under dark-ground illumination it shows a rapid corkscrew motion and periodic angular bending of the body. Its progression is relatively slow. It cannot be gram-stained but will take Giemsa stain and can be demonstrated in tissue sections by silver impregnation methods.

Culture

Despite claims to the contrary, *Tr. pallidum* cannot be cultured on artificial media. Under experimental conditions it can infect apes and rabbits. Serial propagation in the testis of the rabbit is used to prepare suspensions of the organism.

Syphilis

Shortly after Columbus returned from the New World a new disease (syphilis) appeared in Europe and spread with devastating effects. Although the evidence is meagre it is believed that his crew acquired the disease in the West Indies and brought it back to the Old World. In the course of the next century syphilis lost most of its original extraordinary virulence.

Syphilis is nearly always acquired by sexual intercourse. The primary lesion, an indurated ulcer known as the *primary chancre* ('hard chancre'), appears 9—90 days after infection. It is usually on the genitalia but may occur in the mouth, in the rectum or on a finger. Although the lesion is localized, spirochaetes are already widely distributed throughout the body. They probably begin to leave the site of inoculation within a few hours of infection.

The secondary stage begins in 6—12 weeks and takes the form of rashes, lesions of the mucous membranes and painless enlargement of the lymph nodes.

The tertiary stage is often delayed for several years. It is characterized by chronic inflammatory lesions (gummas) which involve the cardiovascular system, brain, skin, internal organs and bones.

Late manifestations of syphilis are degeneration of the spinal cord (tabes dorsalis) and brain (general paralysis of the insane).

Non-venereal syphilis is uncommon. The spirochaete is very susceptible to drying and light and soon dies when outside the body. It is rare for infection to be conveyed by contaminated articles. The lesions of secondary syphilis are highly infectious and the disease is sometimes acquired by close contact with a patient in this stage. The most important type of non-venereal syphilis is congenital syphilis in which the disease is acquired *in utero* from an infected mother.

The human race has limited resistance to *Tr. pallidum* and it is doubtful if the tissues can ever rid themselves of spirochaetes without assistance from chemotherapy. A person suffering from syphilis shows some immunity, e.g. a fresh dose of spirochaetes is unlikely to produce a fresh primary sore. However, the degree of immunity is slight and a person who has been cured can contract a second infection.

Diagnosis of syphilis

The clinical diagnosis is confirmed by demonstrating the spirochaete in the early stages of the disease and by serological tests for syphilis (STS) in later stages.

Demonstration of the spirochaete

Juice is expressed from the primary chancre (p. 172) and examined by dark-ground illumination. Non-pathogenic spirochaetes are sometimes present, but are usually thicker and more irregular than *Tr. pallidum* or show a different type of motility. Some resemble it closely and great experience is needed for differentiation. Spirochaetes can also be found in the lesions of secondary syphilis. In later stages the organisms are very scanty and only prolonged special investigation of post-mortem material is likely to reveal them in gummas or the lesions of late neurosyphilis.

Serological tests using cardiolipin antigens

The particular antibody concerned, often referred to as 'reagin', can be measured by the Wassermann reaction, which is a complement fixation reaction, or by one of several very similar 'flocculation' (precipitation) reactions such as the VDRL test.

Wassermann reaction (WR). Since *Tr. pallidum* could not be grown in culture it occurred to Wassermann in 1906 that an extract of the liver of a fetus with congenital syphilis might provide sufficient spirochaetes to act as the antigen in a complement fixation test. The test was an immediate success. In fact Wassermann was lucky because shortly afterwards the theoretical basis of the WR was shown to be untenable: the test would work just as well with extracts of normal liver or extracts of many other tissues. It is now known that the WR depends on a chance similarity between a normal tissue lipid (a hapten) and a lipid present in *Tr. pallidum*. The lipid can be obtained by ethanol extraction of bovine heart muscle and is available in a purified form known as *cardiolipin*. In practice the 'antigen' used consists of cardiolipin together with suitable proportions of lecithin and cholesterol. The WR, probably the best known serological test of all time, is now obsolete because flocculation tests have proved to be simpler, quicker, cheaper and slightly more sensitive.

Venereal disease research laboratory (VDRL) test. The antigen consists of a colloidal suspension of cardiolipin antigen. A positive serum causes aggregation of the particles and flocculation. The test is usually performed on a slide. By adding carbon particles to the system the result can be read by naked eye. The VDRL test is of value as a rapid screening test for examining large numbers of sera and is the preferred flocculation test in most laboratories. The test should be carried out quantitatively.

Other flocculation tests. These include the *rapid plasma reagin (RPR) card test* and the *Kahn test*.

Results of tests. Positive reactions to tests using cardiolipin antigens begin to appear 2—4 weeks after the appearance of the chancre and by the secondary stage virtually all cases are positive. In tertiary and late syphilis 10—20% of cases give negative reactions. In most cases the reaction becomes negative as a result of treatment. A persistent negative reaction indicates a cure. In cases showing central nervous system involvement antibodies appear in the CSF as well as in the blood. A positive reaction is obtained with the CSF of all cases of general paralysis and most cases of meningovascular syphilis; the reaction is often negative in tabes dorsalis.

Positive reactions are also obtained in yaws, pinta and bejel, which are caused by treponemas closely related to *Tr. pallidum*. So-called 'biological false positive reactions' may occur in malaria, leprosy, infectious mononucleosis, pregnancy and the acute stages of various infectious diseases. In most cases the positive reaction is a temporary phenomenon. Persistent false positive reactions are not common but are often associated with serious conditions such as systemic lupus erythematosus and other auto-immune diseases.

Serological tests using treponemal antigens

By using antigens obtained from spirochaetes a number of highly specific tests have been developed.

Treponema pallidum haemagglutination assay (TPHA). The patient's serum is allowed to react with a suspension of formalinized tanned sheep red cells coated with antigens obtained from *Tr. pallidum*. Syphilitic antibodies cause agglutination of the red cells. The TPHA test is easily performed and is the most suitable specific test for examining large numbers of sera in a general diagnostic laboratory. False positive reactions are occasionally encountered.

Fluorescent treponemal antibody (FTA) test. A smear of killed *Tr. pallidum* is incubated in the presence of the patient's diluted serum. The slide is then washed thoroughly and treated with a fluorescent anti-human globulin serum. If human anti-treponemal globulins have become attached to the treponemal antigens they can be detected by examining the film microscopically for fluorescence in ultraviolet light. In practice the test is complicated by the fact that most normal sera contain low titres of group-reactive anti-treponemal antibodies which react with *Tr. pallidum* to give positive results. However, antibodies specific for *Tr. pallidum* can be detected by making suitable dilutions of the serum or by using special techniques to absorb the group-reactive antibodies. The *absorbed FTA (FTA-ABS) test* is a sensitive and relatively simple test.

Treponema pallidum immobilization (TPI) test. A living suspension of *Tr. pallidum* obtained from infected rabbit testis is incubated under anaerobic conditions, in the presence of complement and the patient's serum, and observed under dark-ground illumination. If the serum contains syphilitic antibodies the spirochaetes are rendered non-motile. Traces of penicillin or other antibiotics in the patient's blood interfere with the test. The procedure is technically difficult.

Reiter protein complement fixation (RPCF) test. This test resembles the WR but the antigen consists of a protein extracted from the Reiter strain of non-pathogenic treponemas. The test is sometimes used as a routine screening procedure.

Results of tests. These are highly specific for treponemal infection When patients give positive reactions with cardiolipin antigen tests but show no clinical evidence of syphilis, tests with treponemal antigens will distinguish latent syphilis from non-specific conditions. The RPCF test, which mainly measures group-reactive anti-treponemal antibodies, occasionally gives false positive reactions. The TPHA, FTA-ABS and TPI tests in which *Tr. pallidum* itself is used as the antigen are the most specific verification tests available, the TPI test being generally accepted as the ultimate standard of reference. The antibody measured by these tests is distinct from the 'reagin' antibody and the antibody giving reactions in the RPCF test. The FTA-ABS test becomes positive in early primary syphilis and the TPHA and TPI tests in the late primary stage. The antibody measured in these tests persists for many years after cure so the results are of limited value in assessing response to treatment. In newborn babies with suspected congenital syphilis, patients with a past history of yaws and some cases of treated syphilis the interpretation of the results can be very difficult. Help can often be obtained by using the FTA-ABS test adapted to measure IgG and IgM antibodies. The presence of IgM antibodies indicates active infection.

Other pathogenic treponemas

Non-venereal treponemal infections are endemic in certain parts of the world. Infection is transmitted by close personal contact and occurs in communities with low standards of hygiene. The lesions closely resemble those found in syphilis and the serological tests for syphilis are positive. The causative organisms are morphologically indistinguishable from *Tr. pallidum*, but minor differences in antigenic properties and pathogenicity have been noted. They are best regarded as subspecies or variants of *Tr. pallidum*.

Yaws, due to *Tr. pertenue*, occurs over wide areas of the tropics. Ulcerative and granulomatous lesions occur in the skin, mucous membranes and bones.

Pinta, due to *Tr. carateum*, is mainly found in Central and South America. It is characterized by depigmentation and hyperkeratosis of the skin.

Bejel is prevalent among Bedouin Arabs in the Middle East. The disease cannot clearly be distinguished from syphilis and yaws. It is representative of a class of diseases which have been regarded as endemic syphilis.

Rickettsiae

*Typhus is not dead. It will live on for centuries, and
it will continue to break into the open whenever
human stupidity and brutality give it a chance...*
                                    H. Zinsser, 1935

The rickettsiae are small obligate intracellular bacteria transmitted
by insect vectors. They cause typhus fever and a group of similar
diseases. They will not multiply on laboratory media but can be
grown in the yolk sac of the developing chick embryo and will
infect animals such as the mouse and the guinea-pig. They contain both deoxyribonucleic acid (DNA) and ribonucleic acid
(RNA), they multiply by binary fission, possess a certain amount
of independent metabolic activity, contain muramic acid in their
cell walls and are susceptible to chemotherapeutic agents such as
chloramphenicol and the tetracyclines. They are visible by the
light microscope as minute coccobacilli inside infected cells. They
are usually about 0.5 μm long and 0.3 μm wide. They are gram-
negative but stain very poorly and are best demonstrated by
Giemsa, Macchiavello or Castaneda stains.

Rickettsia

Rickettsia prowazeki

R. prowazeki is the cause of classical or epidemic (louse-borne)
typhus and the milder Brill-Zinsser disease. The organism is
named after the early workers Ricketts and Prowazek who both
died of the disease. It is a human parasite and is transferred
from man to man by the human louse, *Pediculus humanus*. The
louse becomes infected when it feeds on the blood of a patient or
carrier. The organisms multiply in the intestinal cells and after an
interval of several days are liberated in the faeces. When the
louse transfers its activity to a new human host its infected faeces
are deposited on the skin and the rickettsiae are inoculated into
the tissues by scratching.

Typhus appears after an incubation period of 8–14 days. The

onset is sudden and prostration is severe. A characteristic macular rash appears on about the fifth day. The death rate is 10—20%. Mild and latent infections also occur.

Epidemics are associated with conditions which predispose to an increase in human lousiness, e.g. overcrowding, lack of washing facilities, cold weather and lack of fuel so that clothes are worn continuously. All major epidemics have been associated with wars, revolutions and famines. In the past typhus has probably been the most serious of all pestilential diseases affecting mankind. Epidemics have often been on an enormous scale, e.g. it is estimated that in 1918—22 there were 30 million cases in Russia with some 3 million deaths. In World War II there were severe outbreaks in North Africa, the Middle East and in concentration camps in Europe. The first large epidemic of typhus to be brought under effective control in winter occurred in Naples in 1944. Control was achieved by widespread disinfestation of the population with DDT.

Brill-Zinsser disease is a mild form of typhus first observed in New York among immigrants from eastern Europe. It is due to a recrudescence of infection in persons who have had classical typhus in the past. The rickettsiae have lain dormant in the tissues, sometimes for as long as twenty years.

Rickettsia typhi

R. typhi is the cause of murine (flea-borne) typhus. It is a parasite of the rat and is transmitted from rat to rat by the rat flea and the rat louse. Man is infected when he is bitten by an infected rat flea. Murine typhus occurs in many parts of the world, mainly as a sporadic infection among individuals living or working in heavily rat-infested areas. The disease is rarely fatal.

Rickettsia rickettsi and related species

R. rickettsi is the cause of Rocky Mountain spotted fever, a severe form of tick-borne typhus. The organism is primarily a parasite of wild rodents but it sometimes infects dogs. Human infection is acquired from ticks.

Rickettsiae closely related to *R. rickettsi* cause tick-borne, typhus-like diseases ('spotted fevers') in many parts of the world, e.g. *R. conori*, the cause of African tick-borne typhus and fièvre boutonneuse in Mediterranean countries; *R. australis*, the cause of Queensland tick typhus; *R. sibirica*, the cause of tick-typhus in the USSR. The diseases are characterized by a relatively mild course, a local lesion at the site of the tick-bite, and a maculopapular rash.

R. akari is the cause of rickettsialpox, a mild disease resembling chickenpox. Antigenically it is closely related to the spotted fever group. The natural reservoir of infection is the house mouse. Infection is transmitted to man by mites.

Rickettsia tsutsugamushi

R. tsutsugamushi is the cause of scrub typhus (tsutsugamushi fever) a form of mite-borne typhus occurring in the Far East. The disease resembles epidemic typhus. A small necrotic ulcer usually develops at the site of inoculation. Wild rodents, particularly rats, constitute a reservoir of infection. The disease is transmitted to man by the bite of the larvae of mites parasitic on rats.

Coxiella

Coxiella burneti

C. burneti is the cause of Q fever (from 'Query' fever when the aetiology was unknown), an influenza-like illness of worldwide distribution. Pneumonic changes are usually demonstrable by radiological means, but symptoms and signs referable to the respiratory tract are often slight. Rashes do not occur. *C. burneti* is a rare cause of infective endocarditis and should be considered when routine blood cultures are sterile.

The organism is found in small wild animals, birds, domestic animals and many species of ticks. Ticks probably maintain the disease in wild animals and in a few cases transmit it to domestic animals. Cattle, sheep and goats are the main source of human infection. Infected animals discharge large numbers of organisms in the placenta and birth fluids during parturition and also excrete them in their milk. *C. burneti* is a remarkably resistant organism and survives in the environment for long periods.

Q fever is not common in the UK and most cases are found in rural areas. Infection is mainly acquired by inhalation. Patients often give no history of direct contact with animals and indirect infection from contaminated materials is more important. Sources of infection include infected farm buildings and abattoirs, dust from infected clothes, hay and straw, dried faeces of ticks parasitic on domestic animals, and animal products such as meat, hides, hair and wool. Infection acquired by ingestion is of minor importance but may occur in areas where milk is unpasteurized. With rare exceptions patients with Q fever give no history of tick-bite.

Rochalimaea

R. quintana is the cause of trench fever, an acute febrile illness which has occurred in epidemic form among troops in time of war. It is a human parasite and is transmitted by the human body louse. It is antigenically distinct from the rickettsiae and *C. burneti* and can be grown in cell-free media.

Diagnosis of rickettsial infections

In the acute stages of the disease rickettsiae can be recovered from the patient's blood by intraperitoneal injection of animals. The danger of laboratory-acquired infection is so great that isolation is attempted only in specialist laboratories. Routine diagnosis of rickettsial infections is by serology. Two types of antigen are used:

1 *Rickettsial antigens.* Typhus is commonly diagnosed by means of a complement fixation test using group-specific antigens extracted from rickettsiae grown in the yolk sac. There is antigenic overlap between some of the rickettsiae, but by means of agglutination and complement fixation tests using rickettsial suspensions the different species can be distinguished. Reliable immunofluorescent and haemagglutination tests are also available. Q fever is diagnosed by means of a complement fixation test using suspensions of *C. burneti.* The organism exists in two antigenic forms, phase 1 and phase 2. In ordinary Q fever there is a rise in the level of phase 2 antibodies, but phase 1 antibodies remain at low levels or do not appear at all. In Q fever endocarditis both phase 1 and phase 2 antibodies may reach high levels.

2 *Proteus antigens.* Because of a chance antigenic similarity between various rickettsiae and certain strains of *Proteus* the detection of antibodies which agglutinate *Proteus* can be used in the diagnosis of typhus (Weil-Felix reaction). Thus *Proteus* OX19 is agglutinated in epidemic typhus, murine typhus and the spotted fevers; *Proteus* OXK is agglutinated in scrub typhus but not in the other diseases; *Proteus* OX2 is agglutinated in the spotted fevers but only to a small extent in epidemic and murine typhus. The test is not very reliable. In Q fever and trench fever antibodies against *Proteus* do not develop.

22

Chlamydiae

> *Homo sapiens even offered them the gift of tongues*
> *and encouraged wise old parrots with lumps of sugar.*
> *His instinct in all this was childlike affection.*
> *He hoped for some return of this emotion, and if*
> *occasionally he received a savage peck instead, he*
> *was prepared to put this down to a misunderstanding.*
> *But he never expected psittacosis.*
> A. B. Christie, 1980

The chlamydiae are a group of pathogens causing disease in man and a wide variety of animals. Like the rickettsiae they are bacteria which, due to extreme specialization, lead an obligately intracellular existence. They are larger than viruses, being 300–500 nm in diameter, and can be seen with the light microscope. Unlike viruses they contain both deoxyribonucleic acid (DNA) and ribonucleic acid (RNA); they stain with basic dyes such as Castaneda stain and can be seen inside infected cells as basophilic intracytoplasmic inclusion bodies; they multiply by binary fission and undergo a development cycle in which large bodies 1 μm in diameter are formed; they possess considerable independent metabolic activity; they contain muramic acid in their cell walls; and they are to varying degrees susceptible to chemotherapeutic agents such as tetracyclines, erythromycin and sulphonamides.

The organisms which make up the genus *Chlamydia* show a large amount of overlap in their biological properties, e.g. they share a major complement-fixing antigen. The chlamydiae responsible for human disease are classified into two species:

C. trachomatis includes twelve serotypes of the TRIC agent causing trachoma, inclusion conjunctivitis, genital infection and pneumonia and three serotypes of the LGV agent causing lymphogranuloma venereum. The inclusion bodies are compact and contain glycogen.

C. psittaci includes the agents causing psittacosis and ornithosis. The inclusion bodies are diffuse and do not contain glycogen.

The finer differentiation of chlamydiae into types or strains is mainly based on their possession of type-specific antigens as determined by immunofluorescent tests. Other features used in classification include antibiotic sensitivities, host range, and infectivity in laboratory animals.

Trachoma

Trachoma is a severe form of chronic conjunctivitis producing scarring and deformity of the eyelids, and corneal vascularization and opacities which may lead to blindness. The disease is of world-wide distribution and over 500 million people are infected. It is particularly prevalent in the Middle East, India and China. It is rare in the UK. Trachoma is associated with a low standard of living and poor personal hygiene. The organism is probably transmitted from eye to eye by the fingers and infected articles. In countries where trachoma is endemic, infection is usually acquired in infancy from the mother.

Cytoplasmic inclusion bodies are found in conjunctival scrapings stained with iodine, Giemsa or fluorescent antibodies. *C. trachomatis* can be isolated in special tissue cultures, e.g. non-replicating McCoy cells. Antibodies in the patient's blood can be detected by means of an immunofluorescent test.

Genital infection, inclusion conjunctivitis, pneumonia

Three main types of infection caused by *C. trachomatis* are common in temperate climates.

Genital infection. *C. trachomatis* is primarily a parasite of the human genital tract. In females it usually produces symptomless infection of the cervix but it may cause widespread pelvic infection including salpingitis which may result in blockage of the fallopian tubes and infertility. In males it infects the anterior urethra and is the cause of about 50% of all cases of 'non-specific' (i.e. non-gonococcal) urethritis. Complications include epididymitis and proctitis. Infection is transmitted by sexual intercourse. The incidence of non-gonococcal urethritis has risen in recent years and the disease is now about three times as common as gonorrhoea. It has been suggested that chlamydiae act as a trigger factor for Reiter's syndrome, a combination of urethritis, conjunctivitis and arthritis found most commonly in patients carrying the B27 histocompatibility (HLA) antigen.

Inclusion conjunctivitis. This occurs in two main forms: (1) an acute purulent conjunctivitis in infants occurring 5–12 days after birth and due to infection acquired from the maternal birth canal; (2) a more protracted, non-purulent, follicular conjunctivitis in adults, commonly associated with genital infection in the patient and his or her sexual partner, but in rare cases acquired by swimming in non-chlorinated baths contaminated with discharges from the genital tract of infected swimmers (one type of 'swimming-bath conjunctivitis'). In contrast to trachoma, the disease usually resolves spontaneously in a comparatively short time without corneal lesions or scarring.

Pneumonia. C. trachomatis is a common cause of pneumonia in infants. Chlamydial pneumonia is typically a prolonged, non-fatal, afebrile illness with diffuse X-ray changes in the lungs. Infection is acquired from the mother's genital tract. In adults chlamydial pneumonia is an occasional complication of immuno-suppressive therapy.

Diagnosis

Inclusion bodies can be demonstrated in conjunctival scrapings. They can also be found in smears from the cervix and urethra. The organisms can be rapidly and reliably identified by direct staining of specimens with fluorescein-labelled monoclonal anti-bodies. Enzyme-linked immunosorbent assay (ELISA) can be used for direct detection of chlamydial antigens in material obtained on swabs. *C. trachomatis* can be isolated in non-replicating McCoy cells. The organisms are indistinguishable from those that cause trachoma, although the predominant serotypes are different. In patients with non-specific urethritis type-specific antibodies can usually be detected by a sensitive immunofluorescent IgM test. Chlamydiae can seldom be isolated from affected joints but their presence can often be detected by staining with monoclonal antibodies.

Lymphogranuloma venereum

Lymphogranuloma venereum (LGV) is a sexually transmitted disease caused by particular serotypes of *C. trachomatis*. LGV is of world-wide distribution but is more common in the tropics. The primary lesion is a small, ulcerating papule usually on the genitalia. Suppuration of the regional lymph nodes follows 2–3 weeks later. Finally, chronic granulomatous infection of the lymphatics and adjoining tissues of the pelvis and genital tract may lead to rectal stricture, elephantiasis of the genitalia and pelvic fistulae.

The organisms can sometimes be seen in smears of pus from infected lymph nodes. They can be isolated in special tissue cultures. The diagnosis is usually made by detecting antibodies in the patient's serum by means of a complement fixation test.

As normally performed, the test is also positive in psittacosis and sometimes in other chlamydial infections. Type-specific antibodies can be measured by immunofluorescent tests.

Psittacosis (ornithosis)

C. psittaci is primarily a parasite of the parrot family (psittacine birds), but similar organisms cause infection (ornithosis) among other types of wild and domestic birds including pigeons, hens, ducks, turkeys, canaries, finches and sea birds. The birds usually acquire the organism from their parents while still in the nest and after an inapparent infection remain carriers more or less indefinitely. Latent infection may be converted into overt and highly infectious disease by environmental factors, e.g. capture and transportation of parrots.

Psittacosis in man is almost entirely limited to those in close contact with birds. Psittacine birds are the most dangerous, and newly imported parrots have been responsible for initiating many outbreaks. Control of the importation and quarantine of such birds is therefore of great importance. Ornithosis is particularly common among poultry workers, e.g. in the UK over 60% of workers employed in duck processing plants show serological evidence of past infection. Infection is acquired by inhalation of dried faeces and infected dust. In poultry processing plants evisceration releases infectious aerosols. The disease classically takes the form of severe pneumonia with a high mortality, but mild and inapparent infections are more common. Patients in the acute stages may transmit the disease to those in attendance. Some cases develop infective endocarditis.

The organisms can be identified in sputum by direct staining with fluorescent antibodies or by ELISA and can be isolated from the blood and sputum by using special tissue cultures. Infected cells show characteristic cytoplasmic inclusion bodies. The diagnosis is usually made by means of a complement fixation test on the patient's serum.

Chlamydia psittaci infections in animals

C. psittaci is the cause of enzootic abortion in sheep. Pregnant women helping with lambing may become infected and suffer an influenza-like illness followed by premature labour and fetal death.

TWAR strains

Some strains of *C. psittaci* spread from human to human without an intermediary bird or animal host. These 'human' or 'TWAR' strains (a name derived from the first two isolates: TW=Taiwan, AR=acute respiratory disease) are an important cause of pneumonia and other acute respiratory tract infections in man. Epidemics have occurred in many countries. TWAR strains differ from classical *C. psittaci* strains in serological and cultural properties.

23

Mycoplasmas

. . .neither fish, flesh, fowl, nor good red herring.

Anon.

The genus *Mycoplasma* consists of a group of very small, highly pleomorphic organisms which are capable of growth on cell-free media. They are the smallest free-living organisms known. Many are able to pass through coarse antibacterial filters. They have exacting nutritional requirements but completely independent metabolic activity. They contain both deoxyribonucleic acid (DNA) and ribonucleic acid (RNA). The organisms have a limiting membrane but lack a rigid cell wall. They are susceptible to some chemotherapeutic agents such as the tetracyclines but are unaffected by others, such as penicillin, which act by interfering with cell wall synthesis. The group includes the human pathogens *M. pneumoniae* and *M. hominis*, various commensal and occasionally pathogenic species which infect man, several species which cause diseases of great economic importance in animals, and species which live as saprophytes.

General properties of mycoplasmas

Cultural properties

Mycoplasmas will grow in liquid and solid media that have been enriched with yeast extract and a high proportion (20% or more) of serum. Serum provides a source of cholesterol and other lipids which are essential nutrients for most mycoplasmas. Penicillin and other inhibitors are usually added to the media to suppress bacterial contaminants.

Most mycoplasmas grow best in an atmosphere containing added carbon dioxide and a reduced oxygen concentration. The pathogenic strains grow best at 37°C. The colonies on soft agar media take 2–7 days to develop. They are usually less than 0.5 mm in diameter and occasionally as small as 10–20 μm. Typically, the centre of each colony embeds itself in the agar and the periphery spreads on the surface, giving the colony a characteristic 'fried egg' appearance when examined under the microscope. Mycoplasmas are ubiquitous and frequently contaminate tissue cultures.

Growth and morphology

Reproduction is by binary fission. The smallest viable units are about 200 nm in size. These grow into irregularly shaped bodies which ultimately bud to produce daughter cells. The lack of a rigid cell wall accounts for their extreme pleomorphism.

The organisms are gram-negative but stain poorly. They stain well with Giemsa stain. The smallest forms cannot be seen with the ordinary microscope. Electron microscopy reveals that the individual cells are bounded by a triple-layered membrane enclosing ribosomes and scattered granular or fibrillar nuclear material.

Classification

The different species are distinguished partly on general biological properties, but precise identification is made by serological methods. Growth of mycoplasmas is inhibited by their specific antibodies and growth inhibition tests have proved of great value in identifying species. The test can be carried out by spreading mycoplasmas on an agar plate and noting whether zones of inhibition appear around paper discs dipped in specific antisera. Fluorescent antibody tests in which intact colonies are treated with specific antisera are valuable for rapid diagnosis.

Relation to L-forms

Many properties of mycoplasmas are shared by the L-forms of bacteria, but there is no good evidence that mycoplasmas represent stable (non-reverting) L-forms. Whatever their evolutional origin, the better-defined species of mycoplasmas form a unique and stable group, the genus *Mycoplasma*.

Mycoplasma pneumoniae

M. pneumoniae is distinguished from other species by serological means and by such characteristics as β-haemolysis of sheep red cells, aerobic reduction of tetrazolium, and ability to grow in the presence of methylene blue.

Mycoplasmal pneumonia

M. pneumoniae is the commonest cause of non-bacterial pneumonia. Infection with this organism may also take the form of

bronchitis or a mild febrile respiratory illness. Inapparent infections are common. Family outbreaks are frequently encountered
and large outbreaks of the disease have occurred in military
training centres. The incubation period is about two weeks.

M. pneumoniae can be isolated by culture of sputum and throat
swabs, but the diagnosis is more readily made by serological
methods, usually a complement fixation text. Diagnosis of mycoplasmal pneumonia is assisted by the empirical finding that many
patients produce cold agglutinins to human group O red cells.

Other mycoplasmas affecting man

Mycoplasmas are normal inhabitants of the genital tract of men
and women. One commonly encountered species, *M. hominis*, is
responsible for some cases of vaginal discharge, urethritis,
salpingitis and pelvic sepsis. It is a common cause of postpartum
fever. It may enter the maternal blood during delivery and settle
in joints. A group of mycoplasmas (ureaplasmas) which produce
tiny colonies, so-called T-strains, have been considered as a possible
cause of non-gonococcal urethritis in both sexes, but the evidence
is inconclusive. Other species are normal commensals of the
mouth and nasopharynx.

DNA Viruses

...O'er ladies' lips, who straight on kisses dream;
Which oft the angry Mab with blisters plagues...
[Herpes simplex]

Shakespeare

Poxviruses

This group of deoxyribonucleic acid (DNA) viruses includes small-pox, vaccinia and molluscum contagiosum viruses and numerous animal poxviruses. Chickenpox (varicella) is caused by a herpes-virus not by a poxvirus. Poxviruses are just large enough to be seen with the light microscope. Under the electron microscope most poxviruses are rounded brick-shaped objects 200 × 300 nm in size. The virions have complex symmetry with tube-like structures surrounding a central core (Fig. 12C, p. 35). The viruses of orf and milker's nodes are smaller and more elongated and have an internal structure resembling a ball of yarn (Fig. 49, p. 329). Poxviruses have an envelope, but most are moderately resistant to ether. Smallpox, vaccinia and cowpox viruses grow readily in the chick embryo (Fig. 17, p. 53) and in a variety of tissue cultures.

Smallpox (variola)

This once dreaded disease is now extinct. At one time smallpox was endemic in many parts of the world, particularly in Asia. From time to time it was imported into nearly all countries and caused devastating epidemics. As recently as 1967 smallpox was endemic in 33 countries and caused 10−15 million cases with two million deaths. The disease existed in two main forms: classical smallpox (variola major), a virulent disease with a mortality of 20−30%, and the less common alastrim (variola minor), a mild form of smallpox with a mortality of about 1%. Strains inter-mediate in their pathogenicity also occurred, suggesting that smallpox virus is genetically unstable. However, outbreaks of alastrim never gave rise to classical smallpox.

In 1967 the World Health Organization launched a massive

programme to eradicate smallpox. This was a feasible objective because most cases of the disease were clinically obvious, there was no such thing as a carrier, there were no non-human reservoirs, and widespread vaccination of populations was reasonably easy and highly effective. Progress was remarkable and country after country was cleared of infection. The world's last known case of naturally occurring endemic variola major was a three-year-old girl who had the disease in Bangladesh in October 1975. The last known case of variola minor was a 23-year-old male hospital cook who had the disease in Somalia in October 1977.

Now that human beings no longer harbour the virus the sole remaining source of infection is virus kept in laboratories. Smallpox virus has escaped twice in recent years: in 1973 from the London School of Hygiene and Tropical Medicine causing three cases with two deaths and in 1978 from Birmingham University Medical School causing two cases with one death. Officially, smallpox virus is now stored in only two laboratories, one in the USA and one in the USSR, where rigid safety precautions are enforced. However, in 1985 ampoules of the virus were unexpectedly found at the London School of Hygiene and Tropical Medicine!

Vaccinia

Vaccinia virus is the name given to the strains of virus which have been propagated in calves and other animals for the production of vaccine used in human vaccination. It differs in minor respects from naturally occurring cowpox virus.

Cowpox

Cowpox is a naturally occurring disease in cows. The eruption usually appears on the udder and teats and infection can be transferred to the hands of milkers. Human cowpox is rare. In the UK some cases are probably acquired from infected cats. Cowpox virus was the organism originally used for vaccination by Jenner.

Other animal pox diseases

Pox diseases occur in most species of animal, e.g. monkeypox, mousepox (ectromelia), rabbitpox, horsepox, fowlpox, etc. Most of these are not transmissible to man, but a few cases of human monkeypox have occurred in Africa. The illness closely resembles smallpox but person-to-person spread is almost unknown. Whitepox virus, so called because it produces white (non-haemorrhagic) lesions when growing on the chorio-allantoic membrane of the chick embryo, has been isolated from monkey kidney tissues. It is indistinguishable from smallpox virus in all laboratory tests. It is probably a natural variant of monkeypox virus. So far there is no evidence that whitepox constitutes a serious threat to man.

Orf or contagious pustular dermatitis of sheep is caused by a virus of this same general group and human infection is not uncommon among farmers and butchers. The characteristic lesion is usually on a finger where it is often mistaken for a whitlow and incised. Orf virus is difficult to isolate. The appearances of orf and paravaccinia viruses in the electron microscope are characteristic (Fig. 49).

Paravaccinia virus causes lesions on the udders of cows. Human infection takes the form of milker's nodes, small non-ulcerating nodules on the hands. The virus closely resembles orf virus.

Molluscum contagiosum

Man is the only known host of the poxvirus causing this disease. The virus produces multiple nodules in the epidermal layer of the skin. Infected cells contain large, hyaline, acidophilic intracytoplasmic inclusion bodies. The virus can be grown in tissue culture with difficulty.

Herpesviruses

This group of DNA viruses includes herpes simplex virus, Epstein-Barr virus, varicella-zoster virus and cytomegalovirus. They are 100–180 nm in diameter and the capsid has the form of a regular icosahedron and is composed of 162 capsomeres. The virions have an envelope and are ether-sensitive (Fig. 12A, p. 35).

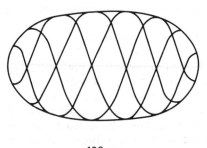

100 nm

Fig. 49 Orf virus, showing the characteristic internal structure.

All herpesviruses can be grown in tissue culture and many of them will grow in the chick embryo. Herpes simplex virus produces pocks on the chorio-allantoic membrane. Herpesviruses produce characteristic eosinophilic intranuclear inclusion bodies.

Herpes simplex virus (HSV)

This highly successful and well-adapted parasite is more constantly present in man than any other virus. By the age of five over 60% of the population have been infected. The proportion may exceed 95% among adults living in cities. The upper socioeconomic groups show a much lower incidence of infection. People who acquire the virus remain carriers for the rest of their lives.

Primary herpes usually occurs in the first few years of life. It characteristically takes the form of vesicular stomatitis often associated with febrile illness but it is more often overlooked. In some cases the primary lesions are on the skin or involve the eye. Infants with eczema may develop a widespread vesicular eruption (eczema herpeticum). Herpetic whitlows due to contamination of abrasions by the virus are not uncommon among doctors, dentists and nurses. Traumatic herpes is also seen among rugger players and wrestlers. In rare cases primary herpes leads to generalized infection or encephalitis. These conditions are often fatal and early diagnosis is essential as they are potentially treatable with acyclovir. Herpes meningitis is a benign self-limiting illness. Herpes infections are acquired by contact with patients with obvious herpetic lesions or with symptomless salivary carriers. Kissing is probably the most important method of transmission.

Recurrent herpes occurs in adult life. Following the primary infection naked virus travels up the sensory nerves and lies dormant in the sensory ganglia of nerves supplying particular areas. From time to time it becomes active and, clothed with an envelope, it travels down the nerves and produces a vesicular eruption, 'cold sores', most commonly in a small localized area on the lips or around the nostrils. The virus can be isolated from these lesions. Recurrent herpes may also involve the genital mucous membranes or the eye. In each attack the eruption usually occurs in the same area. Factors which stimulate the virus to activity include colds, influenza, other fevers, sunlight, cold and menstruation. Most cases of herpes encephalitis probably represent reactivation of a latent infection. Generalized herpes may occur during immunosuppressive therapy.

Genital herpes is a sexually transmitted disease. It commonly affects the glans and shaft of the penis and the vulva, vagina and cervix. The main reservoirs of the virus are the cervix and the male genital tract. Herpes virus is often associated with carcinoma of the cervix and is thought to play some part in the development of this condition.

Viral particles can be demonstrated by electron microscopy and viral antigens can be stained with a fluorescent antibody. These techniques are of special value when a diagnosis is required urgently, e.g. for examining brain tissue from patients with suspected herpes encephalitis. Herpes virus can be isolated from vesicle fluid and swabs from lesions, but is seldom recoverable from the cerebrospinal fluid. Fully infective virus is not present in sensory ganglia, but it can be readily isolated if ganglia explants are first grown in culture for several days.

Two types of herpes virus are distinguished on the basis of their antigenic, biological and biochemical properties. HSV-1 mainly attacks 'above the belt' and is responsible for lesions in the mouth and on the face; HSV-2 is much less common, mainly attacks 'below the belt' and causes genital and neonatal infections. In recent years there has been an increase in the incidence of HSV-1 isolated from genital lesions. Viruses of both types can be classified into many different strains by restriction endonuclease mapping (DNA fingerprinting). This technique is of value in tracing outbreaks of herpes virus infection. There is little cross-immunity between the two types, e.g. a patient with existing type 1 infection can be infected with a type 2 virus or, rarely, with a different strain of type 1. Antibodies can be measured by neutralization or complement fixation tests. Primary herpes is associated with a rising titre of antibodies, but the detection of antibodies in a single specimen of adult serum is of no diagnostic significance unless specific IgM antibodies can be demonstrated. Type 1 antibodies normally begin to appear in the population in early childhood but type 2 antibodies seldom appear before adolescence.

B virus (Herpesvirus simiae)

This virus is the monkey equivalent of human herpes simplex virus. In man it produces a severe and usually fatal form of encephalomyelitis. A few cases have occurred among laboratory workers who have been bitten by monkeys or who have been in contact with monkeys, monkey tissues or monkey tissue cultures.

Pseudorabies virus (Herpesvirus suis)

This virus causes a neurological disease ('mad itch') in animals. Very rarely it has caused a minor illness in laboratory workers.

EB (Epstein-Barr) virus

This herpesvirus will not grow in ordinary tissue cultures, but can be maintained in human lymphoid cell lines. Viral antigens in infected cells can be detected by immunofluorescent techniques. Human infection with EB virus is extremely common and antibodies against the virus can be detected in 40—95% of adults. The virus sets up a persistent latent infection of B-lymphocytes and is spontaneously reactivated in a few cells. Infectious viral particles are periodically released into the saliva ensuring spread of infection to non-immune individuals. EB virus is the cause of infectious mononucleosis and is associated with the development of Burkitt's lymphoma and nasopharyngeal carcinoma.

Infectious mononucleosis (glandular fever)

This disease ('kissing disease') mainly affects teenagers and young adults and takes the form of fever, sore throat and enlargement of lymph nodes and spleen. Rashes may occur. Hepatitis is almost invariably present as judged by liver function tests. In a few cases there is jaundice. The disease is not very infectious, but small outbreaks have occurred in closed communities. Kissing is important in transmission. A few patients develop a chronic mononucleosis syndrome in which symptoms persist or recur for several years. Cytomegalovirus, *Toxoplasma gondii*, *Chlamydia psittaci*, AIDS virus (HIV) and secondary syphilis sometimes cause an illness closely resembling infectious mononucleosis.

The disease is diagnosed by finding abnormal mononuclear cells and an increase in lymphocytes in the blood and by detecting antibodies to EB virus and antibodies which agglutinate sheep red cells (Paul-Bunnell test). These heterophile antibodies are absorbed by bovine red cells but not by an emulsion of guinea-pig kidney. In these respects they differ from similar antibodies sometimes encountered in normal persons and in patients who have had injections of horse serum, e.g. antitetanus serum. Heterophile antibodies are of the IgM class and usually disappear within 1—2 months. Specific IgM antibodies to the viral capsid antigen (VCA) of EB virus appear shortly after infection but are soon replaced by IgG antibodies which persist indefinitely. Antibodies to EB nuclear antigen (EBNA) appear late after infection (often several months) and also persist indefinitely.

Burkitt's lymphoma

This is a malignant tumour of the jaw prevalent among children regardless of race in high-rainfall, low-altitude areas of equatorial Africa. This unusual geographical distribution is similar to that of mosquito-borne diseases such as malaria. There is substantial evidence linking Burkitt's lymphoma with EB virus. EB viral DNA is almost always present in lymphoma cells obtained by biopsy. When the cells are cultured the daughter cells produce EB viral antigens or undergo lysis liberating infectious virus which is capable of transforming lymphocytes in cultures. EB virus produces lymphomas in monkeys, although the tumours differ in several respects from those in man. Patients with Burkitt's lymphoma usually have higher levels of antibodies than healthy children and the patterns of antibodies against different EB viral antigens are characteristic. The levels of these antibodies can be correlated with the prognosis. Additional factors, such as infection with malaria parasites, are thought to contribute to the development of malignancy.

Nasopharyngeal carcinoma

This is a malignant tumour mainly affecting adults. It is common in southern China, Tunisia and East Africa. There is a close association between the carcinoma and EB virus. Viral DNA is invariably present in the carcinoma cells. Cells in culture can be activated to produce viral antigens or infectious virus. Patients with the disease produce a characteristic pattern of antibodies, distinct from the patterns found in Burkitt's lymphoma.

Chickenpox and herpes zoster

These two conditions are caused by the same virus, the varicella-zoster virus (VZV). The virus does not infect laboratory animals or the chick embryo, but can be grown in human tissue culture. Strains from chickenpox and herpes zoster are identical.

Chickenpox (varicella) occurs mainly in young children. It represents a primary infection with VZV. It is highly infectious with a generalized itching rash, papular at first but very soon vesicular.

Herpes zoster (shingles) occurs mainly in adults. It represents infection of an individual who has some immunity to VZV and is due to the reactivation of a virus that has lain dormant in the tissues since an earlier attack of chickenpox. Restriction endonuclease analysis of viral DNA has been used to prove the identity of virus from chickenpox and subsequent shingles in the same patient. The virus becomes active in the posterior root ganglia or the sensory ganglia of the cranial nerves and produces a localized eruption and often severe pain in the area of distribution of a sensory nerve. Children who have been in contact with cases of shingles may develop chickenpox, but shingles is much less important as a source of infection, probably because the virus is seldom present in the upper respiratory tract. Shingles cannot be caught from patients with shingles or chickenpox.

In patients undergoing immunosuppressive therapy chickenpox and shingles can be life-threatening infections.

Cytomegalovirus (CMV)

This is an extremely common human parasite. Normally it produces no symptoms but sets up a persistent latent infection, particularly in the salivary glands and kidneys.

Congenital infection usually occurs during a symptomless infection in the mother. A young child is a common source of maternal infection. In the UK about 2% of pregnant women develop a primary infection during pregnancy and in 5% there is reactivation of a latent virus. Primary infections are usually more damaging to the fetus. In most cases the fetus suffers no harm and the newborn baby remains healthy but excretes the virus in its urine. In a few cases the results of infection are disastrous. Infection in early pregnancy may cause abortion or congenital defects. Infection late in pregnancy may result in severe fetal disease and stillbirth or the child may be born alive and develop 'cytomegalic inclusion disease', a severe and often fatal generalized illness with jaundice, thrombocytopenic purpura, anaemia, choroidoretinitis and enlargement of the liver and spleen. Infected infants who do not succumb to this syndrome commonly show evidence of severe brain damage with microcephaly, intracranial calcification and hydrocephalus. CMV probably causes 200−600 cases of mental retardation every year in the UK or about 10% of the total number, compared with 2−3% caused by rubella and toxoplasmosis.

Acquired infection is usually inapparent but the virus occasionally produces an illness resembling infectious mononucleosis. Some cases follow blood transfusion and tissue transplantation. Fever is the commonest symptom and atypical mononuclear cells often appear in the blood. Sometimes there is enlargement of lymph nodes. Hepatitis is common as judged by liver function tests and jaundice occurs occasionally. Severe generalized CMV infection is seen as a complication of immunosuppressive therapy. It is also one of the commonest features in the acquired immunodeficiency syndrome (AIDS). CMV may play a role in the development of the malignant tumour, Kaposi's sarcoma. Serological tests indicate that 50−95% of the adult population have been infected. The virus is excreted in large amounts in the saliva and urine and has been found in cervical secretions and breast milk. It rapidly loses its infectivity and close contact and kissing are important in transmission.

CMV can be isolated from throat swabs or urine in cultures of human embryonic fibroblasts. Antibodies can be measured by a complement fixation test. CMV infections are characterized histologically by the presence in various organs, particularly the salivary glands, of large cells with prominent ('owl's eye') intranuclear inclusion bodies. These can be found in tissue biopsies and in cells from the urinary deposit.

Human B-cell lymphotropic virus (HBLV)

This herpesvirus has been isolated from patients with lymphomas. It may have an oncogenic role.

Adenoviruses

These DNA viruses are among the most common and well-adapted of all viruses affecting man. Their existence was first recognized because of the frequent occurrence of degenerative changes in tissue cultures prepared from surgically removed adenoids and tonsils. Adenoviruses are about 70–90 nm in diameter. The capsid has the form of a regular icosahedron. It is composed of 252 capsomeres: 12 hollow pentagons (*pentons*) at the vertices and 240 hollow hexagons (*hexons*) covering the rest of the surface. A fine fibre with a terminal knob projects from each of the 12 pentons. The virions have no envelope and are ether-resistant.

Adenoviruses will grow and produce cytopathic effects in continuous cell lines such as HeLa cells. They do not normally cause disease in animals, but some types produce tumours in newborn hamsters. Nearly all adenoviruses cause haemagglutination with red cells from suitable species. About 40 serological types of adenoviruses have been isolated from human sources. They share a soluble complement-fixing antigen, but can be distinguished by neutralization tests in tissue culture and by haemagglutination-inhibition tests. Some 'fastidious' adenoviruses, provisionally designated types 40 and 41, cannot be grown in ordinary tissue cultures.

Infections

Antibodies against adenoviruses are highly prevalent in human sera. By the age of five many children show serological evidence of infection, particularly with types 1, 2, 5 and 6. Most of these infections are inapparent or take the form of mild respiratory illnesses. These adenoviruses commonly set up a persistent latent infection in the adenoids and tonsils.

Other adenoviruses, particularly types 3, 4, 7, 14 and 21, are more frequently found in association with outbreaks of respiratory tract infection and conjunctivitis. Large outbreaks occur when children and young adults live in closed communities. Various overlapping clinical syndromes are recognized:

Acute respiratory disease. Epidemics with fever, sore throat and cough have often occurred in recruit training establishments. The attack rate may exceed 50%. Some cases develop viral pneumonia. Conjunctivitis is a feature of some outbreaks. Most outbreaks have been caused by types 4 and 7.

Pharyngo-conjunctival fever. Outbreaks of sore throat, conjunctivitis and fever have occurred in schools and holiday camps. Types 3 and 7 have been mainly responsible. Adenoviruses are the cause of one type of 'swimming-bath conjunctivitis'.

Pneumonia. Severe and sometimes fatal viral pneumonia can occur in infants. Epidemics have occurred. Adults may also be affected. Types 4 and 7 are often responsible.

Pertussis-like illness. An illness resembling whooping cough may occur in infants and young children. Various types are responsible.

Follicular conjunctivitis. This disease mainly affects adults. Types 3 and 7 are often responsible.

Epidemic kerato-conjunctivitis. This disease is particularly associated with types 8, 19 and 37. Outbreaks have occurred among factory workers whose trade exposes them to risk of corneal abrasions. Transmission in the course of ocular examination is probably important.

Meningitis. This mainly occurs in young children. Types 1, 2 and 5 are often responsible.

Acute haemorrhagic cystitis. This is a rare disease of children usually associated with types 11 and 21.

Other diseases. Hyperplasia of intestinal lymphoid tissue is thought to be responsible for some cases of intussusception in infancy. Adenoviruses are also suspected of causing some cases of mesenteric adenitis and acute thyroiditis. They are often present in very large numbers in the faeces of healthy individuals and there is evidence that some types, particularly types 40 and 41, cause gastroenteritis.

Papovaviruses

The papovaviruses are mainly animal viruses. The name is derived from the initial letters of the three main types: *pa*pilloma, *po*lyoma and *va*cuolating viruses. The virions are 30–55 nm in diameter. They have icosahedral symmetry, no envelope and are ether-resistant.

Human warts

Common, plantar and genital warts are benign, infectious, epithelial tumours. Warts can be transmitted to human beings, but not to animals, by cell-free filtrates. Human papillomavirus (HPV) is an icosahedral structure about 55 nm in diameter. It cannot be grown in ordinary tissue cultures. Restriction endonuclease mapping and nucleic acid hybridization techniques have shown that there are many types of HPV. Genital warts is the commonest sexually transmitted viral disease. Infection of the cervix often occurs. It has been suggested that some types of HPV play a role in the aetiology of carcinoma of the cervix. Other types of HPV are associated with unusual skin cancers.

Progressive multifocal leucoencephalopathy

This rare demyelinating disease occurs in patients whose immune mechanisms have been severely depressed by malignant disease or immunosuppressive therapy. Characteristic intranuclear bodies can be detected by electron microscopy of brain tissue and a papovavirus (JC virus) can be isolated in tissue culture.

BK virus

Human infection with this virus is widespread. Antibodies usually appear in childhood. Most infections are subclinical but mild upper respiratory tract symptoms may occur in young children. The virus is often found in the urine of patients undergoing immunosuppressive therapy.

Papovaviruses in animals

These are of medical interest because of their bearing on the relation between viruses and tumours.

Papilloma virus of rabbits (Shope papilloma virus) produces warty growths which may become malignant.

Polyoma virus (Stewart-Eddy or SE virus) which normally causes inapparent infections of mice produces malignant transformation of cells in tissue culture. Polyoma virus is unusual: it produces a great variety of tumours; it is contagious, being transmitted by contact with saliva, faeces and urine; and it produces tumours when inoculated into suckling mice, rats, guinea-pigs or hamsters.

Vacuolating virus (Simian virus 40 or SV40) causes malignant transformation in human and animal cells in tissue culture and

produces malignant tumours in some animals. SV40 may contaminate tissue cultures of monkey kidney cells used to make
vaccines for man, and special precautions have to be taken to
ensure that the virus has been inactivated. SV40 can cause silent
infections in man, with production of antibodies and excretion of
the virus in the faeces.

Parvoviruses

These are probably the smallest viruses to infect man. They are
minute (about 20 nm), non-enveloped, icosahedral viruses containing single-stranded DNA. The DNA is in two complementary
forms present in separate viral particles and capable of uniting
to form double-stranded DNA.

Human parvovirus (B19) frequently infects man without causing
significant illness. It is the cause of erythema infectiosum (fifth
disease), a mild illness occurring mainly among children, characterized by a malar flush ('slapped cheeks') and a generalized rash.
Arthralgia is common in adults. The virus can also cause aplastic
crises in patients with chronic haemolytic anaemia, e.g. sickle cell
anaemia or hereditary spherocytosis.

Adeno-associated viruses are sometimes isolated with adenoviruses from clinical material. They are *defective* viruses that
replicate only in the presence of *helper* adenoviruses. They have
not yet been associated with illness but antibodies against them
may appear in man.

RNA Viruses

A family is a unit composed not only of children, but of men, women, an occasional animal, and the common cold.

Ogden Nash

Picornaviruses

The picornaviruses are a group of very small ribonucleic acid (RNA) viruses (pico=very small, plus RNA). The group contains over 160 different viruses affecting man and includes the enteroviruses, namely hepatitis A virus (p. 364), polio, coxsackie and echoviruses, which are primarily inhabitants of the intestinal tract; the rhinoviruses which are inhabitants of the respiratory tract and a cause of common colds; and various animal viruses such as encephalomyocarditis and foot-and-mouth disease viruses which on rare occasions have been known to infect man.

The virions are 20–30 nm in diameter. They have icosahedral symmetry, no envelope and are highly resistant to ether. The capsids of poliovirus and rhinovirus 14 have been shown to consist of 60 identical subunits, each made up of four proteins.

Poliovirus

Poliovirus is an exclusively human parasite and is the cause of poliomyelitis. The virus grows readily in many types of tissue culture, e.g. monkey kidney, human amnion and HeLa cells. Three antigenically distinct types are recognized: type 1 is responsible for most epidemics; type 2 is mainly associated with inapparent endemic infections; type 3 occasionally causes epidemics. Infection with one type does not confer immunity against the other types, and second attacks with paralysis, though rare, do occur.

Results of infection

In most cases there are no symptoms at all, but in some there is a mild febrile illness lasting a day or so with headache and vomiting (abortive poliomyelitis). In a few cases after premonitory symptoms for 5–7 days there is a second rise in temperature and the patient develops symptoms and signs of meningitis (non-paralytic poliomyelitis). In a very few cases, less than 1% of those infected during epidemics, the disease progresses further: the virus produces degenerative changes in the anterior horn cells of the spinal cord and the motor nuclei of the cranial nerves, and the patient develops flaccid paralyses.

In some tropical and subtropical countries with overcrowding and low standards of hygiene, infection is endemic and most individuals come into contact with the virus in infancy. In these countries paralytic poliomyelitis is rare, but when it does occur it almost invariably affects infants or very young children.

In Europe and North America at the beginning of this century paralytic poliomyelitis was mainly a disease of children under five (infantile paralysis). In later years social and hygienic improvements diminished the opportunities for infection in early life and a higher proportion of the population possessed no immunity. In these circumstances the disease spread in epidemic form and tended to attack older children, particularly those aged 6–12 years, as well as adults. The proportion of paralytic cases in such epidemics is higher than in communities where the disease is endemic. Routine immunization has almost eliminated the disease, but immunization levels have fallen to 50–60% in parts of the UK and further outbreaks may occur.

Transmission

Poliovirus is present in the pharynx and stools a few days before the onset of symptoms. It remains in the pharynx for only the first few days of illness, but it persists in the faeces for several weeks or even months. Spread is by close personal contact with overt or subclinical cases of the disease. The virus is found in the stools of a high proportion of family contacts. In temperate climates epidemics usually occur in summer and autumn, times when gastrointestinal diseases spread by excreta are at their height. Transmission by flies, food, milk and water is important in countries with low standards of hygiene. The virus enters by the mouth, multiplies in the pharynx and intestinal tract and gains access to the nervous system by way of the blood.

Diagnosis

The presence of the virus in faeces and washings or swabs from the throat can be detected by cytopathic effects in tissue cultures. The serological type is determined by neutralization tests with specific antisera. The virus is hardly ever isolated from the cerebrospinal fluid (CSF).

Antibodies against the virus can be detected by neutralization and complement fixation tests.

Coxsackieviruses

Coxsackieviruses are so named because the first strains were isolated from the faeces of two children living in Coxsackie, NY.

A characteristic of the group is that although ordinary laboratory animals cannot be infected the viruses can be grown in suckling mice and hamsters. These animals rapidly lose their susceptibility and when they are more than five days old they can no longer be infected.

Many serologically distinct types of coxsackieviruses have been described. They are divided into two groups on the basis of the lesions they produce in mice. Group A, consisting of at least 23 types, produces generalized myositis. Group B, consisting of at least six types, produces necrotic lesions in the interscapular fat pad, pancreas, liver, brain and myocardium. All group B and some group A viruses can be grown in tissue cultures. HeLa and monkey kidney cells are suitable for routine purposes.

Human infections

These are extremely common. They are usually mild and often pass unrecognized. Various types of illness are recognized:

Herpangina is a febrile illness with vesicular lesions usually on the anterior pillars of the fauces. It is mainly a disease of young children and occurs in epidemic form in the summer. It is caused by viruses of group A.

Bornholm disease (epidemic myalgia, pleurodynia) is characterized by fever and severe pain ('devil's grip') in the lower thorax and abdomen. It is caused by viruses of group B. Epidemics are common and the island of Bornholm in the Baltic is only one of many places where the disease has occurred.

Meningitis (meningoencephalitis, etc.) may be caused by viruses of groups A and B. A paralytic disease indistinguishable from paralytic poliomyelitis has occurred in a few cases, particularly in children infected with coxsackievirus A7.

Myocarditis. Intrauterine or neonatal infection with group B viruses has caused small outbreaks of fatal myocarditis in the newborn. Group B viruses are also responsible for some cases of benign myocarditis and pericarditis in older children and adults.

Hepatitis is sometimes the most prominent feature of generalized neonatal infection with group B viruses. The babies often die.

Respiratory illness. Coxsackievirus A21 has caused large outbreaks of cold-like illnesses. Viruses of group B have been associated with bronchitis and pneumonia in children.

Rashes. Some viruses of groups A and B cause febrile illnesses with rashes. Hand-foot-and-mouth disease, a syndrome of painful stomatitis and a vesicular rash on the hands and feet, and on the buttocks in young children, is mainly caused by coxsackievirus A16.

Conjunctivitis. Coxsackievirus A24 has caused large outbreaks of acute haemorrhagic conjunctivitis.

Diabetes. Some cases of acute-onset juvenile diabetes are thought to be caused by group B viruses.

Postviral fatigue syndrome (myalgic encephalitis, 'Royal Free disease') is a chronic illness characterized by extreme exhaustion after exercise and ill-defined neurological and psychological symptoms. Various viruses have been suspected as being responsible. Several outbreaks are thought to have been caused by group B coxsackieviruses.

Diagnosis

An attempt is made to isolate the virus from the faeces, throat and, in cases of viral meningitis, the CSF by inoculation of tissue cultures and litters of suckling mice. The virus is identified by neutralization tests. Coxsackieviruses can often be isolated from the faeces and throats of normal persons.

A rise in antibody titre in the patient's serum can be detected by neutralization, fluorescent antibody and complement fixation tests.

Echoviruses

The introduction of tissue culture methods drew attention to the existence of large numbers of previously unrecognized viruses in human faeces. They were named echo or *e*nteric *c*ytopathogenic *h*uman *o*rphan viruses. They were 'orphans' because at first their relationship to human disease was unknown.

Most echoviruses grow well and produce cytopathic effects in cultures of monkey kidney cells. With rare exceptions animals are not susceptible. At least 31 distinct serological types can be recognized by neutralization and complement fixation tests.

Infections

Most infections are inapparent. Echoviruses can frequently be isolated from normal individuals and a high proportion of the population possess neutralizing antibodies to some types. Clinical syndromes associated with echovirus infection include various combinations of the following:

Meningitis. Echoviruses are the commonest cause of viral

meningitis and encephalitis. Types 4, 6, 9, 19 and 30 have caused large outbreaks. In rare cases, particularly with types 9 and 16, there has been paralysis, usually transient.

Gastroenteritis. Many types can cause febrile illness associated with mild gastroenteritis, particularly in infants and children. Type 6 has caused large outbreaks.

Respiratory illness. Mild upper respiratory tract infections and cold-like illnesses have been associated with several types. Large outbreaks have been caused by type 20.

Rashes. Maculopapular rashes are caused by several types, and have been a special feature of outbreaks caused by types 9 and 16.

Diagnosis

Faeces provide the best material for virus isolation. The virus may also be isolated from the pharynx in the early stages of the illness and the CSF in the acute stages of meningitis.

Antibodies can be detected by neutralization and complement fixation tests. Because of the complexity of the echovirus group, serological tests are usually restricted to a neutralization test against the strain of virus isolated from the particular patient.

Other enteroviruses

Coxsackieviruses and echoviruses have overlapping properties and the more recently discovered enteroviruses have been simply assigned numbers, e.g. enterovirus type 68, enterovirus type 69, etc.

Conjunctivitis. Enterovirus type 70 has caused large outbreaks of acute haemorrhagic conjunctivitis.

Poliomyelitis-like illness. A paralytic illness occasionally follows the conjunctivitis in patients infected with enterovirus type 70.

Rhinoviruses

The rhinoviruses or common cold viruses are a large group of picornaviruses. Their natural habitat is the nose and throat and, unlike the enteroviruses, they are not found in the faeces.

Growth and classification

Rhinoviruses will grow and produce cytopathic effects in primate tissue cultures. For primary isolation of most strains it is essential to use a lower temperature (33°C) and a more acid medium than is normally used in virus isolation, and ensure oxygenation by rotating the cultures. Rhinoviruses are divided into two groups: H strains, the most commonly encountered, grow only in human embryonic tissue; M strains grow in monkey kidney tissue as well as in human embryonic tissue and other human cells. Most strains can be adapted to grow in cultures such as HeLa cells. Some rhinoviruses can be grown only in organ cultures of ciliated nasal or tracheal epithelium. Over 100 types of rhinoviruses can be distinguished by neutralization tests in tissue cultures. There is almost no antigenic overlap between the different types.

Common colds

Intranasal instillation of rhinoviruses will produce typical colds in individuals who do not possess antibodies against that particular type. The susceptibility of the human race to repeated colds is explained by the existence of many types of rhinoviruses. This multiplicity of types makes it unlikely that an effective vaccine can be devized. There is no evidence that chilling predisposes to colds.

Cold-like illnesses

Colds or cold-like illnesses are occasionally caused by parainfluenza viruses, respiratory syncytial virus, coxsackieviruses (particularly coxsackievirus A21), echoviruses, reoviruses, adenoviruses and coronaviruses.

Encephalomyocarditis viruses

These viruses are parasites of rodents and other animals, but on rare occasions they have caused encephalitis in man.

Foot-and-mouth disease

This highly contagious virus disease of cattle, sheep and pigs is rarely transmitted to man, but should be considered as a possible cause of vesicular lesions in persons having contact with infected animals.

Reoviruses

Reoviruses or *r*espiratory *e*nteric *o*rphan viruses are double-stranded RNA viruses, 60—90 nm in diameter. The RNA is made up of ten separate segments. The virions have icosahedral symmetry, no envelope and are ether-resistant. The viruses grow readily in monkey kidney tissue culture. Three main types of reoviruses are recognized. They share a complement-fixing antigen but can be distinguished by haemagglutination-inhibition tests.

Reoviruses are ubiquitous and are frequently isolated from man and animals. Serological surveys confirm that human infections are widespread. The relation of reoviruses to disease is uncertain, but they are probably responsible for some mild upper respiratory tract infections. Reoviruses have been isolated from a few cases of hepatitis with encephalitis.

Orbiviruses

Orbiviruses are a group of arthropod-borne viruses (arboviruses) which resemble reoviruses in containing double-stranded RNA. Man is seldom a host to these viruses.

Colorado tick fever virus causes a febrile illness and encephalitis in the north-western USA and Canada.

Rotaviruses (infantile gastroenteritis viruses)

Rotaviruses are the most important cause of acute gastroenteritis in infants and young children. This disease is a major cause of childhood mortality, particularly in underdeveloped countries.

The viral particles are about 60 nm in diameter with a central core and a double-layered capsid which gives them a characteristic wheel-like appearance under the electron microscope. The capsid is composed of 32 capsomeres. Rotaviruses resemble reoviruses in containing double-stranded RNA. Rotavirus RNA is made up of 11 separate segments. Several serotypes of human rotaviruses are recognized. Other serotypes cause disease in calves, piglets and other animals.

Gastroenteritis caused by these viruses is most common in infants and children under three but may occur up to the age of six. Rotaviruses are responsible for 25–75% of all cases of gastroenteritis in children admitted to hospitals. The peak frequency occurs in winter. Mild or asymptomatic infections are very common as judged by serological methods. Antibodies can be detected in over 80% of children by the age of three and in nearly all children by the age of six.

The diagnosis in the acute stage of the disease can be made in a few hours by electron microscopy of faecal extracts. The viral particles may be present in vast numbers. Enzyme-linked immunosorbent assay (ELISA) techniques provide a sensitive and rapid method for detecting rotavirus antigens in faeces. Rotaviruses can be grown in certain tissue cultures and the presence of virus can be demonstrated by immunofluorescent techniques.

There remain many cases of gastroenteritis ('winter vomiting disease', 'non-bacterial gastroenteritis', etc.) in which no bacterial or viral cause can be identified. Some of these may be infections caused by various poorly characterized viruses which have been seen in faecal extracts under the electron microscope, e.g. astroviruses, caliciviruses, Norwalk virus and the 'small round viruses' which are often associated with shellfish poisoning.

Orthomyxoviruses

This group of RNA viruses includes the viruses responsible for influenza in man and various animals. They are named myxoviruses because of their affinity for mucoproteins (protein-polysaccharide complexes) present on the surface of mammalian cells.

The viruses consist of particles 80–120 nm in diameter. They are typically spheroidal but filamentous forms are often present. The virions comprise an envelope surrounding the nucleocapsid which is a helical arrangement of protein and RNA. The envelope bristles with regularly spaced radial projections (Fig. 12B, p. 35). These are of two kinds: (1) haemagglutinins by which the virus attaches itself to the mucoprotein receptors of red cells, and (2) the enzyme neuraminidase (p. 41). The RNA is single-stranded and has negative-strand polarity, i.e. it is complementary to messenger RNA. Replication of viral RNA requires an RNA-dependent RNA polymerase which being absent from the uninfected host cell needs to be packaged within the virion in order to initate viral nucleic acid synthesis. The RNA of orthomyxoviruses is unusual in that it is composed of eight separate segments. Reassortment of these segments during replication probably accounts for the ease with which genetic recombination occurs in influenza viruses.

Influenza virus

There are three types of influenza virus, A, B and C, each possessing type-specific soluble S antigens which can be recognized by complement fixation tests. The S antigens are nucleoproteins. They are minute particles about 10 nm in diameter and can be obtained free from the intact virus. Antibodies to S antigens play no part in the development of immunity to influenza. Strain-specific viral V antigens can be recognized by haemagglutination-inhibition, neutralization and, provided precautions are taken to exclude S antigens, complement fixation tests. The V antigens are protein components of the viral surface, namely the haemagglutinin (H) and neuraminidase (N) antigens. Antibodies to V antigens, particularly the H antigens, are responsible for immunity to influenza. A standard nomenclature is used to describe strains of influenza virus, e.g. A/Hong Kong/1/68 (H3N2) is the first type A strain isolated in Hong Kong in 1968 and it possesses H antigen 3 and N antigen 2. Influenza type A includes four subtypes, each consisting of a family of antigenically distinct strains which possess a particular combination of the main H and N antigens: H0N1 (also known as subtype A0) was in existence when influenza virus was first isolated in 1933, H1N1 (A1) appeared in 1946, H2N2 (A2 or Asian) in 1957 and H3N2 (Hong Kong) in 1968. Influenza type B includes minor antigenic variants. Type C is more or less homogeneous.

Influenza in man

The virus is transmitted from person to person by infected nasopharyngeal secretions. It is assumed that the first stage of infection is adsorption of virus to mucoprotein receptors on the cells of the upper respiratory tract. Influenza typically takes the form of an acute general illness with fever, prostration, headache, pains in the muscles and relatively minor respiratory symptoms. In severe cases pneumonia may occur. This can usually be attributed to colonization of the damaged respiratory epithelium by bacteria such as *Staphylococcus aureus* or *Haemophilus influenzae*, but in some cases the virus alone seems to be responsible for the lung lesions. *Staph. aureus* is known to produce a protease which activates the haemagglutinin of influenza virus. Various viral infections, including influenza and chickenpox, are occasionally associated with encephalopathy and hepatic failure (Reye's syndrome). Aspirin may be a contributory factor. It should not be given to children.

Epidemiology

Influenza viruses are widespread throughout the world and produce recurrent epidemics usually during the winter months. Type A shows the greatest tendency to spread through the community and has produced epidemics roughly every two years. Type B has tended to produce less extensive outbreaks at intervals of 3–6 years. Type C is much less important and has so far produced no large epidemics.

From time to time world-wide pandemics occur, e.g. the 1918 pandemic which killed some 20 million people, particularly young adults, and the 1957 pandemic of Asian influenza which had a very high incidence of infection but low mortality. Most major outbreaks represent the emergence of new antigenic variants against which the population possesses little or no immunity. Influenza type A has been the most prolific source. Minor changes in its H and N antigens ('antigenic drift') are common. Occasionally there is a sudden major change ('antigenic shift') and a new subtype is produced, e.g. in the Asian (H2N2) strain which appeared in 1957 both the H and N antigens were completely unlike those of earlier strains. It has been suggested that new subtypes arise as a result of genetic recombination between a human strain and a strain from an animal or bird. Strains of type A have been isolated from pigs, horses and other animals and from a variety of wild and domestic birds. The prevalence of different variants in the history of the community is mirrored by the antibodies currently found in persons of different ages.

Diagnosis

In the first three days the virus can be isolated from garglings or throat swabs by inoculation of the amniotic cavity of the chick embryo or by growth in tissue culture. Rolled cultures of monkey kidney cells are suitable for primary isolation. The virus can be both detected and identified in infected tissue cultures by immunofluorescent techniques. Alternatively it can be detected by haemagglutination and haemadsorption techniques and identified by the inhibition of these effects by specific antisera. Haemagglutination-inhibition and complement fixation tests can be used to identify antibodies in the patient's serum.

Prevention

Killed vaccines prepared in chick embryos are available but their effectiveness is limited by the antigenic variability of influenza virus.

Swine influenza virus

Swine influenza virus is a type A influenza virus. There is serological evidence that this or an antigenically related virus caused the pandemic of 1918. In recent years occasional human cases have occurred, usually in persons in contact with pigs. In 1976 alarm was caused by a small outbreak among military personnel at Fort Dix, NJ, in which person-to-person spread was clearly demonstrated. Over 40 million people were immunized in the USA. Unfortunately over 500 of them developed severe polyneuritis (Guillain-Barré syndrome) and there were 25 deaths. Meanwhile the outbreak fizzled out on its own.

Paramyxoviruses

This group of RNA viruses includes parainfluenza, mumps, Newcastle disease, measles and respiratory syncytial viruses. Their normal habitat is the respiratory tract.

Paramyxoviruses resemble orthomyxoviruses in having a nucleocapsid with helical symmetry and an envelope with haemagglutinins. However, they are larger (150–200 nm), rarely or never produce filaments, and are antigenically stable. The RNA is not segmented. Measles and respiratory syncytical virus are smaller than other paramyxoviruses, do not possess neuraminidase and are antigenically distinct.

Parainfluenza viruses

These viruses are an important cause of acute respiratory illness in the first few years of life. Severe infections such as croup, bronchiolitis and pneumonia may occur in infants and young children. Parainfluenza viruses are the commonest cause of croup.

The viruses grow relatively poorly in the chick embryo, but can be readily isolated in human or monkey kidney cells. The viruses can be detected by haemagglutination and haemadsorption techniques. Four serological types are recognized: types 1 and 2 are associated with severe infections but types 3 and 4 usually cause only minor illness.

Mumps virus

Mumps is a world-wide disease caused by a human virus with a special affinity for the salivary glands. The virus closely resembles influenza virus, e.g. it grows readily in the chick amniotic cavity, causes haemagglutination and possesses S and V antigens. Serologically it is a distinct and homogeneous virus. Infection is usually limited to the parotid glands, but other salivary glands may also be enlarged and tender. In males after puberty orchitis occurs in up to 20% of cases; in a few cases the orchitis is bilateral and causes sterility. Minor involvement of the central nervous system is common and mumps virus accounts for 10–20% of all cases of viral meningitis and meningoencephalitis. Pancreatitis, oophoritis and mastitis are other results of infection with mumps virus. About 30% of all mumps infections are inapparent. In special cases an attempt can be made to isolate the virus from saliva, urine or CSF using chick embryos or tissue culture. Serological tests, usually a complement fixation test, are of help in diagnosing mumps meningitis when attempts to isolate the virus have failed.

Newcastle disease virus

Newcastle disease is a generalized infection occurring in chickens and turkeys. Human infection is uncommon and is largely confined to poultry workers and laboratory staff. It takes the form of an influenza-like illness with conjunctivitis.

Measles

Measles virus is an RNA virus about 140 nm in diameter. It can be grown in human and monkey tissue cultures. Infected cultures show multinucleate giant cells and syncytial masses containing vacuoles and acidophilic intranuclear inclusion bodies. The virus can be identified by neutralization or complement fixation tests.

Measles is the most infectious of all the specific fevers and until vaccines became available few children escaped it. Large epidemics tended to occur every other year. The virus is a strictly human parasite. It is acquired by inhalation and produces a catarrhal infection of the upper respiratory tract, Koplik's spots and a rash. The rash represents a delayed hypersensitivity reaction, i.e. the action of T-lymphocytes on cells containing measles antigen. Measles is more serious in children under three or suffering from other diseases. Bronchopneumonia is the most common complication and accounts for most of the deaths. Otitis media is also common. Measles encephalitis is rare but has a mortality of 15%. Giant cell pneumonia is a rare and usually fatal disease occurring in children whose immune mechanisms are defective.

Measles virus is also responsible for a rare, slowly progressive, fatal neurological disease known as subacute sclerosing panencephalitis which affects children and young adults. The patients usually give a history of typical measles several years previously and have extremely high levels of measles antibodies. Measles antigen can be demonstrated by immunofluorescent techniques in cerebral biopsy specimens and in cells of the CSF. By using special techniques measles virus can be isolated from brain tissue. The mechanism of the disease is obscure. The virus is probably acquired during an attack of ordinary measles and then persists in the central nervous system in some altered or defective form. Persistent measles virus RNA in lymphocytes and high levels of measles antibody are also associated with some cases of chronic active hepatitis.

Laboratory diagnosis of measles is rarely required. Up to one day after the appearance of the rash the virus can sometimes be isolated from the nasopharynx or the blood, but the success rate is low. Examination of nasopharyngeal secretions by an immunofluorescent technique is quicker and more sensitive. Giant cells can be found in sputum and nasal secretions in the early stages of measles.

Human normal immunoglobulin can be used to prevent or attenuate measles in very young or debilitated children. Effective living attenuated vaccines are available. In the USA indigenous measles has been almost eliminated by enthusiastic use of these vaccines.

Respiratory syncytial virus (RSV)

This RNA virus is roughly spherical, 120–130 nm in diameter, but filamentous forms also occur. It can be grown in human tissue cultures, such as certain strains of HeLa cells, where it produces a characteristic cytopathic effect with formation of giant cells and syncytia. RSV can be rapidly identified in nasopharyngeal secretions by direct staining with fluorescent antibodies.

RSV is one of the most important causes of acute lower respiratory tract infection in young children. In infants under six months the disease is often severe with acute bronchiolitis and bronchopneumonia. Death is not uncommon. In older children the disease is usually milder. Brief localized outbreaks are common. Serological studies show that 80% of children have been infected by the age of four. Second attacks of infection occur. These often take the form of a minor respiratory illness with cough and running nose.

Togaviruses

These RNA viruses are 30–70 nm in diameter and possess a polyhedral nucleocapsid surrounded by a lipid envelope (hence the 'toga') and are sensitive to ether. On the basis of their serological and general biological properties togaviruses of medical significance are classified into two large groups of arthropod-borne viruses (arboviruses) known as alphaviruses (formerly group A arboviruses) and flaviviruses (group B arboviruses). Rubella virus is also classified as a togavirus.

In infections caused by alphaviruses and flaviviruses the arthropod vector (mosquito or tick) is more than a mechanical transmitter of infection. After the vector has acquired the virus by feeding on the blood of an infected host the virus multiplies in the body of the vector and several days usually elapse before the vector can transmit infection. It often remains infected for life. In mosquitoes and ticks there may be transovarian passage of the virus to the next generation.

Human diseases caused by togaviruses include many types of encephalitis and tropical fevers but the viruses are primarily parasites of animals and birds. Man is an occasional host of little or no importance in the perpetuation of the viruses. The diseases are most common in tropical and subtropical countries and often have a very restricted geographical distribution. More than 200 togaviruses are recognized. Other arboviruses which infect man belong to a number of virus families, namely bunyaviruses, orbiviruses, rhabdoviruses and arenaviruses.

Togaviruses are pathogenic for mice and produce encephalitis on intracerebral inoculation. Many of them can also be grown in the chick embryo and in tissue culture. Most togaviruses cause haemagglutination of the red cells of day-old chicks. Antigenic overlap between togaviruses is common as judged by haemagglutination-inhibition and complement fixation tests. Neutralization tests are more specific.

In human infections the most satisfactory material for virus isolation is usually blood taken in the early stages of the disease. In cases of encephalitis the virus is rarely found in the CSF but may be isolated from brain tissue in fatal cases. Serological diagnosis can be made by haemagglutination-inhibition, complement fixation, immunofluorescent and neutralization tests.

Togaviruses causing encephalitis

The large family of togaviruses causing encephalitis can be classified into three groups:

1 *Equine encephalitis viruses.* This group includes eastern, western and Venezuelan equine encephalitis viruses, three closely related alphaviruses mainly affecting horses in the eastern and western parts of the USA and in South America. Birds are probably the main reservoir of infection and mosquitoes are the main vectors. Human infections are often inapparent, but there have also been serious outbreaks.
2 *St Louis encephalitis and related viruses.* St Louis, Japanese and Australian encephalitis viruses are closely related flaviviruses. Birds are the main reservoir and mosquitoes are the vectors. Domestic pigs are an important reservoir for Japanese encephalitis virus. Inapparent human infections are common, but there have also been serious outbreaks, e.g. in 1975 St Louis virus caused hundreds of cases in the USA.
3 *Tick-borne encephalitis viruses.* Louping-ill, Russian spring-summer encephalitis and Powassan viruses are flaviviruses. Louping-ill is the only arthropod-borne encephalitis indigenous to the UK. It is a disease of sheep and is found mainly in Scotland and the North of England. The affected animals show ataxia and leaping movements which give the disease its name. The vector is the sheep tick. Human infection is rare, but a few cases of encephalitis have occurred among those working with infected sheep. Louping-ill or similar viruses also occur in various countries in Europe. Russian spring-summer encephalitis is a tick-borne disease mainly found in humid, wooded areas in the USSR. The reservoirs include small rodents, birds and ticks themselves. Powassan virus is a rare cause of encephalitis in North America.

Yellow fever

Yellow fever is endemic over large areas of tropical Africa and Central and South America. It has caused devastating epidemics.

The virus is a flavivirus. It is primarily a parasite of mosquitoes, in which infection persists throughout life and is passed trans-ovarially through infected eggs. The virus is transmitted from monkey to monkey by jungle-living mosquitoes. Man becomes an occasional and incidental host when he ventures into the jungle and is bitten by an infected mosquito. This type of the disease is known as jungle yellow fever.

If the infected person returns to a town the virus can be transmitted from man to man by domesticated mosquitoes. This was clearly demonstrated by Walter Reed of the US Yellow Fever Commission using human volunteers. This type of the disease is known as urban yellow fever.

The disease classically takes the form of a severe illness with fever, vomiting, haemorrhages, jaundice and a fatal outcome. Serological surveys in areas where the disease occurs indicate that overt cases are greatly outnumbered by mild or inapparent infections.

Urban yellow fever has been largely eradicated by mosquito control and human immunization with a living attenuated vaccine. However, in an outbreak in Nigeria in 1986 there were over 5000 cases and 500 deaths. Strict precautions are necessary to ensure that no infected mosquitoes or non-immunized human beings are allowed to travel by aeroplane, boat, etc., from endemic areas to regions where the disease might take hold.

Dengue

Dengue is an acute, rarely fatal, febrile illness associated with severe headache, excruciating pains in the bones and joints ('breakbone fever') and a maculopapular or scarlatiniform rash on the third to fifth day. Dengue haemorrhagic fever (dengue shock) is a serious illness affecting children in south-east Asia. It is caused by deposition of immune complexes produced as a result of reinfection with dengue virus. Dengue is the most widely distributed of all arbovirus infections and has occurred in all tropical and subtropical countries.

In some tropical countries monkeys form a reservoir of infection, the virus being transmitted by mosquitoes from monkey to monkey with man as an occasional host. In other areas man appears to be the only host. Infection is transmitted from man to man by domestic mosquitoes. The virus is a flavivirus. Four serological types are recognized.

Dengue-like diseases

Mosquito-borne fevers caused by togaviruses occur in various parts of the world. Ross River virus, an alphavirus, causes epidemics of polyarthritis with a rash and sore throat in Australia and the South Pacific. Chickungunya virus, an alphavirus, causes a dengue-like illness in parts of Africa and Asia. West Nile virus, a flavivirus, causes a mild febrile illness in Egypt, Israel and India.

Tick fevers

Omsk haemorrhagic fever in the USSR and Kyasanur Forest fever in India are tick-borne haemorrhagic fevers without encephalitis. They are caused by flaviviruses which in their main features belong to the louping-ill and Russian spring-summer encephalitis group. Colorado tick fever is caused by an orbivirus and Crimean (Congo) haemorrhagic fever by a bunyavirus.

Rubella (German measles)

This RNA virus is 50—75 nm in diameter and has an envelope. In some tissue cultures, such as a line of rabbit kidney cells, the virus produces cytopathic effects and can be identified by neutralization tests. Growth of rubella virus in tissue culture yields a haemagglutinin active against red cells of newly-hatched chicks. Haemagglutination-inhibition tests provide a reliable method for estimating rubella antibodies. Antibodies can also be estimated by complement fixation, radial haemolysis, radioimmunoassay and ELISA techniques.

Rubella is normally a mild disease. Transient arthralgia, most commonly affecting the joints of the hand, is common. Persistent arthritis occurs occasionally. The virus can be isolated from the synovial fluid of chronically infected joints. The main importance of rubella is that when infection is contracted by women during the first three months of pregnancy the fetus may develop congenital defects including deafness and deaf-mutism, microcephaly and mental retardation, cataracts and other eye defects, heart disease and dental abnormalities. The reported incidence of these defects has varied in different surveys from 10% to over 70%. Infection of the fetus is usually widespread and may also result in purpura, enlargement of the liver and spleen, bone lesions, myocardial necrosis and interstitial pneumonitis. Because of these risks young girls should be immunized with a rubella vaccine before they reach child-bearing age. Deliberate exposure of young girls to natural rubella is still practised but entails a slight risk to the rest of the population. If pregnant women are exposed to rubella a careful history should be taken of the time and nature of the exposure and a sample of blood should be tested for rubella antibodies. A past history of clinical rubella is an unreliable guide to immune status and what appear to be second attacks are not uncommon. To interpret the results of the serological tests it is necessary to understand the time-scale of rubella virus infection (Fig. 50).

When a patient is infected with rubella the virus can be isolated from the patient's throat from the fifth or sixth day onwards, i.e. the patient is infective for at least nine days before the appearance of the rash which usually occurs between the fifteenth and twenty-first day. The patient remains infective until about the twenty-second day. Haemagglutination-inhibiting antibody is first detectable on the fifteenth day, rises rapidly during the next week and remains detectable for the rest of the patient's life. Complement-fixing antibody appears on about the twenty-second day, rises slowly for the next three weeks and gradually disappears over the next two or three years. By measuring both types of antibody, repeating the tests if necessary after an interval of a few days, it is usually possible to distinguish active or very recent infection from past infection. Help can also be obtained by

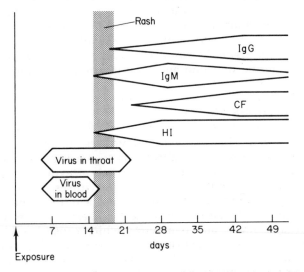

Fig. 50 Time-scale of events in rubella. The diagram shows the relation between the appearance of the rash, the presence of rubella virus in the throat and blood and the appearance of haemagglutination-inhibiting (HI), complement-fixing (CF), IgM and IgG antibodies.

using special techniques to determine the classes of immuno-globulin responsible for the antibody activity. Nearly all the anti-body appearing on the fifteenth day is IgM. This is present in significant amounts for only the next 8–12 weeks, being gradually replaced by IgG, i.e. the presence of IgM indicates active or very recent infection.

By correlating the history of exposure with the serological results most cases will fall into one of three categories:

1 Patients who have had rubella in the past. These are not at risk and can be reassured.
2 Patients with active or very recent infection. These should be referred to a gynaecologist who will consider the advisability of therapeutic abortion.
3 Patients with no detectable antibodies. These may or may not develop rubella. The serological tests should be repeated at intervals until five weeks after the date of exposure. By this time antibodies will have appeared if the patient has been infected. If no antibodies appear the patient has not been infected and can be advised to have a rubella vaccine after delivery.

Rubella virus can be isolated from fetuses aborted in the early months of pregnancy, from infants born with congenital defects, and from normal infants whose mothers have had rubella late in pregnancy. Since the virus often persists in the throat, blood and urine for several months after birth, congenitally infected infants are important in ensuring the survival of the virus. Rubella reinfection in pregnant women is only very rarely associated with intrauterine infection and is of minimal risk to the fetus.

Bunyaviruses

This large group of enveloped RNA viruses are arthropod-borne viruses (arboviruses). They differ from togaviruses in their larger size (diameter 90–100 nm) and the helical symmetry of their capsids. They include the true bunyaviruses ('Bunyamwera supergroup'); phleboviruses which cause sandfly fever and Rift Valley fever; the nairovirus which causes Crimean (Congo) haemorrhagic fever; and hantavirus which cause haemorrhagic fever with renal syndrome (Korean haemorrhagic fever).

Bunyamwera supergroup

This group includes more than 80 different arboviruses serologi-cally related to Bunyamwera virus, named after a region in Africa.

Ten subgroups are distinguished on serological grounds. Several members of the Bunyamwera subgroup cause febrile illness in man, particularly in Africa. California encephalitis is caused by members of the California subgroup. Small animals are the normal hosts. Infection is transmitted to man by mosquitoes.

Sandfly fever (Phlebotomus fever)

Sandfly fever is a non-fatal, influenza-like illness with conjunctival injection found in Mediterranean countries and parts of Asia and Africa. The virus is transmitted by the bite of the female sandfly, *Phlebotomus papatasi*, which is mainly active at night. No animal reservoir of infection has been discovered. Several serological types of the virus are recognized.

Rift Valley fever

Rift Valley fever is a mosquito-borne disease of sheep and cattle in Kenya and other parts of Africa. There is almost certainly a reservoir of infection among wild animals. In man the disease resembles influenza. A large epidemic occurred in Egypt in 1977 and caused many deaths. The virus is transmitted to man by mosquito bites and by handling sick and dead animals.

Crimean (Congo) haemorrhagic fever

This is a severe haemorrhagic fever found in the USSR, eastern Europe, the Middle East, Pakistan and tropical Africa and caused by a distinct tick-borne virus. Several deaths have occurred among laboratory workers.

Haemorrhagic fever with renal syndrome

This important human disease, also known as Korean haemorrhagic fever, occurs in many parts of the Far East, the USSR and, usually in a milder form, in Europe. The causative agent, hantavirus (Hantaan virus), has been isolated from rodents. Infection is transmitted to man by aerosols. Serological evidence of infection is occasionally found in the UK. Laboratory workers in contact with rodents are at special risk.

Rhabdoviruses

These are rod or bullet-shaped RNA viruses. The virion has helical symmetry and a lipoprotein envelope covered with spikes.

Rhabdoviruses are primarily parasites of animals. Man is affected by rabies virus and occasionally by vesicular stomatitis virus.

Rabies

Rabies virus is a bullet-shaped RNA virus measuring 75 × 180 nm. The virion is enveloped and has helical symmetry (Fig. 51). The virus is most easily isolated by intracerebral inoculation of mice, but it will also grow in chick embryos and in various tissue cultures.

Rabies chiefly affects dogs, wolves, foxes and, in Trinidad, vampire bats, but may occur in many other wild and domestic animals. In some countries various species of bats suffer from latent rabies and are an important reservoir of infection. In the last decade foxes have been mainly responsible for an alarming spread of rabies westwards across Europe. Dogs are by far the most important source of human infection.

The virus is present in the saliva and is transmitted by biting. It multiplies locally in the wound and travels to the central nervous system mainly by the sensory nerves. After a very variable incubation period, usually 3−12 weeks, it produces a characteristic syndrome of pain around the bite, restlessness, gross difficulty in swallowing (hydrophobia) due to pharyngeal spasms, generalized convulsions and death. Before 1970 no patient had ever recovered from established rabies. Since then at least three survivors have been reported.

Diagnosis in dogs and man can be confirmed in life by isolating the virus from saliva. After death characteristic eosinophilic inclusions (Negri bodies) can be found inside nerve cells, particularly in the hippocampus. The rabies antigen in Negri bodies and in the salivary glands can be specifically identified within a few hours by staining with a fluorescent antibody. The virus can also be isolated from brain tissue and salivary glands. If the dog is alive when first seen it should be kept in captivity for ten days: if it survives it has not got rabies; if it dies the brain is examined for Negri bodies.

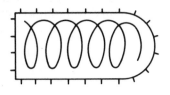

100 nm

Fig. 51 Rabies virus, showing the envelope and helical internal structure.

Rabies has been eradicated from the UK and is kept out by strict quarantine of all imported dogs and other animals. Rigidly enforced legislation to control this horrible disease is entirely justifiable. Vaccination of domestic dogs and elimination of strays is important in countries where rabies is endemic. Persons bitten by rabid animals should be given human antirabies immuno-globulin (or horse antirabies serum), injected partly into the wound and partly intramuscularly, and a course of rabies vaccine.

Vesicular stomatitis virus

This virus causes disease in cattle. A mild influenza-like illness or an inapparent infection is not uncommon in farmers, veterinary surgeons and laboratory workers.

Coronaviruses

This group of enveloped RNA viruses derives its name from the characteristic fringe of projections which surrounds the virus particles when viewed with the electron microscope. The viruses are 80–160 nm in diameter. Coronaviruses are mainly found in the nose and throat and are responsible for colds and cold-like illnesses. They can be grown on human embryonic cell lines.

Arenaviruses

These RNA viruses have a characteristic appearance when viewed with the electron microscope. The interior of the virus consists of a central area containing a number of granules giving a sand-strewn appearance. The viruses are 50–80 nm in diameter and have an envelope covered with short projections. Members of the arenavirus group share a major antigen.

Lymphocytic choriomeningitis virus

This virus is a parasite of mice, in which it produces latent infection. It is an occasional cause of viral meningitis in man. Transmission occurs via the respiratory tract and does not depend on an insect vector.

Lassa fever

This highly lethal disease occurs in Nigeria and adjoining parts of West Africa. In some areas mild or subclinical infections are common. It is spread by close contact and by material such as blood, faeces and infected tissues. Deaths have occurred among doctors, nurses and laboratory workers. Investigation of suspected cases is hazardous and is best left to institutions specially equipped to deal with highly dangerous pathogens. A rat-like rodent is the natural reservoir.

Junin and Machupo viruses

These viruses cause severe haemorrhagic fever in Argentina (Junin virus) and Bolivia (Machupo virus). Rodents are the normal host. The animals excrete large quantities of virus in their urine and saliva. The viruses are extremely hazardous to laboratory workers.

Retroviruses

These RNA viruses are 100–120 nm in diameter. They have helical symmetry and possess an envelope. The viruses contain an RNA-dependent DNA polymerase (reverse transcriptase) and transfer genetic information from RNA to DNA which is integrated into the chromosomal DNA of the host cell. The group includes: (1) human immunodeficiency viruses (HIV), the cause of acquired immunodeficiency syndrome (AIDS), (2) human T-cell lymphotropic virus type 1 (HTLV-1) which is associated with the development of some types of T-cell leukaemia and lymphoma in man, (3) HTLV-2 which is of doubtful importance and (4) Rous sarcoma virus and other RNA tumour viruses.

Acquired immunodeficiency syndrome (AIDS)

The acquired immunodeficiency syndrome (AIDS) is the occurrence of life-threatening opportunistic infections and malignant tumours associated with severe defects of cell-mediated immunity occurring without obvious cause in previously healthy individuals. The patients develop infections such as *Pneumocystis carinii* pneumonia, generalized cytomegalovirus infection, progressive herpes and mucocutaneous candidiasis and tumours, particularly a tumour of the skin and viscera known as Kaposi's sarcoma and various types of lymphoma. The patients lose weight ('slim disease') and the outcome is usually fatal. AIDS was first recognized in the USA in 1979. Subsequently the number of cases increased rapidly and the disease has been reported in most countries. A majority of the patients are promiscuous male homosexuals. Intravenous drug abusers, haemophiliacs and other recipients of blood products and multiple transfusions are also at risk. As the disease spreads in the community, transmission by heterosexual intercourse has become increasingly common. In central Africa AIDS is almost entirely a heterosexual disease affecting men and women in equal numbers. It probably first emerged as a human disease in this part of the world. Kaposi's sarcoma is common in this area. In AIDS patients the disease occurs in a highly aggressive form. It has been suggested that the African green monkey may have been the original source of the virus that causes AIDS.

The primary cause of AIDS is infection with human immunodeficiency virus (HIV). The virus has also been called 'lymphadenopathy-associated virus' (LAV) and HTLV-3. Although HIV is a retrovirus that attacks T-cells, it is unlike HTLV-1 or 2 in most of its biological, structural, immunological and genetic properties. It is closely related to a lentivirus (slow virus) which causes visna and maedi, two lethal diseases of sheep. HIV shows frequent variations in its antigenic make-up. It has been isolated from blood, semen, vaginal secretions, breast milk, tears and saliva of AIDS patients. The levels of virus in tears and saliva are very low and infection from these sources is highly unlikely. HIV has been isolated from vaginal secretions from apparently healthy women with antibodies to the virus and male heterosexuals can contract AIDS from such women. Mosquitoes and other blood-sucking insects may carry HIV but there is no evidence that they transmit it to man. Virtually all AIDS patients have antibodies against HIV. Such antibodies are common among healthy homosexuals but are still uncommon among the general population. In the UK over 1200 haemophiliacs (about 30% of the total) are seropositive following the use of contaminated factor VIII. Possession of HIV antibodies indicates past exposure to the virus. Seroconversion takes several months and a negative result soon after exposure must be treated with caution. Detection of HIV antigens by means of a DNA probe provides the most reliable method of diagnosis. Infection is probably life-long and the patient is likely to remain an excreter of the virus and a danger to others. To begin with, most individuals infected with HIV show no symptoms. Later many of them develop *persistent generalized lymphadenopathy* or an *AIDS-related complex* of fever, loss of weight, weakness and other symptoms, signs and immunological abnormalities consistent with AIDS. These two conditions often progress to AIDS. Children born to seropositive women are commonly infected and may develop AIDS. HIV-infected children may be antibody-negative. In addition to its effect on the immune system HIV can cause brain damage. At least 50% of AIDS patients develop encephalopathy with loss of memory, impaired speech and dementia. The incubation period of AIDS is usually very long, e.g. about two years for transfusion-associated AIDS. The prevention and control of AIDS is considered elsewhere (p. 203).

The immunological mechanisms underlying AIDS are obscure. HIV infects and replicates in helper T-lymphocytes. The virus blocks the ability of these T-cells to recognize foreign antigens. The total number of lymphocytes in the peripheral blood falls with a reversal of the helper:suppressor (T4:T8) ratio. Patients with AIDS give negative results in tests for delayed hyper-sensitivity.

Other AIDS viruses

A second AIDS virus known as HIV-2 is endemic in parts of Africa. It is radically different from the original AIDS virus (HIV-1) and serological tests for HIV-1 may fail to pick up antibodies against HIV-2.

Other RNA viruses

Marburg and Ebola viruses

These are pleomorphic rod-shaped viruses 80 nm in diameter and varying greatly in length. Very long filamentous forms are common. Marburg virus is highly lethal to man. In 1967 seven laboratory workers handling African vervet monkeys died of the infection in Marburg in Germany. Ebola virus is morphologically indistinguishable from Marburg virus but is antigenically distinct. It has caused outbreaks of severe and often fatal haemorrhagic fever in tropical Africa. The natural reservoir of these viruses is unknown.

---------- 26 ----------

Miscellaneous Viruses

*...the diseases of the liver have continued to remain
to the present day a subject of extreme difficulty.*
                              Karl von Rokitansky, 1846

It is not yet known whether certain viruses contain deoxyribonucleic acid (DNA) or ribonucleic acid (RNA). In particular there
are some diseases almost certainly caused by viruses in which it
has not yet been possible to isolate a virus. In other diseases such
as viral hepatitis, a number of different DNA and RNA viruses
are known to play a causative role.

Hepatitis viruses

Viral hepatitis is typically associated with prodromal symptoms
such as anorexia, nausea, vomiting and fever followed after a few
days by jaundice. Such cases are greatly outnumbered by those
in which jaundice does not develop. In all cases there is hepatic
damage as judged by biochemical tests of liver function and by
histological examination of biopsy specimens. A few patients die
of acute hepatic failure but most make an uninterrupted recovery.
Attempts to isolate viruses by conventional techniques are rarely
successful, the usual laboratory animals are not susceptible, and
for many years there were no serological tests. Hepatitis viruses
can be assigned to one of four categories:

1 Hepatitis A virus, causing hepatitis type A (infective hepatitis
   or short incubation hepatitis).
2 Hepatitis B virus, causing hepatitis type B (serum hepatitis or
   long incubation hepatitis).
3 Hepatitis delta virus, dependent on hepatitis B virus for
   replication.
4 Non-A, non-B hepatitis viruses, causing hepatitis that cannot
   be ascribed to either type A or B viruses.

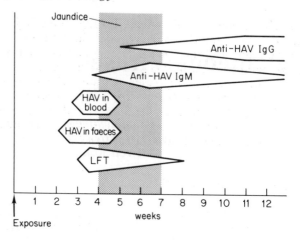

Fig. 52 Time-scale of events in hepatitis A. The diagram shows the relation between the appearance of jaundice, the development of abnormal liver function tests (LFT), the presence of hepatitis A virus (HAV) in the faeces and blood and the appearance of IgM and IgG antibodies against the virus (anti-HAV IgM and anti-HAV IgG).

Hepatitis A (infective hepatitis)

Hepatitis A virus (HAV) is an icosahedral RNA virus about 27 nm in diameter. It does not possess an envelope and is considered to be an enterovirus (enterovirus type 72). It grows slowly in various cell lines. It does not produce cytopathic effects but can be identified by immunofluorescent techniques.

The incubation period is usually three to five weeks (Fig. 52). The virus is present in the faeces and blood for 1–2 weeks before the onset of symptoms. Towards the end of the incubation period large numbers of viral particles can be detected in the faeces by immune electron microscopy and radioimmunoassay (RIA). The virus disappears at about the time of onset of jaundice and the patient ceases to be infectious. This stage coincides with the appearance of IgM antibodies which can be measured by RIA and enzyme-linked immunosorbent assay (ELISA) techniques. Chronic carriers of the virus are unknown and hepatitis A does not progress to chronic hepatitis or cirrhosis. The mortality rate of hepatitis A is less than 0.1%. The new host acquires infection by mouth; very rarely the virus may be transmitted parenterally. The disease is endemic in most countries and small localized outbreaks occur in families and institutions. Most cases occur in children and young adults. Subclinical infections in childhood are extremely common and produce lasting immunity. In communities with high standards of hygiene children are less likely to be infected and a higher proportion of adults remain susceptible. Large explosive outbreaks due to faecal contamination of water, milk and food are fairly common. Incriminated foods have included frozen raspberries (e.g. these caused 53 cases among 142 guests dining at Apothecaries' Hall in London in 1980!) and shellfish. Chimpanzees and some other primates are susceptible to hepatitis A and have occasionally been the source of human infection.

Hepatitis B (serum hepatitis)

Hepatitis B virus (HBV) is a DNA virus about 42 nm in diameter. Much of our information about this virus has been derived from study of its surface antigen.

Hepatitis B surface antigen (HBsAg), originally known as *Australia (Au) antigen* because it was first found in the serum of an Australian aborigine, can be detected by gel-diffusion methods and highly sensitive passive haemagglutination, RIA and ELISA techniques.

Electron microscopy of HBsAg-positive blood reveals structures of three types: small (22 nm) spherical particles, long rod-shaped particles 22 nm in diameter and large (42 nm) spherical particles with an outer coat and an inner core (Fig. 53, p. 366). The large particles are the complete hepatitis B virus and contain a lipoprotein surface antigen HBsAg and a DNA-containing core antigen, HBcAg. The corresponding antibodies are designated anti-HBs and anti-HBc. The other particles represent excess viral coat and contain only HBsAg. Total counts of 10^{12} viral particles/ml may occur in blood. In infected liver cells HBcAg is found in the nuclei and HBsAg in the cytoplasm. Four main subtypes of HBsAg are recognized. They share a common antigen but can be distinguished by the possession of other antigens. Individuals who carry HBsAg may also carry another antigen known as e antigen (HBeAg) which is associated with the presence of large numbers of complete viral particles and DNA polymerase which is present in core particles. Carriers of HBeAg are highly infectious. DNA hybridization tests for hepatitis B virus DNA provide the most reliable method for detecting infectious virus.

The incubation period is usually two to three months (Fig. 54, p. 367). Rarely, it may be as long as six months. HBsAg appears in the blood about one month before the onset of symptoms and usually disappears 2–3 months later at the end of the acute stage of the illness. Anti-HBc appears at the beginning of the acute stage and anti-HBs during convalescence. In patients who develop chronic hepatitis anti-HBs does not appear and HBsAg persists

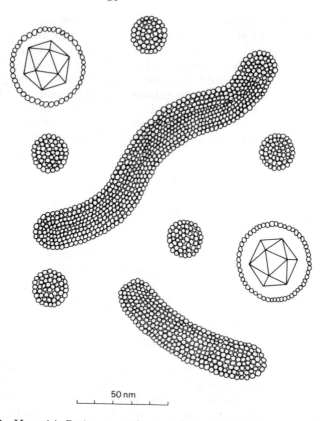

Fig. 53 Hepatitis B virus particles in infected blood. The rods and small spheres contain surface antigen (HBsAg). The large spheres contain core antigen (HBcAg) surrounded by an outer coat of HBsAg.

in the blood. HBsAg occurs in about 0.1% of apparently healthy blood donors in the UK and the USA but the incidence is as high as 5–10% in certain tropical and subtropical countries. Symptom-free carriers rarely give a history of acute hepatitis. There is a very high incidence of HBsAg in patients with primary carcinoma of the liver. HBsAg is also found in saliva and seminal fluid. In parts of Africa the antigen is found in mosquitoes and bedbugs (*Cimex* spp.). Patients who are transfused with blood containing HBsAg frequently develop hepatitis, but this rarely occurs if they already possess anti-HBs.

In the past hepatitis B was regarded as an entirely artificial disease occurring as a result of injection or transfusion of human blood, plasma, serum or blood products. It is now clear that infection acquired by other routes must be common. The disease

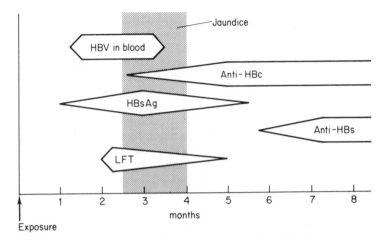

Fig. 54 Time-scale of events in acute hepatitis B. The diagram shows the relation between the appearance of jaundice, the development of abnormal liver function tests (LFT), the presence of complete hepatitis B virus (HBV) and hepatitis B surface antigen (HBsAg) in the blood and the appearance of antibodies against the surface and core antigens (anti-HBs and anti-HBc).

is more serious than hepatitis A. Rarely, outbreaks have been associated with mortality rates as high as 20%. A few patients suffer from chronic hepatitis which may progress to cirrhosis. Polyarteritis nodosa, arthritis and nephritis due to deposition of antigen-antibody complexes are common, particularly in persistent infections. Some apparently healthy people with no history of jaundice carry the virus in their blood, sometimes for years. Women who are highly infectious carriers, i.e. HBsAg positive and either HBeAg positive or HBeAg and anti-HBe negative, usually transmit infection to their infants at the time of birth. Such infants become persistent symptomless carriers with a greatly increased incidence of chronic hepatitis, cirrhosis and primary liver carcinoma in later life. The risk seems to depend on genetic factors, e.g. most Chinese carrier women are HBeAg-positive and 40–70% of their children become carriers whereas European carrier women are usually HBeAg-negative and their children rarely become carriers. If infected infants are given a course of hepatitis B vaccine and anti-HBsAg immunoglobulin starting within a few hours of birth it is possible to prevent the development of the carrier state in over 90% of cases.

The incidence of hepatitis B following transfusion of blood and plasma has been almost eliminated by careful screening of donors.

At one time an important cause of infection was the practice of using the same needle and syringe, without intervening sterilization, to inject a number of patients. Syringe-transmitted hepatitis accounted for many outbreaks among patients attending clinics dealing with sexually transmitted diseases, diabetes and immunization. Today there is a high incidence among drug addicts. In World War II thousands of cases of hepatitis (the largest point-source outbreak ever recorded) followed injection of yellow fever vaccine containing traces of contaminated human serum. Dentists, chiropodists, acupuncturists, tattooists, barbers and ear-piercers may use improperly sterilized equipment and transmit the disease. Hepatitis B is an occupational hazard among health workers. Laboratory workers, surgeons, and staff of institutions for the mentally handicapped are at special risk. They usually produce antibodies without developing overt hepatitis. Haemodialysis units present special problems. Everyday articles such as razors, scissors, sewing needles, toothbrushes and towels may be important in the home. The incidence of hepatitis B is high in the sexual partners (especially male homosexuals) of cases or carriers. The disease is also common in institutions for the mentally handicapped. It is assumed that the low standards of personal hygiene and poor immune responses of some of the patients encourage spread of the virus. Patients with Down's syndrome are particularly liable to become carriers. In the UK hepatitis B is most common among teenagers and young adults but in underdeveloped countries infection is often acquired in infancy. The control of outbreaks is considered elsewhere (p. 202).

Delta virus

Delta virus is a defective RNA virus which depends on hepatitis B virus (a DNA virus) for its replication. The outer coat of delta virus consists of hepatitis B surface antigen (HBsAg). Simultaneous infection with delta virus and hepatitis B virus usually produces an illness which is no more serious than infection with hepatitis B virus alone. However, when carriers of hepatitis B virus are infected with delta virus they may develop severe acute hepatitis and chronic liver disease. The presence of delta virus always indicates active hepatitis. In the UK infection is mainly found in drug addicts.

Non-A, non-B hepatitis

Many cases of hepatitis are caused by agents unrelated to hepatitis A or B viruses. Now that blood for transfusion is routinely screened for HBsAg, non-A, non-B hepatitis viruses cause about 90% of all cases of post-tranfusion hepatitis. Blood products prepared from large pools of plasma are particularly liable to be infectious. The viruses are responsible for 10−25% of cases of sporadic hepatitis and have also caused large water-borne outbreaks. There is usually a long incubation period of 35−70 days. The clinical picture is similar to hepatitis B and chronic hepatitis and cirrhosis of the liver are common. At least three distinct viruses have been recognized: two are transmitted parenterally and one orally.

Kuru and slow virus infections

Kuru is a fatal familial cerebellar ataxia occurring among the Fore people in New Guinea ('Kuru' = shivering or trembling in Fore language). The disease affects adult women and younger people of both sexes. Epidemiological evidence suggested that an infective agent was responsible. Until suppressive legislation was enforced in 1957 the Fore people indulged extensively in cannibalism of an unusual type; they ate their relatives and friends but not their enemies. This was a ceremonial act of mourning performed by women and young children. Correlation between the occurrence of cases of kuru and the gastronomic habits of individual members of the tribe leaves no doubt that cannibalism was the most important mode of transmission. The incubation period ranged from five to more than 25 years. The number of cases of kuru has declined steadily since the 1960s and the disease will probably disappear completely in a few years.

A kuru-like illness can be transmitted to chimpanzees by intra-cerebral inoculation of brain tissue from patients who have died of kuru. Provisionally the agent of kuru is assigned to a class of 'slow viruses' which cause disease only after an extremely long incubation period. Creutzfeldt-Jakob disease, and uncommon form of human presenile dementia associated with spongy degeneration of the brain, and scrapie, a disease of sheep, are probably caused by similar agents. Their small size, lack of immunogenicity and extreme resistance to heat and radiation suggest that slow viruses are fundamentally different from ordinary viruses. They may be *prions*, a unique class of pathogens consisting of rod-shaped proteinaceous infectious particles, but no-one really knows! Instances strongly suggesting human-to-human transmission of Creutzfeldt-Jakob disease by corneal transplant, brain electrodes and human growth hormone have been described.

Other diseases caused by viruses

Encephalitis lethargica

This disease, possessing the characteristics of a severe virus encephalitis, appeared during World War I, became world-wide in the early 1920s and then disappeared. No specific virus was isolated. Many non-fatal cases later developed chronic neurological symptoms (Parkinsonism).

Roseola infantum (exanthem subitum)

This is a mild febrile illness with a rubella-like rash which occurs almost exclusively in children aged from 6 months to 3 years. Small outbreaks may occur. The causative agent is thought to be a virus.

Paget's disease of bone

There is evidence that this disease is caused by a chronic paramyxovirus infection of osteoclasts. Measles virus, respiratory syncytial virus and canine distemper virus have been considered as possible causal agents.

Kawasaki disease

Kawasaki disease (mucocutaneous lymph node syndrome) is characterized by fever, rash, conjunctival injection, strawberry tongue and cervical lymphadenopathy. The illness mainly affects young children and is particularly common in Japan. The cause is unknown but a virus is suspected.

Viruses and tumour formation

Viruses can undoubtedly cause certain tumours in animals. These tumour viruses may contain DNA or RNA.

DNA tumour viruses include the papovaviruses which produce tumours in animals and malignant transformation of cells in tissue culture. Some adenoviruses which infect man (such as types 12, 18 and 31) produce malignant tumours when inoculated into newborn hamsters and malignant transformation of rodent cells *in vitro*. In monkey kidney tissue cultures some adenoviruses grow well only if the culture also contains a *helper virus*, the vacuolating virus SV40. In such cultures hybrid viruses are produced with an SV40 core and an adenovirus capsid. The tumours produced by such hybrids have the antigenic properties of SV40 tumours.

RNA tumour viruses (oncornaviruses) belong to the retrovirus group. They include Rous sarcoma virus which can be isolated from Rous sarcomas of fowls. This virus can be grown in tissue culture or the chick embryo and will produce tumours in fowls, other birds and some newborn animals. Some strains are defective and the ability of cells to release infectious virus depends on the presence of a helper virus known as Rous-associated virus. Other conditions in which RNA viruses are implicated include leukaemia and a variety of tumours in fowls, and leukaemia, sarcomas and mammary gland carcinoma in mice. It must be stressed that virus tumours constitute only a very small proportion of all tumours studied.

The relevance of these observations to the causation of the majority of mammalian tumours and particularly human tumours, is controversial. Viruses have often been isolated from human tumours but usually there is little to suggest they are more than passengers. However, certain cancers appear to be associated with particular viruses, e.g. primary hepatocellular carcinoma (primary liver cancer) and hepatitis B virus (p. 367); carcinoma of the cervix and herpes virus type 2 (p. 331); carcinoma of the cervix and certain skin cancers and human papillomavirus (p. 337); some types of leukaemia and lymphoma and human T-cell lymphotropic virus type 1 (p. 360); lymphomas and human B-cell lymphotropic virus (p. 335); Kaposi's sarcoma and cytomegalovirus (p. 334) and human immunodeficiency virus (p. 360); and Burkitt's lymphoma and nasopharyngeal carcinoma and Epstein-Barr virus (p. 332).

A major advance in our understanding of malignant disease in man has been gained by the study of *oncogenes*, i.e. genes that cause cancer. Most RNA tumour viruses are thought to owe their tumour-producing properties to genes they have picked up from normal cells in the course of evolution, e.g. the RNA viral oncogene of Rous sarcoma virus (v-*src*) is closely related to a DNA cellular oncogene (c-*src*) found in normal cells of all vertebrates, including man. When a virus carrying an oncogene infects another cell the viral genes become integrated into the chromosome of the cell where the oncogene functions as a slightly altered version of a normal gene and encodes for a slightly altered version of a normal protein. These oncogenic proteins somehow transform normal cells into malignant cells.

Bacteriophages

Bacteriophages or phages are viruses which infect bacteria. The great majority are DNA viruses, but a few are RNA viruses. The number of different phages is enormous since, with a few exceptions, every bacterial species has its own set of phages. Each phage attacks only that particular species or in many cases only certain types or strains within that species.

Structure

A typical phage is a tadpole-shaped particle with a polyhedral head consisting of DNA surrounded by a thin protein membrane and a long straight tail consisting of protein (Fig. 55A). Structural distinction between the nucleic acid and protein components is well illustrated by phages in which loss of DNA from the head leaves an otherwise well-preserved hollow-headed *ghost*. Polyhedral (i.e. tailless) and filamentous phages have been reported.

Antigenic properties

Phages are antigenic and antibodies against them neutralize phage activity. Most phages contain at least two antigenic components, corresponding to head and tail proteins.

Mutation

A phage may produce mutants which differ from the parent in host range, appearance of the plaques (see below) and many other properties. When a bacterium is infected with two closely related phages, some of the phage offspring may possess properties derived from both phages (genetic recombination).

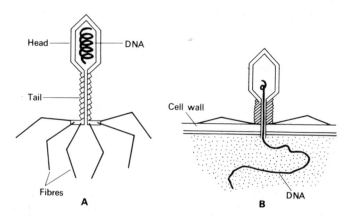

Fig. 55 A large phage. A, Free phage particle (a phage of *Escherichia coli*). B, After attachment to a bacterial cell, showing injection of nucleic acid (DNA).

Effect on bacteria

On the basis of the relationship they establish with their host, phages are divided into two groups: (1) virulent or lytic phages grow within and lyse the organism that they infect; (2) temperate phages may grow in the organism that they infect; alternatively, they may produce a *lysogenic* response, in which the potentiality to produce phages which will grow in and lyse the cell is transmitted to the progeny of the bacterium.

1 *Virulent phages.* The clear-cut holes or nibbled-out areas which are often seen in colonies of *Staphylococcus aureus* are an example of the lytic activity of phage. Normally, phage is demonstrated by special methods. In the tube method the phage preparation is added to a young broth culture of the bacterium. If the bacterium is susceptible the culture shows clearing after incubation for 30–60 minutes. In the plate method a plate is evenly spread with a broth culture of the bacterium, dried for 1–2 hours, inoculated with the phage preparation, dried again and incubated overnight. Phage in high concentration produces confluent lysis, but at a suitable dilution it produces discrete, circular islands or *plaques* of lysis (Fig. 56). Each plaque is caused by the progeny of a single phage particle, i.e. a plaque is analogous to an isolated colony obtained by plating out a bacterial culture. Phage can be obtained in pure culture from an isolated plaque. Unlysed bacteria are destroyed by heat (phages are often relatively heat-resistant) or removed by filtration.

Most phages have a similar mechanism of infection. They attach themselves to the surface of the bacterium by means of minute fibres at the tips of their tails. The nucleic acid in the

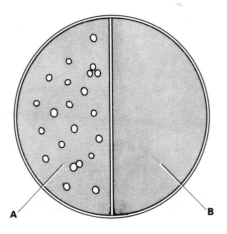

Fig. 56 Phage plaques.
A, Film of bacterial growth showing plaques of lysis.
B, Control film without phage.

head of the phage is then injected into the bacterium. The proteins comprising the tail and head membrane remain outside (Fig. 55B, p. 372). For some time after infection no infective phage is detectable. During this *eclipse phase* the phage nucleic acid and the phage protein are being synthesized independently. Finally the components are assembled to form mature or infective phage. When the number of mature phages in the cell reaches a critical *burst size*, e.g. 200 phage particles, the cell bursts and the phage is liberated. The whole cycle may take as little as 20 minutes. Cultures that have undergone lysis are seldom sterile. A few bacterial cells survive and on further incubation they will produce cultures which are resistant to the phage.

2 *Temperate phages.* Adsorption and penetration is the same as with virulent phages, but instead of immediately multiplying and destroying the bacterium, the phage nucleic acid may, under certain conditions, become integrated with the host genetic apparatus as *prophage*. The prophage is reproduced in step with the bacterial chromosome and is transmitted to the daughter bacterial cells. Cultures infected in this way are described as lysogenic. The phage usually causes no perceptible change in the host cell but in some cases it confers heritable properties, e.g. ability to produce toxin by *Corynebacterium diphtheriae* and the presence of certain *Salmonella* O antigens depend on lysogenic infection. Although lysogenic cultures do not normally undergo mass lysis, the organisms have the potentiality to produce phage. This occurs normally as a spontaneous event in a few individual bacteria, but may occur in a high proportion of cells when these have been *induced* by ultraviolet light or certain chemical mutagens. The production of lytic phage can be recognized by the ability of the supernatant fluid of lysogenic cultures to cause lysis when added to uninfected cultures of susceptible strains.

Phage-typing

The susceptibility of bacteria to known phages provides a precise means of classification which can be of great value in epidemiological investigations, e.g. phage-typing of *Staph. aureus*, *Salmonella typhi* and *S. typhimurium*.

Fungi

There are a multitude of other shapes of which these microscopical mushrooms are figured...
Robert Hooke, 1665

Fungi can be divided into four groups:

1 *Yeasts* are round or oval bodies which reproduce by budding, e.g. *Cryptococcus neoformans*.
2 *Yeast-like fungi* grow mainly as yeasts, but may also grow in the form of chains of elongated, filamentous cells (pseudomycelium) which give rise to yeast cells by budding, e.g. *Candida albicans* and *Pityrosporum orbiculare*.
3 *Filamentous fungi* grow as filaments (*hyphae*) which interlace to form a tangled mass or *mycelium*. They reproduce by asexual spores, e.g. fungi of the genera *Microsporum*, *Trichophyton*, *Epidermophyton*, *Aspergillus*, *Mucor*, *Rhizopus* and *Penicillium*.
4 *Dimorphic fungi* have a filamentous form (saprophytic phase) when growing at room temperature and a yeast form (parasitic phase) when growing in the body or at 37°C, e.g. fungi of the genera *Histoplasma*, *Blastomyces*, *Coccidioides*, *Paracoccidioides* and *Sporothrix*.

Diagnosis of fungal infections

Yeasts and fungi will often be detected in stained films during routine examination of sputum, swabs, etc. In other cases, e.g. ringworm infections, unstained wet preparations are examined.

Yeasts and fungi grow on ordinary bacteriological media but, apart from a few fast-growing species such as *C. albicans*, the colonies will not appear in the 24–48 hours used for incubation of routine specimens. Special cultures are set up and examined at intervals for 2–3 weeks. Sabouraud glucose agar is most widely used. It is highly acid (pH 5.5) and inhibits most bacteria. Blood agar containing added antibiotics is also valuable. Sabouraud medium (in slopes or plates sealed with tape) incubated at 28°C is adequate for isolation of the common filamentous fungi and

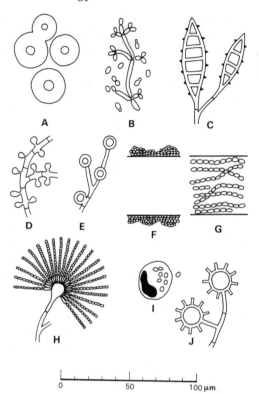

Fig. 57 Morphological features of some fungi. A, *Cryptococcus neoformans*, showing capsules. B, *Candida albicans*, showing yeast forms and pseudomycelium. C, *Microsporum canis*, showing hypha and macroconidia. D, *Trichophyton mentagrophytes*, showing hyphae and microconidia. E, *Epidermophyton floccosum*, showing hypha and chlamydospores. F, Ringworm infection of the hair, showing arthrospores (small-spored ectothrix). G, Ringworm infection of the hair showing arthrospores (large-spored endothrix). H, *Aspergillus* sp., showing hypha, terminal conidiophore and chains of spores (conidia). I, *Histoplasma capsulatum* (parasitic phase), showing yeast forms inside macrophage. J, *Histoplasma capsulatum* (saprophytic phase), showing hypha and tuberculate chlamydospores in culture at 26°C.

yeasts. For full investigation of generalized fungal diseases and to exclude the rarer dimorphic fungi it is best to inoculate two plates of Sabouraud medium, at 28 and 37°C, two plates of blood agar and two tubes of Sabouraud glucose broth.

Identification of fungi is mainly made on morphological grounds. A small portion of the sporing surface growth is removed with a needle and examined as a wet preparation stained with lactophenol blue. If no characteristic features are seen the organism can be grown on a small block of agar in slide culture and stained *in situ*.

Detection of antibodies by precipitation, complement fixation and immunofluorescent tests is useful in the diagnosis of systemic mycoses.

Yeasts and yeast-like fungi

Cryptococcus neoformans

This yeast has a thick, gelatinous capsule (Fig. 57A). It produces mucoid white colonies on blood agar and is pathogenic for mice. Human cryptococcosis is rare but often fatal. It usually takes the form of meningitis. Capsulated yeasts can be seen in the cerebrospinal fluid (CSF). Infection may also occur in the lungs, skin and other organs. In the UK cryptococcosis is almost unknown except in patients with severe immunodeficiency. The yeast is common in the soil and this is probably the main source of infection in man. Several cases have been traced to infected pigeon droppings. A latex agglutination test can be used to detect cryptococcal antigen in serum or CSF.

Candida albicans

This yeast-like fungus (Fig. 57B) is a normal inhabitant of the mouth and intestinal tract. Human candidiasis is common. The organism causes thrush, a condition mainly occurring in infants, in which white patches develop on the mucous membrane of the mouth. It is the commonest cause of vaginitis, giving rise to vaginal irritation and discharge. Diabetes and pregnancy are important predisposing factors. It sometimes infects the skin and nails and occasionally causes pulmonary and generalized infections, including endocarditis. Chronic mucocutaneous candidiasis is an intractable infection of the mouth, skin and nails occurring in patients with defective cell-mediated immunity. Proliferation of *C. albicans* and other yeasts in the upper respiratory and intestinal tracts is an almost inevitable complication of therapy with broad-spectrum antibiotics. In most cases the yeasts cause little harm and disappear rapidly when treatment is stopped.

In direct films the organism can be seen as large, gram-positive, oval, budding cells sometimes with short strands of pseudo-mycelium. It grows well on blood agar and Sabouraud medium. It can be distinguished from other *Candida* species often present in clinical material by production of germ-tubes on incubation for 1–2 hours in serum, production of round, thick-walled chlamydospores when grown on corn-meal agar and by fermentation reactions.

Antibodies against *C. albicans* are present in small amounts in most normal people. High levels are often associated with serious conditions such as chronic mucocutaneous candidiasis, generalized infections and endocarditis. Circulating antigens of *C. albicans* can be detected in these illnesses.

Pityrosporum orbiculare (Malassezia furfur)

This yeast-like fungus is a normal skin commensal and the cause of tinea versicolor (pityriasis versicolor), a common superficial scaly infection of the skin. Characteristic thick-walled budding cells and short bent hyphae are found in skin scrapings.

Filamentous fungi

Dermatophytes (ringworm fungi)

Fungi of the dermatophyte group infect the keratinized surface of the body producing the conditions known collectively as tinea or ringworm. Three genera are distinguished:

Microsporum. This genus attacks hair and skin but not nails. *M. audouini* is a human parasite and is the cause of epidemic ringworm of the scalp, tinea capitis, in children. *M. canis* (Fig. 57C, p. 376) is a parasite of dogs and cats but not infrequently causes ringworm in children. *M. gypseum* is found in the soil and occasionally causes human infection.

Trichophyton. This genus attacks skin, hair and nails. *T. mentagrophytes* (Fig. 57D, p. 376), which includes a human variety, *T. interdigitale*, and varieties found in cattle and horses, is the organism most commonly responsible for 'athlete's foot', or tinea pedis. Over half the population is infected with this fungus. *T. rubrum*, a human parasite, causes severe and intractable infections of the skin and nails but rarely infects the scalp. *T. schoenleini*, a human parasite, is the main agent of favus, a chronic infection of the scalp. *T. sulphureum* (*T. tonsurans*) and *T. violaceum* are human parasites. *T. verrucosum* causes ringworm in cattle from which man becomes infected.

Epidermophyton. There is only one species, *E. floccosum* (Fig. 57E, p. 376). It is a human parasite and attacks skin and nails but not hair. It is the commonest cause of ringworm of the groin, or tinea cruris.

Diagnosis of ringworm

Scrapings are taken from the active periphery of skin lesions with a blunt scalpel. Hairs which fluoresce under ultraviolet light (characteristic of infections caused by *M. audouini, M. canis* and *T. schoenleini*) or which show abnormality (lustreless, broken stumps, etc.) are extracted with forceps. Full-thickness clippings or thick shavings are taken from affected nails. Samples should be sent to the laboratory in folded squares of black paper secured with a paperclip. Small pieces of skin, hair or nail are placed in a drop of 30% KOH on a slide. A coverslip is placed on top and the slide is gently warmed until the specimen is cleared.

The diagnosis of fungal infection is confirmed by finding hyphae which may or may not show fragmentation into chains of spores (arthrospores). With specimens of hair the size and arrangement of the spores may afford some indication of the type of fungus involved (Fig. 57F and 57G, p. 376). Thus *Microsporum* spp. and *T. mentagrophytes* show small spores outside the hair (ectothrix infection); *T. verrucosum* shows large-spored ectothrix infection; *T. schoenleini, T. sulphureum* and *T. violaceum* show large-spored endothrix infection; *T. schoenleini* also produces small air bubbles in the hair.

Cultures on Sabouraud medium are incubated at room temperature. Identification of the different species depends on rate of growth, colonial appearance and the microscopical appearance of various types of spores (macroconidia, microconidia, chlamydospores) and other specialized structures which are formed by fungi when they are grown in culture.

Other filamentous fungi

Aspergillus

Fungi of this genus (Fig. 57H, p. 376) are common saprophytes and frequently contaminate cultures. *A. fumigatus* is the most important species causing human infection (aspergillosis). It not infrequently establishes itself in the lungs of patients with pre-existing pulmonary disease such as bronchiectasis, tuberculosis and cystic fibrosis. It sometimes produces a large mycelial mass (aspergilloma) which may require surgical removal. Generalized aspergillosis may arise as a complication of immunosuppressive therapy, e.g. cerebral aspergillosis is an important cause of death in patients who have recently had renal transplants. The fungus is also responsible for a crippling asthma-like illness, extrinsic allergic alveolitis, among individuals who are repeatedly exposed to organic dust contaminated with its spores, e.g. workers with mouldy barley. Chronic infections of the ear are frequently caused by aspergilli, including *A. fumigatus*, *A. niger* and *A. flavus*. When *A. flavus* grows in certain foodstuffs it produces *aflatoxins* which are carcinogenic and potent hepatic poisons. Aflatoxin poisoning has occurred in animals such as turkeys fed on contaminated groundnuts and it is strongly suspected that it has also occurred in man, e.g. aflatoxins are probably responsible for cirrhosis and cancer of the liver in parts of India.

Mucor and other zygomycetes

In recent years there has been an increase in generalized infections caused by fungi normally regarded as harmless saprophytes, e.g. species of *Mucor* and *Rhizopus*. The disease is known as zygomycosis (mucormycosis, etc.). The lungs and brain are most commonly attacked and the outcome is often fatal. Prolonged antibiotic therapy and use of immunosuppressive agents have been predisposing factors in most cases.

Penicillium

This large genus of saprophytic fungi is of note in that one species, *P. notatum*, first provided penicillin. *P. chrysogenum* is now mainly used.

Other genera

There are other filamentous fungi of minor medical importance and a vast number of saprophytic fungi from which they must be distinguished. The subject is a specialized branch of biology.

Dimorphic fungi

Fungi of this group can cause serious deep-seated and generalized infections. The diseases are almost unknown in the UK.

Histoplasma capsulatum (Fig. 57I and 57J, p. 376) causes histoplasmosis, a pulmonary or generalized disease occurring in the USA and many other parts of the world. The fungus is found in the soil, particularly when this contains bird or bat droppings. Human infection is acquired by inhalation. The patient may give a history of clearing out a hen house or exploring a bat-infested cave. Person-to-person infection does not occur. Subclinical infection in early life is extremely common in endemic areas. Severe forms of histoplasmosis are rare. Histoplasmosis occurs in dogs, cats and various other animals in endemic areas.

Blastomyces dermatitidis causes blastomycosis, a cutaneous, pulmonary or generalized granulomatous disease occurring in parts of the USA, Canada, South America and Africa. The epidemiology is obscure. Man is probably infected by inhalation. Blastomycosis occurs in dogs and other animals in endemic areas.

Coccidioides immitis causes coccidioidomycosis, an acute pulmonary or progressive generalized granulomatous disease occurring in the south-western states of the USA and Central and South America. The fungus lives in the hot dry soils of these regions and man is infected by inhalation. The usual result is a subclinical infection or a mild self-limiting illness. A high proportion of residents in endemic areas acquire immunity in this way. Newcomers are more likely to develop severe forms of the disease. Progressive coccidioidomycosis is rare but often fatal. Immunosuppression by drugs or disease is sometimes a predisposing factor. Person-to-person infection does not occur. Laboratory cultures of *C. immitis* (and other dimorphic fungi) release clouds of spores and are highly infectious.

Paracoccidioides brasiliensis causes paracoccidioidomycosis, a chronic granulomatous disease occurring in rural areas in South America. Ulceration of the mucous membranes of the nose and mouth with extension to local lymph nodes is a characteristic feature.

Sporothrix schenki causes sporotrichosis, an uncommon disease of world-wide distribution characterized by chronic granulomatous and ulcerative lesions of the skin, particularly along the course of lymphatics. The fungus grows on timber and in soil and man is usually infected by inoculation of cuts and abrasions.

Protozoa

> ...some of 'em a bit bigger, others a bit less, than a
> blood-globule, but all of one and the same make.
> Their bodies were somewhat larger than broad, and
> their belly, which was flatlike, furnisht with sundry
> little paws, wherewith they made such a stir in the
> clear medium...
> [Giardia lamblia]
>
> Antony van Leeuwenhoek, 1681

Plasmodium

The name malaria expresses the association of this disease with
bad air, particularly the damp night air in marshy places. The
danger is not the air itself but the mosquitoes which fly in the
air, and they are dangerous only when they carry a small protozoon of the genus *Plasmodium*. Only female mosquitoes of the
genus *Anopheles* are able to transmit infection.

Malaria

Malaria usually takes the form of an intermittent fever with
anaemia due to destruction of red blood cells. The fever is often
remittent, particularly in the early stages. Enlargement of the
spleen is common. The possible clinical manifestations are legion.
This diversity of symptoms is most marked in malignant malaria
in which there is localized slowing or even complete blocking of
the capillary circulation caused by enormous numbers of parasit-
ized red cells.

Four species of malaria parasite infect man. *P. falciparum* causes
malignant malaria, the most severe type of the disease and the
predominant type in the tropics; paroxysms of fever occur every
two days or less. *P. vivax* causes the most widely distributed type
of malaria and is the predominant type in temperate zones; fever
occurs every two days. *P. malariae* causes a disease of patchy
distribution mainly in the subtropics; fever occurs every three
days. *P. ovale* is a relatively uncommon parasite of limited distribution; fever occurs every two days. The intervals between the

paroxysms of fever depend on the length of time the organisms take to complete their asexual cycle in the blood.

The chances of dying in a particular attack of malaria are small but the disease is so widespread, particularly in the tropics, and so likely to take a chronic relapsing course, that it kills more people than any other specific infectious disease. At least a million children die of malaria in Africa every year. In the UK the number of fatal cases is higher than it should be because doctors fail to think of malaria as a cause of fever. 'Airport malaria' (mainly *P. falciparum*) due to infected mosquitoes carried in aircraft has occurred in several European countries, including the UK.

Cycle in man (schizogony or asexual cycle)

1 *Pre-erythrocytic phase.* The parasite is introduced into the body by the bite of the mosquito, as a thin, motile, spindle-shaped *sporozoite*. These rapidly disappear from the blood and enter parenchymal cells of the liver. Here they develop into large multinucleate *schizonts* which mature and liberate small, round, mononucleate *merozoites*.

2 *Exo-erythrocytic phase.* Some merozoites enter fresh liver cells and repeat the cycle by producing further schizonts and merozoites. In *P. vivax* malaria this phase may persist for long periods and relapses may occur although the parasites have been eliminated from the peripheral blood.

3 *Erythrocytic phase.* This is the main asexual cycle. The merozoites enter red cells and grow as *trophozoites*. Those of *P. vivax* show lively amoeboid movement. At first the trophozoites produce *ring forms*, small, round structures, clear in the centre with a chromatin dot at one side (Fig. 58A, p. 384). These develop into *mature trophozoites*, large, irregular structures, usually containing dark granules of altered blood pigment and occupying much of the red cell volume. When fully developed the nucleus of the trophozoite begins to segment and it becomes a *schizont*. Pigment accumulates towards the centre of the red cell. The mature schizont consists of 6–32 small, round or oval merozoites, the number varying with the species. In *P. falciparum* malaria the infected red cells usually disappear from the peripheral blood before the trophozoites are mature and schizogony occurs in the capillaries of internal organs. Finally the merozoites are liberated into the blood where they attack new red cells and repeat the asexual cycle. The paroxysms of fever occur when the merozoites are liberated. Malaria parasites undergo antigenic variation during the course of the disease, enabling them to escape the action of antibody.

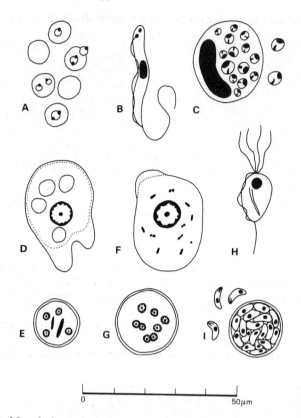

Fig. 58 Morphological features of some protozoa. A, *Plasmodium falciparum*, ring forms inside red blood cells. B, *Trypanosoma gambiense*. C, *Leishmania donovani* inside splenic macrophage. D, *Entamoeba histolytica* with ingested red blood cells. E, *Entamoeba histolytica*, mature cyst with chromatoid bodies and four nuclei. F, *Entamoeba coli* with ingested bacteria. G, *Entamoeba coli*, mature cyst with eight nuclei. H, *Trichomonas vaginalis*. I, *Toxoplasma gondii*, individual protozoa and cystic stage.

4   *Gametocyte production.* When parasitaemia has been present for several days some merozoites, instead of developing into schizonts, develop into sexual cells or gametocytes. These may be male (*microgametocytes*) or female (*macrogametocytes*). The gametocytes of *P. falciparum* are large banana-shaped bodies known as *crescents*. Those of other malaria parasites are round bodies about the size of a mature trophozoite. No further development of these cells occurs in the human body.

Cycle in mosquito (sporogony or sexual cycle)

If the blood is sucked by a female anopheline mosquito the gametocytes start a sexual cycle in the stomach of the insect. The macrogametocyte matures to form a female *macrogamete* and the microgametocyte develops 4–8 coarse flagellum-like structures which break off and swim away as male *microgametes*. The male and female gametes unite to form a *zygote* which rapidly becomes a motile cell known as an *ookinete*. This penetrates the muscle of the stomach wall where it becomes a rounded *oocyst* inside which thousands of *sporozoites* develop. The cyst ultimately ruptures, liberating the sporozoites into the body cavity, whence they find their way to the salivary gland. The cycle in the mosquito takes about ten days, or longer if the weather is cold. In the interval the mosquito is not infectious.

Immunity

Repeated attacks of malaria produce considerable immunity against the particular species or strains of *Plasmodium* responsible, but this mainly depends on persistence of the parasite in the body (infection-immunity). In areas of high endemicity adults have a low parasite rate and rarely suffer from acute attacks of the disease, but young children have a high parasite rate and are severely afflicted, as are visitors from non-malarial districts.

Diagnosis

Films of blood are stained by Leishman or Giemsa stains and the red cells are examined for parasites. Thin films are usually satisfactory but thick films which have first been haemolysed are time-saving, particularly when the parasites are scanty. DNA probes have been used to screen populations for *P. falciparum* malaria. Serological tests are of no help in the diagnosis of acute malaria. Immunofluorescent tests are occasionally of value for retrospective diagnosis.

Control

There is no animal reservoir of infection for human malaria. Since *Anopheles* mosquitoes are the sole vectors, prevention mainly depends on anti-mosquito measures. Breeding places can be removed by draining stagnant water and covering wells. Larvae can be killed by covering the surface of ponds, puddles and water-butts with a thin layer of oil and stocking open water with fish. Some mosquitoes find unusual breeding places such as footprints or ruts from vehicles. *Anopheles* mosquitoes can be recognized by their habit of resting with their bodies in a straight l at an angle to the supporting surface; other mosquitoes hold themselves parallel to the surface. Spraying the inside of houses with insecticides is the most important method of destroying adult mosquitoes. Individual protection is provided by insect repellents, mosquito-proof clothing, mosquito-screened houses, mosquito-nets at night and the regular prophylactic use of anti-malarial drugs such as chloroquine or proguanil. In the 1960s a few optimists hoped that with the help of DDT malaria would soon be eradicated. Figures tell another story, e.g. in India there were 40 000 reported cases in 1966, 1.4 million in 1972 and 5.8 million in 1976. Premature abandonment of conventional methods of malaria control and the increasing resistance of mosquitoes to DDT were mainly to blame. Malaria parasites themselves have fought against eradication as shown by the relentless spread of chloroquine-resistant strains of *P. falciparum* in South East Asia, South America and much of tropical Africa. In these areas various combinations of drugs should be used, e.g. chloroquine plus proguanil or chloroquine plus dapsone/pyrimethamine. Up-to-date information should be obtained from specialist centres.

Trypanosoma

Three species of trypanosomes are pathogenic for man: *T. gambiense* and *T. rhodesiense* causing African sleeping sickness, and *T. cruzi* causing South American trypanosomiasis.

Sleeping sickness

Sleeping sickness has spread devastation in parts of Africa. *T. gambiense* and *T. rhodesiense* are almost identical.

Morphology

Typical trypanosomes seen in human blood are sinuous, motile protozoa 12−40 μm long and 1.5−3.5 μm wide. Along one margin they have an *undulating membrane* which projects at the front end of the organism as a *flagellum*. There is a large *nucleus* near the middle of the organism and a small *kinetoplast* at the rear end near the origin of the undulating membrane (Fig. 58B, p. 384). Morphological variants are common, e.g. non-motile forms.

)n

kness is transmitted from person to person by the flies, e.g. *Glossina palpalis* transmits *T. gambiense* and transmits *T. rhodesiense*. The tsetse fly does not become infective until about 20 days after an infected feed. Wild animals are known to be reservoirs of infection for *T. rhodesiense*.

Disease in man

A local lesion forms at the site of the bite. After two weeks trypanosomes appear in the blood. Fever, skin eruptions and enlargement of lymph nodes are common. The fever shows characteristic periodicity due to the emergence of new antigenic variants of the organism. A single trypanosome has several hundred genes each coding for different surface antigens (variable surface glycoproteins). Later the parasites may invade the brain and cerebrospinal fluid (CSF) producing a chronic disease characterized by lethargy, increasing drowsiness and a fatal outcome.

Diagnosis

Trypanosomes can usually be found in Leishman-stained films of fluid aspirated from lymph nodes, less regularly in fluid from the primary lesion and in thin or thick films of blood, and occasionally in the CSF in advanced cases. Inoculation of rats and detection of trypanosomes in their blood is of value in identifying *T. rhodesiense*.

South American trypanosomiasis (Chagas' disease)

Chagas' disease is common in Brazil. The causative organism, *T. cruzi*, is transmitted by blood-sucking bugs. Armadillos and opossums are important reservoirs of infection. Human infection is usually acquired in childhood and takes the form of an acute febrile illness often followed by a chronic progressive disease in which the trypanosomes grow in an intracellular non-motile leishmania form in the heart, voluntary muscle and internal organs.

Leishmania

Protozoa of the genus *Leishmania* are closely related to the trypanosomes. Four species cause disease in man: *L. donovani*, *L. tropica*, *L. brasiliensis* and *L. mexicana*.

Leishmania donovani

L. donovani is the cause of kala-azar, a severe generalized disease prevalent in parts of India, Africa and the Far East and characterized by fever, anaemia, hyperglobulinaemia, wasting, enlargement of the liver and spleen, and a high mortality.

Morphology

The parasites, *Leishman-Donovan bodies*, are round or oval cells about 3 μm in diameter with a round *macronucleus* and a rod-shaped *kinetoplast* (Fig. 58C, p. 384). When cultured on special media or when growing in sandflies they develop into motile flagellates.

Transmission

Blood-sucking sandflies (*Phlebotomus* spp.) are the vectors of kala-azar. Dogs act as a reservoir of infection in some areas.

Diagnosis

Leishman−Donovan bodies can sometimes be found inside monocytes in blood films stained by Leishman stain, but are more likely to be found inside macrophages in material aspirated from bone marrow, lymph nodes or the spleen. The protozoa grow readily on special media. An immunofluorescent test on the patient's serum is a useful aid to diagnosis.

Other species of Leishmania

L. tropica causes cutaneous leishmaniasis (Aleppo sore, Baghdad button, Delhi boil, etc.) but does not invade the viscera. Sandflies are important vectors.

L. brasiliensis causes espundia, a granulomatous and ulcerative disease found in South America and mainly affecting the skin and mucous membranes of the mouth, nose and throat.

L. mexicana causes chiclero's ulcer, a form of mucocutaneous leishmaniasis mainly affecting the face and ears, found in chicle (gum) collectors in Central America.

Entamoeba

Entamoeba histolytica

E. histolytica is a pathogenic amoeba and is the cause of amoebic dysentery. It lives in the intestinal tract where it burrows into the mucosa of the large intestine, infiltrates the underlying tissues and produces local necrosis and ulceration. Typical ulcers have extensively undermined edges. The intervening mucosa is usually normal. Deeper penetration may result in perforation. Ulcers sometimes progress to the formation of an amoeboma, a granulomatous mass which may be confused with a carcinoma. In some cases the amoebae gain access to the blood and produce liver abscesses. The fluid in a typical abscess consists of necrotic tissue and altered blood and its appearance is said to resemble anchovy sauce.

Amoebic dysentery mainly occurs in tropical and subtropical countries. It typically has a more insidious onset and runs a more chronic course than bacillary dysentery. Acute attacks of diarrhoea sometimes occur, but it is more characteristic for the patient to produce three or four bulky stools each day.

As the disease settles down to a chronic form the amoebae tend to encyst. Cysts may be excreted in the faeces for years after clinical recovery. Healthy persons who have never had an attack of dysentery may also excrete cysts.

Cysts are very resistant and can survive outside the body for long periods. Amoebic dysentery is transmitted by the ingestion of cysts in contaminated food, particularly raw vegetables and fruit, and water. The use of human faeces as fertilizer is largely responsible for heavy infestation in some areas. Flies and dust may contribute to the spread of infection. Sexual transmission of *E. histolytica* is common among male homosexuals.

Morphology

The amoebae vary from 10 to 40 μm in diameter. They show flowing movements and elongated pseudopodia may be suddenly protruded and retracted. Ingested red cells are frequently present. The ectoplasm of the organism is usually distinct from the endoplasm. The nucleus is seldom visible in unstained preparations (Fig. 58D, p. 384).

The cysts are 10–20 μm in diameter. 'Small race' cysts with a diameter of less than 10 μm are non-pathogenic and are referred to as *E. hartmanni*. Cysts of *E. histolytica* are round, thin-walled and usually contain four nuclei. Immature cysts contain one or two nuclei. The cysts usually contain conspicuous, refractile, rod-like *chromatoid bodies* which stain with iron haematoxylin (Fig. 58E, p. 384).

Diagnosis

The stools tend to be large, offensive, relatively normal in consistency and flecked with blood and mucus. This is in contrast to the numerous, scanty, odourless, watery stools consisting almost entirely of blood and mucus, typical of patients with acute bacillary dysentery. Leucocytes are scanty in the stools in amoebic dysentery but very numerous in bacillary dysentery.

To demonstrate amoebae a fleck of blood-stained mucus selected from a *freshly passed* specimen of stool is emulsified in a drop of normal saline on a warm slide (a special *warm stage* can be used if desired) and examined for active amoebae containing red cells. Scrapings taken from ulcers during sigmoidoscopy often reveal amoebae when they cannot be found in the stools. In liver abscesses the amoebae are located in the walls of the cavity and are virtually never found in the fluid. For identification of cysts the nuclei can be rendered prominent by staining with iodine solution.

E. *histolytica* grows readily in special cultures. Isoenzyme analysis shows that only certain zymodemes are responsible for amoebic dysentery and liver abscess. Other zymodemes are mainly found in symptom-free cyst passers.

Antibodies against E. *histolytica* regularly appear in the course of the disease and can be detected by immunofluorescent, gel-diffusion, indirect haemagglutination and complement fixation tests. Serological tests are of particular value in cases of suspected amoebic abscess and when amoebae or cysts cannot be found in faeces. Serological tests are often positive in apparently healthy subjects who carry pathogenic zymodemes.

Other amoebae

Diagnosis of amoebic dysentery is complicated by the frequent presence in normal stools of harmless species of amoebae of which *Entamoeba coli* is the most common. This organism shows sluggish movements, has blunt pseudopodia and never contains red cells, although it is often full of bacteria and other debris (Fig. 58F, p. 384). Its cysts are relatively thick-walled, have eight nuclei when they are mature, and contain inconspicuous needle-like chromatoid bodies (Fig. 58G, p. 384). Reliable differentiation of E. *histolytica* and E. *coli* requires great experience.

Some normally free-living amoebae, e.g. *Naegleria fowleri* and *Acanthamoeba* spp., are on rare occasions pathogenic for man. Primary amoebic meningitis is an acute and usually fatal infection occurring in previously healthy children and young adults. The patients give a history of bathing in ponds and lakes. Granulomatous amoebic encephalitis usually occurs in debilitated or immunocompromized patients and there may be a primary infection in the lung, skin or eye. Motile amoebae can be found in the CSF in both conditions.

Amoebae growing in the water of air-conditioning systems are one cause of 'humidifier fever', a respiratory illness due to hypersensitivity to inhaled antigens. Other outbreaks are caused by bacterial contaminants.

Toxoplasma

Toxoplasma gondii

T. gondii is primarily a parasite of the domestic cat and other members of the cat family. Schizogony and gametogony occur in the mucosal cells of the intestine of the cat. Oocysts are produced and excreted in the faeces. In warm moist conditions oocysts can survive for more than a year. When ingested by animals they give rise to extraintestinal forms of the parasite. These are the forms seen in man as well as in a wide variety of wild and domestic animals and some birds. The proliferative parasites are small, 5 × 2 μm, non-motile, oval or crescentic bodies with a single nucleus and are mainly found inside macrophages and endothelial cells. In chronic infections cysts are formed containing large numbers of the parasites (Fig. 58I, p. 384). Man is mainly infected by ingesting oocysts in soil contaminated with cat faeces. Raw or undercooked meat containing extraintestinal forms is not an important source of infection.

Human infection is world-wide. In the great majority of cases *T. gondii* causes a latent infection which can be recognized only by serological tests. In the UK 30–40% of the adult population possess antibodies against the organism; in some parts of the world the figure exceeds 95%. Overt infection is rare. Congenital toxoplasmosis is acquired *in utero* from a mother suffering from an inapparent infection, usually acquired during that pregnancy. The manifestations include encephalitis, hydrocephalus, cerebral calcification and choroidoretinitis and the outcome is often fatal. In France serological tests for toxoplasmosis are carried out routinely on women during pregnancy and those found to be infected are treated. The effectiveness of this regime in reducing the incidence of congenital toxoplasmosis is uncertain. Acquired toxoplasmosis, which is mainly seen in children and young adults, commonly resembles infectious mononucleosis and takes a benign course with pyrexia, lymphocytosis and enlargement of lymph nodes. Chronic latent infections may develop into severe and fatal forms of the disease in patients undergoing immunosuppressive therapy.

Diagnosis

T. gondii can be isolated from lymph nodes, CSF or blood by intraperitoneal or intracerebral inoculation of mice. Toxoplasmosis is normally diagnosed by serological methods, usually a fluorescent antibody test, a haemagglutination test or a dye test which depends on the fact that staining of *T. gondii* by methylene blue is inhibited by specific antibodies. Active infection is indicated by rising titres but is usually present when the titres are high, e.g. more than 256 in the dye test. Confirmation is provided by specific IgM tests, e.g. an enzyme-linked immunosorbent assay (ELISA) IgM test.

Miscellaneous protozoa

Trichomonas vaginalis (Fig. 58H, p. 384) is an oval or pear-shaped flagellate about 15 μm long with four flagella projecting from the broad end. It is a common inhabitant of the vagina, where its presence is often associated with irritation and discharge. It frequently infects the male urethra. The infected male is commonly symptomless but is capable of infecting his sexual partner and should be treated at the same time. Similar organisms are sometimes encountered in the mouth and faeces.

Giardia lamblia (Fig. 59) is a pear-shaped flagellate about 15 μm long with a large ventral sucker, two nuclei and eight flagella arising in pairs from various regions in its midline. It lives mainly in the duodenum and duodenal aspiration may reveal the organism when faecal specimens are negative. It is a common cause of chronic diarrhoea and is the most frequently identified intestinal parasite in the UK. Symptomless carriers are often encountered. Infection is usually acquired by ingesting cysts of the organism in faecally contaminated food or drink. Large waterborne outbreaks of giardiasis have occurred. Adequate filtration of drinking water is important in prevention as cysts may survive chlorination.

Balantidium coli is a large oval ciliate, 40 × 60 μm, with an obvious groove leading to its mouth. It is a rare cause of a dysentery-like illness in man. It is a common parasite of pigs, and human infection is probably derived from these animals.

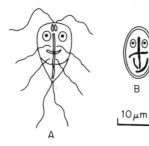

10 μm

Fig. 59 *Giardia lamblia.*
A, Trophozoite.
B, Cyst.

Pneumocystis carinii causes symptomless infections in early life. Serological tests indicate that over 95% of children are infected by the age of four. It is a rare cause of severe and often fatal pneumonia in infants and young children with defective immune mechanisms and in adults undergoing immunosuppressive therapy. It is one of the commonest opportunistic infections in the acquired immunodeficiency syndrome (AIDS). Such infections usually represent reactivation of a latent infection. A fluorescent antibody test on the patient's serum may help in diagnosis if there are rising titres or if the titres are high, e.g. 64 or more. The presence of *P. carinii* antigens in the blood indicates active infection. Spherical bodies, about 10 μm in diameter and containing 1–8 nuclei, are found in sections of lung tissue obtained by biopsy or at autopsy.

Cryptosporidium is a widely distributed parasite related to *Toxoplasma*. Human cryptosporidiosis is common and usually presents as an attack of diarrhoea lasting several days. Children are mainly affected. Severe persistent infections may occur in immunocompromized patients, e.g in AIDS. Thick-walled oocysts 3–5 μm in diameter and containing up to four sporozoites can be demonstrated in the faeces by special staining methods. Transmission is by the faecal-oral route. Human infection is sometimes acquired from animals, usually indirectly via food, milk and water.

Helminths

'Is it weakness of intellect, birdie?' I cried,
'Or a rather tough worm in your little inside?'
                                        W. S. Gilbert

A great variety of helminths or 'worms' may on occasions infect man. In the UK only three species are commonly encountered: *Enterobius vermicularis, Ascaris lumbricoides* and *Taenia saginata*. A few other species are encountered from time to time and a few more are imported from abroad by their human host. The total contribution to ill-health is small.

In some tropical and subtropical countries the picture is entirely different and helminth infection presents a major medical problem. Multiple infections are common and several species are responsible for serious diseases affecting large populations.

Most of the helminths encountered in the UK are intestinal parasites and diagnosis usually depends on demonstrating the parasites or their ova in the faeces. The more important ova are shown in Fig. 60 (p. 396). Eosinophilia occurs at some stage in nearly all helminth infections and a blood count is often of great value in suggesting the possibility of such infections. Eosinophils are important in antibody-dependent destruction of helminths (especially larval forms), phagocytosis of immune complexes and damping down type 1 (anaphylactic) hypersensitivity reactions. A history of residence abroad may suggest the need to look for some particular worm.

With a few rare exceptions the helminths which infect man belong to three classes: nematodes, cestodes and trematodes.

Nematodes (roundworms)

These are round unsegmented worms usually tapering at both ends.

Ascaris lumbricoides

A. lumbricoides, the roundworm, looks like a large pale earthworm. The mature female is 15—30 cm long; the male is shorter and has a curved tail. They live in the human intestinal tract, commonly in pairs. Fertilized ova are passed in the faeces but do not become infective until they have undergone development in moist soil. Man is infected by eating food contaminated with fully embryonated ova. Larvae hatch out in the duodenum and make their way by the blood stream to the lungs where they develop further. After several days they ascend the bronchi and trachea and are swallowed. The larvae mature in the small intestine. In heavy infections respiratory symptoms may occur as the larvae migrate through the lungs. In most cases the adult worms cause minimal symptoms. Sometimes a worm is vomited or passed in the faeces. This may cause alarm. Occasionally as a result of heavy infection or because a worm wanders up the bile duct or into the appendix surgical complications arise. The ova have a characteristic corrugated outline (Fig. 60A, p. 396).

Toxocara canis

T. canis is a roundworm of dogs. The ova are found in about 25% of soil samples from public parks in the UK. Infants and young children who play with infected dogs are particularly liable to ingest the ova. The subsequent migration of the larval forms can cause allergic symptoms but a serious complication is that the larvae occasionally settle in the eye and cause blindness. The worms never mature in the human host. Enzyme-linked immunosorbent assay (ELISA) and immunofluorescent tests on the patient's serum are used in diagnosis.

Enterobius vermicularis

E. vermicularis, the threadworm or pinworm, is very common throughout the world. The worms look like small white threads 0.5–1 cm long. They mainly inhabit the small intestine and can sometimes be seen wriggling in freshly passed stools. At night the female emerges from the anus to lay her eggs. This may cause intense itching. The ova are oval and flattened on one side (Fig. 60B, p. 396). They may be found in the faeces but the most reliable method of demonstrating them is by applying a length of cellophane tape to the perianal skin in the morning. The ova adhere to the tape which is then stuck on a slide for examination.

Trichuris trichiura

T. trichiura, the whipworm, is occasionally found in rural districts in the UK but is more common in warm moist regions of the world. The mature worm is 3–5 cm long and has a thin coiled anterior end resembling a whip. The ova are passed in the faeces

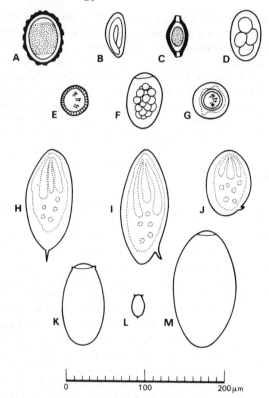

Fig. 60   Helminth ova. A, *Ascaris lumbricoides*. B, *Enterobius vermicularis*. C, *Trichuris trichiura*. D, *Ancylostoma duodenale*. E, *Taenia saginata* or *T. solium*. F, *Diphyllobothrium latum*. G, *Hymenolepis nana*. H, *Schistosoma haematobium* (found in urine). I, *Schistosoma mansoni*. J, *Schistosoma japonicum*. K, *Paragonimus westermani* (found in sputum). L, *Clonorchis sinensis*. M, *Fasciolopsis buski*.

and undergo development in moist soil. Man is infected by eating food contaminated with soil containing the mature ova. Whipworms do not usually give rise to symptoms but heavy infections can cause diarrhoea and anaemia. The ova are barrel-shaped with terminal knobs (Fig. 60C).

Trichinella spiralis

T. spiralis is primarily a parasite of rats which carry on the infection by cannibalism. Pigs become infected by eating dead rats. Human trichinosis results from eating raw or imperfectly cooked pork, particularly sausage meat, containing encysted larvae. The larvae are set free and mature to adults in the small intestine. At this stage heavy infection may give rise to abdominal pain, nausea and diarrhoea. After fertilization the female deposits larvae which penetrate the intestinal wall and find their way to striated muscle. This stage of larval invasion begins one to two weeks after infection and is associated with fever, oedema of the face and eyelids, and pain and tenderness in affected muscles. After several weeks encysted larvae can be demonstrated by muscle biopsy. An immunofluorescent test is also of value in diagnosis.

Hookworms

Ancylostoma duodenale and the related species *Necator americanus* are hookworms. Infection is widespread in tropical and subtropical countries. The adult worms are about 1 cm long and live attached to the intestinal mucous membrane by four hooked teeth (four semilunar cutting plates in *N. americanus*). They feed on mucosal cells, tissue fluids and blood and cause local bleeding. The ova are passed in the faeces but are not infective until they have undergone development in suitable moist surroundings. The fully developed larvae can bore their way through human skin and man usually acquires infection by walking barefoot on infected soil. The larvae pass to the lungs and find their way to the small intestine where they mature. In countries where most of the population is living on an inadequate diet the additional burden of hookworm infection leads to severe anaemia, general ill-health, inability to work and great economic loss to the community. Well-fed Europeans seldom show anaemia even when heavily infected. Adult worms are rarely seen in faeces and the diagnosis is made by finding the ova (Fig. 60D).

Strongyloides stercoralis

S. stercoralis is common in tropical countries. Female worms live in the mucous membrane of the small intestine and lay eggs which develop into larvae. These are either excreted in the faeces and undergo freeliving development in the soil to become infective larvae which enter a new host through the skin or they change into the infective form within the intestine of the original host and cause autoinfection. Repeated autoinfection can go on for a very long time and may, for example, be the cause of urticarial eruptions and abdominal symptoms in ex-servicemen who acquired their original infection more than 40 years previously. Chronic infection is particularly dangerous if the patient is given immunosuppressive therapy as an overwhelming and fatal dissemination of larvae throughout the body may result. Diagnosis of strongyloidiasis mainly depends on finding motile larvae in the faeces or duodenal contents. The patient's serum often gives positive results in serological tests for filariasis.

Filarial worms

Wuchereria bancrofti is the most important of the filariae. It has a widespread tropical distribution, being especially common in the West Indies, India, southern China and the Pacific Islands. The adult worms are thread-like creatures 4–10 cm long. They live in the lymphatics of the trunk and limbs where they set up a hyper-sensitivity reaction with recurrent lymphangitis and fever. Obstruction of the lymphatic circulation may give rise to elephantiasis of the limbs and genitalia and sometimes to chyluria. The larval forms, known as microfilariae, appear in large numbers in the peripheral blood at night. They are highly motile worm-like creatures about 300 μm in length and are enclosed in a thin transparent sheath. Filariasis is diagnosed by taking a sample of blood at night and looking for microfilariae. Group immuno-fluorescent, ELISA and complement fixation tests for *W. bancrofti* and other filarial worms are of value. The disease is transmitted from man to man by mosquitoes, the microfilariae undergoing further development in the insect host.

Brugia malayi is similar to *W. bancrofti* and is found in the Far East.

Mansonella perstans is common in certain parts of the tropics. The adult worms live in the peritoneal and pleural cavities. Symptoms are few. The disease is transmitted by biting midges.

Loa loa is found in West Africa. The adult worms move about under the skin and produce so-called 'Calabar swellings' which may be as large as a hen's egg and usually last for two or three days. Sometimes the worms migrate across the front of the eye. Microfilariae appear in the peripheral blood in the day-time and blood for examination should be taken at mid-day. The disease is transmitted by blood-sucking flies.

Onchocerca volvulus occurs in West Africa and parts of Central America and is the cause of 'blinding filariasis' or 'river blindness'. The adults mainly live in subcutaneous nodules. The micro-filariae migrate to various parts of the body. In heavy infections they often invade the eye where they may produce blindness. They rarely enter the blood. The diagnosis is usually made by finding the microfilariae in skin biopsies. Sometimes microfilariae may be observed in the eye. The disease is transmitted by blood-sucking flies.

Dracunculus medinensis

D. medinensis, the Guinea worm, is common in Africa and India. The worms live in the subcutaneous and interstitial tissues and take up to a year to reach maturity. The adult female is a thread-like worm 40–120 cm long. After fertilization by the much smaller male worm it makes its way to the skin which blisters and then ulcerates. On contact with water the female worm discharges her embryos through the ulcer. The embryos undergo a developmental cycle in water fleas. Man acquires infection by swallowing these crustaceans in drinking water. Diagnosis is made by detecting the embryos in the exudate from the ulcer. Classically, the patient extracts the intact worm by daily douching the ulcer with water and very, very gradually winding the worm round a small stick! Septic complications are frequent. Theoretically, global eradication of dracunculiasis could be achieved by providing clean drinking water.

Cestodes (tapeworms)

Cestodes or tapeworms are flat segmented worms.

Taenia saginata

T. saginata, the beef tapeworm, is the only tapeworm commonly found in man in the UK. Infection is acquired by eating insufficiently cooked beef infected with the cystic larval stage (*Cysticercus bovis*) of the worm. The head, or scolex, is about the size of the head of a large pin and has four suckers but is devoid of hooklets (Fig. 61A, p. 400). From the scolex arises a series of progressively larger segments, or proglottides, so that the mature worm is a white ribbon-shaped creature 5–10 m long. Mature segments measure about 20 × 7 mm and the uterus has 15–25 lateral branches (Fig. 61B, p. 400). The terminal gravid segments become separated from time to time and are passed in the faeces where they may move about for several hours. The presence of the adult worm seldom produces intestinal symptoms but the discovery of segments in the stool may alarm the patient. When examining the faeces, particularly after treatment designed to expel the worm, every effort must be made to identify the head because if it is still attached to the host the tapeworm will regenerate. The whole specimen of stool should be meticulously examined under running water in a bed-pan. The ova of *T. saginata* have a thick radially striated capsule and contain an embryo armed with six hooklets (Fig. 60E, p. 400).

T. solium and cysticercosis

T. solium, the pork tapeworm, is now rare in the UK. Infection is acquired by eating raw or undercooked pork containing the larval form (*Cysticercus cellulosae*) of the worm. The head of the worm is the size of a pin head and has four suckers and a circle of long and short hooklets (Fig. 61C). The worm reaches a length of 2–5 m. The uterus of mature segments has about ten lateral branches (Fig. 61D). Symptoms attributable to the adult worms are minimal. The ova are indistinguishable from those of *T. saginata* (Fig. 60E, 396).

The importance of *T. solium* is that the larval stage, which normally occurs in the pig, occasionally develops in man and produces human cysticercosis. Ova gain access to the stomach in contaminated food or by regurgitation from the intestines. The larvae are liberated and penetrate the intestinal mucosa and develop into cysticerci. These are commonly located in the sub-cutaneous tissues and the skeletal muscles and are palpable as

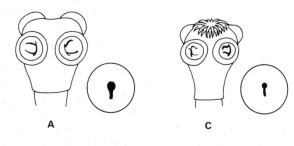

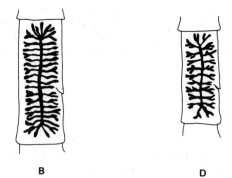

Fig. 61 Tapeworms. A, *Taenia saginata* scolex (natural size in circle). B, *T. saginata* mature segment, × 2. C, *T. solium* scolex (natural size in circle). D, *T. solium* mature segment, × 2.

tense ovoid swellings 5—10 mm in size. They usually cause little trouble but cysts may develop in the brain and cause epilepsy. Diagnosis of such cases is greatly assisted by immunofluorescent and complement fixation tests.

Echinococcus granulosus and hydatid disease

Man is a host for the cystic stage of this tapeworm. Hydatid cysts usually occur in sheep and cattle and the human disease is most common in sheep-rearing countries such as Australia, New Zealand, Argentina and Iceland. Dogs are the most important host for the adult tapeworm, a small parasite only 3—6 mm long. Man acquires the disease, usually in childhood, by eating food contaminated with ova excreted by dogs. Embryos are liberated from the ova in the small intestine, gain access to the blood and develop into cysts in the tissues. The cysts grow slowly for many years and may reach a tremendous size. In 75% of patients a single large cyst is found in the right lobe of the liver. In other patients cysts may be found in the lung, brain or elsewhere. As they grow, one or two generations of daughter cysts containing scolices are produced from the inner walls. The cysts may rupture spontaneously and their contents escape into the abdominal cavity or the bronchi. Severe anaphylactic reactions may occur. In aspirating or removing a hydatid cyst care must be taken to avoid spilling the contents into the tissues because any scolices present will develop into cysts later on. The diagnosis of hydatid disease is confirmed by the structure of the cysts and by finding hooklets and scolices in their contents. ELISA, complement fixation, indirect haemagglutination, latex agglutination and immuno-electrophoresis tests are valuable aids to diagnosis.

E. *multilocularis* closely resembles E. *granulosus*. It causes an alveolar (multilocular) type of hydatid disease in man. The disease occurs in North America and Europe but not in the UK. Foxes and rodents are important hosts.

Diphyllobothrium latum

D. *latum*, the fish tapeworm, is common in Iceland, northern Scandinavia and parts of the USA. It is 3—10 m in length with a long narrow head provided with two slit-like suckers. The ova (Fig. 60F, p. 396) undergo development in water fleas before being eaten by freshwater fish. Human infection is acquired by eating raw or undercooked fish. Symptoms are usually slight but occasionally a patient develops severe macrocytic anaemia.

Hymenolepis nana

H. nana, the dwarf tapeworm, is only 2−4 cm long. It is common in parts of southern Europe, southern USA and India. The ova are shown in Fig. 60G (p. 396).

Trematodes (flukes)

Flukes are flat unsegmented worms. On clinical grounds they may be divided into those which inhabit the blood, the lungs, the liver or the intestines.

Blood flukes

Schistosoma haematobium is particularly common in Egypt and also occurs in many other parts of Africa and the Middle East. It causes the important disease schistosomiasis or bilharzia. The adult flukes live in the veins of the portal system and in the venous plexuses of the bladder and rectum. They may survive for 20−25 years, evading the immune mechanisms of the host by incorporating host antigens into their own outer layers. The ova escape from the veins and pass through the bladder wall into the urine. Haematuria, frequency and dysuria are common symptoms. The bladder wall may undergo ulceration and papilloma formation. Later complications include carcinoma of the bladder and back-pressure effects in the renal tract. The ova (Fig. 60H, p. 396) have a terminal spine and bilharzia is normally diagnosed by finding them in the urine, particularly in the last drops at the end of micturition. They are rarely found in the faeces. Biopsies of the rectal and bladder mucosa are often positive. ELISA and complement fixation tests are useful in screening for infection with *S. haematobium* and other species. The tests become positive about three months before excretion of ova begins. When ova are deposited in water the embryos escape and undergo a development cycle in freshwater snails. Minute larvae known as cercariae escape from the snails and enter the human body by penetrating the skin. Infection is usually acquired by bathing or wading in infected water.

  S. mansoni is a similar fluke found in Egypt, other parts of Africa, South America and the Caribbean. The adults live mainly in the mesenteric veins and mild dysentery is a common symptom. Rectal polyps, periportal fibrosis of the liver and splenomegaly may develop later. The ova (Fig. 60I, p. 396) have a lateral spine and are found in the faeces. Freshwater snails are intermediate hosts.

S. japonicum causes schistosomiasis in the Far East. The symptoms are similar to those caused by *S. mansoni*, but there is often involvement of the central nervous system resulting in fits and nerve lesions. The ova (Fig. 60J, p. 396) have a lateral knob-like hook and are found in the faeces. Amphibious snails are intermediate hosts.

Lung flukes

Paragonimus westermani is the cause of endemic haemoptysis in the Far East. The adult flukes live mainly in the lungs and the diagnosis is made by finding ova (Fig. 60K, p. 396) in the sputum. Ova are also found in the faeces because people swallow their sputum. Less often the flukes inhabit the intestinal tract and the abdominal organs. The ova hatch and the resulting larvae develop first in freshwater snails and then in crayfish and crabs. Man is infected by eating uncooked crustacea.

Liver flukes

Clonorchis sinensis is a common parasite in the Far East. The adult flukes live in the bile ducts. Repeated infection may cause enlargement and fibrosis of the liver with jaundice and ascites. The ova (Fig. 60L, p. 396) are found in the faeces. Freshwater snails and fish are the intermediate hosts. Uncooked fish is the most important source of human infection.

Fasciola hepatica, the sheep liver fluke, rarely affects man. Freshwater snails are the intermediate host and man is infected by chewing grass or eating raw vegetables contaminated with the larval forms of the fluke. A few cases caused by eating infected watercress have been reported from sheep-rearing regions in the UK. An immunofluorescent test is of value in diagnosis.

Intestinal flukes

Fasciolopsis buski, the giant intestinal fluke, is found in the Far East. It inhabits the duodenum and may give rise to diarrhoea, abdominal pain, oedema and ascites. The ova (Fig. 60M, p. 396) are passed in the faeces and undergo development in freshwater snails. The resulting larvae encyst on water plants and man is infected by eating in the raw state such foods as the corms of water chestnuts.

Suggestions for Further Reading

To copy from one book is plagiarism:
to copy from two books is research.
Received wisdom

General

Baron, S., Cerny, J., Albrecht, T.B. *et al.*, ed. (1986) *Medical Microbiology: Principles and Concepts*, 2nd ed. Menlo Park, Calif.: Addison-Wesley.

Bulloch, W. (1938) *The History of Bacteriology*. London: Oxford University Press. (A classic, reprinted 1960)

Burnet, F.M. & White, D. O. (1972) *Natural History of Infectious Disease*, 4th ed. Cambridge: Cambridge University Press.

Christie, A.B. (1987) *Infectious Diseases: Epidemiology and Clinical Practice*, 4th ed. Edinburgh: Churchill Livingstone.

Communicable Disease Report. London: PHLS. (Compiled in the PHLS Communicable Disease Surveillance Centre; published weekly with 4-weekly summaries, quarterly tabulations and short topical articles)

Davis, B.D., Dulbecco, R., Eisen, H.N., Ginsberg, H.S. *et al.* (1980) *Microbiology: Including Immunology and Molecular Genetics*, 3rd ed. New York: Harper & Row International.

Dobell, C. (1932) *Antony van Leeuwenhoek and his 'Little Animals'*. London: John Bale (reprinted 1960, New York: Dover).

Duerden, B.I., Reid, T.M.S., Jewsbury, J.M. & Turk, D.C. (1987) *A New Short Textbook of Microbial and Parasitic Infection*. London: Hodder & Stoughton.

Foster, W.D. (1970) *A History of Medical Bacteriology and Immunology*. London: Heinemann Medical.

Jawetz, E., Melnick, J.L. & Adelberg, E.A. (1987) *Review of Medical Microbiology*, 17th ed. Los Altos, Calif.: Lange Medical Publications. (Comprehensive, up-to-date and down-to-earth)

MacFarlane, R.G. (1979) *Howard Florey: The Making of a Great Scientist*. Oxford: Oxford University Press.

MacFarlane, R.G. (1984) *Alexander Fleming: The Man and the Myth*. London: Chatto & Windus.

Mandell, G.L., Douglas, R.G., Jr., & Bennett, J.E., ed. (1985) *Principles and Practice of Infectious Diseases*, 2nd ed. New York: John Wiley.

Milgrom, F. & Flanagan, T.D., ed. (1982) *Medical Microbiology*. New York: Churchill Livingstone.

Mims, C.A. (1987) *The Pathogenesis of Infectious Disease*, 3rd ed. London: Academic Press.

Proctor, R.A., ed. (1987) Fibronectin and the pathogenesis of infections. *Rev. Infect. Dis. 9* (Suppl.): S317−430.

Shanson, D.C. (1982) *Microbiology in Clinical Practice*. Bristol: Wright/ PSG.

Stahl, F.W. (1987) Genetic recombination. *Sci. Am. 256* (2): 52−63.

Stanier, R.Y., Ingraham, J.L., Wheelis, M.L. & Painter, P.R. (1987) *General Microbiology*, 5th ed. London: Macmillan. (Non-medical)

Watson, J.D., Tooze, J. & Kurtz, D.T. (1983) *Recombinant DNA: A Short Course*. New York: Scientific American Books.

Weinberg, R.A. (1985) The molecules of life. *Sci. Am. 253* (4): 34−43.

Wilson, G.S., Miles, A.A. & Parker, M.T., ed. (1983) *Topley and Wilson's Principles of Bacteriology, Virology and Immunity*, 7th ed., vol. 1 & 2; (1984) vol. 3 & 4. London: Edward Arnold. (One of the great texts of medicine, giving references to the more important original papers and monographs: disappointing index)

Woese, C.R. (1981) Archaebacteria. *Sci. Am. 244* (6): 94−106. (The tree of life updated: *three* primary kingdoms?)

Zinsser, H. (1942) *Rats, Lice and History*. London: Routledge.

Bacteria

Anderson, W.F. & Diacumakos, E.G. (1981) Genetic engineering in mammalian cells. *Sci. Am. 245* (1): 60−93.

Bartlett, C.L.R., Macrae, A.D. & Macfarlane, J.T. (1986) *Legionella Infections*. London: Edward Arnold.

Budd, W. (1873) *Typhoid Fever: Its Nature, Mode of Spreading and Prevention*. London: Longmans. (A classic.)

Cohen, S.N. & Shapiro, J.A. (1980) Transposable genetic elements. *Sci. Am. 242* (2): 36−45.

Darougar, S., ed. (1983) Chlamydial disease. *Br. Med. Bull. 39*: 107−208.

Gilbert, W. & Villa-Komaroff, L. (1980) Useful proteins from recombinant bacteria. *Sci. Am. 242* (4): 68−82.

Glover, D.M. (1980) *Genetic Engineering: Cloning DNA*. London: Chapman & Hall.

Habicht, G.S., Beck, G. & Benach, J.L. (1987) Lyme disease. *Sci. Am. 257* (1): 60−65.

Hardy, K. (1981) *Bacterial Plasmids*. Walton-on-Thames, England: Nelson.

Hobbs, B.C. & Gilbert, R.J. (1978) *Food Poisoning and Food Hygiene*, 4th ed. London: Edward Arnold.

John, J.F., Jr., & Twitty, J.A. (1986) Plasmids as epidemiologic markers in nosocomial gram-negative bacilli: experience at a university and review of the literature. *Rev. Infect. Dis. 8*: 693−704.

Lupski, J.R. (1987) Molecular mechanisms for transposition of drug-resistance genes and other movable genetic elements. *Rev. Infect. Dis. 9*: 357−368.

Macdonald, A. & Smith, G., ed. (1981) *The Staphylococci*. Aberdeen: Aberdeen University Press.

Mandelstam, J., McQuillen, K. & Dawes, I., ed. (1982) *Biochemistry of Bacterial Growth*, 3rd ed. Oxford: Blackwell Scientific.

Muhlemann, M.F. & Wright, D.J.M. (1987) Emerging pattern of Lyme disease in the United Kingdom and Irish Republic. *Lancet, i: 260−262*.

Novick, R.P. (1980) Plasmids. *Sci. Am.* 243 (6): 76—90.

Report (1986) *The Report of the Committee of Inquiry into an Outbreak of Food Poisoning at Stanley Royd Hospital.* London: HMSO. (Lessons for everyone who works in hospitals)

Report (1986) *First Report of the Committee of Inquiry into the Outbreak of Legionnaires' Disease in Stafford in April 1985.* London: HMSO.

Robins-Browne, R.M. (1987) Traditional enteropathogenic *Escherichia coli* of infantile diarrhea. *Rev. Infect. Dis.* 9: 28—53.

Rose, A.H. (1976) *Chemical Microbiology*, 3rd ed. London: Butterworths.

Schaberg, D.R. & Zervos, M. (1986) Plasmid analysis in the study of the epidemiology of nosocomial gram-positive cocci. *Rev. Infect. Dis.* 8: 705—712.

Shlaes, D.M. & Currie-McCumber, C.A. (1986) Plasmid analysis in molecular epidemiology: a summary and future directions. *Rev. Infect Dis.* 8: 738—746.

Smith, H. (1984) The biochemical challenge of microbial pathogenicity. *J. Appl. Bacteriol.* 57: 395—404.

Stephen, J. & Pietrowski, R.A. (1981) *Bacterial Toxins.* Walton-on-Thames, England: Nelson.

Stokes, E. J. & Ridgway, G.L. (1987) *Clinical Microbiology*, 6th ed. London: Edward Arnold. (Well-tried practical procedures)

Wachsmuth, K. (1986) Molecular epidemiology of bacterial infections: examples of methodology and investigations of outbreaks. *Rev. Infect. Dis.* 8: 682—691.

Viruses

Andrews, C., Pereira, H.G. & Wildy, N. P. L. (1978) *Viruses of Vertebrates*, 4th ed. London: Baillière Tindall. (For reference only)

Banatvala, J.E. (1987) The appropriate use of diagnostic services: (xiv) How to make best use of a clinical virology laboratory. *Health Trends 19*: 1—8.

Bishop, J.M. (1982) Oncogenes. *Sci Am.* 246 (3): 68—78.

BMA (1987) *AIDS and You.* London: BMA. (All the answers for the layman!)

Evans, A.S., ed. (1982) *Viral Infections of Humans: Epidemiology and Control*, 2nd ed. London: John Wiley.

Fenner, F., McAuslan, B.R., Mims, C.A., Sambrook, J. & White, D.O. (1974) *The Biology of Animal Viruses*, 2nd ed. London: Academic Press.

Fields, B.N. *et al.*, ed. (1985) *Virology.* New York: Raven Press.

Gallo, R.C. (1986) The first human retrovirus. *Sci. Am.* 255 (6): 78—88.

Gallo, R.C. (1987) The AIDS virus. *Sci Am.* 256 (1): 38—48.

Haywood, A.M. (1986) Patterns of persistent viral infections. *N. Engl. J. Med.* 315: 939—948.

Hogle, J.M., Chow, M. & Filman, D.J. (1987) The structure of poliovirus. *Sci. Am.* 256 (3): 28—35.

Horne, R.W. (1978) *The Structure and Function of Viruses.* London: Edward Arnold.

Jeffries, D. *et al.*, ed. (1987) *Current Topics in AIDS*, vol. 1. Chichester, England: John Wiley.

Jenner, E. (1798) *An Inquiry into the Causes and Effects of the Variolae Vaccinae, etc.*, London: Sampson Low (reprinted 1966, London: Dawson).

Johnson, R.T. (1982) *Viral Infections of the Nervous System*. New York: Raven Press.

Kaplan, M. M. & Koprowski, H. (1980) Rabies. *Sci. Am.* 242 (1): 104–113.

Laurence, J. (1985) The immune system in AIDS. *Sci. Am.* 253 (6): 70–79.

Luria, S.E., Darnell, J.E., Jr., Baltimore, D. & Campbell, A. (1978) *General Virology*, 3rd ed. New York: John Wiley. (Non-medical, for the mentally agile)

Miller, D., Weber, J. & Green, J., ed. (1986) *The Management of AIDS Patients*. London: Macmillan.

Mims, C.A., ed. (1985) Virus immunity and pathogenesis. *Br. Med. Bull.* 41: 1–97.

Mims, C.A. & White, D.O. (1984) *Viral Pathogenesis and Immunology*. Oxford: Blackwell Scientific.

Mortimer, P.P., ed. (1986) *Public Health Virology: 12 Reports*. London: PHLS.

Pinching, A.J., ed. (1986) *Aids and HIV Infection* (Clinics in Immunology and Allergy 6, No. 3). London: Baillière Tindall/W.B. Saunders.

Simons, K., Garoff, H. & Helenius, A. (1982) How an animal virus gets into and out of its host cell. *Sci. Am.* 246 (2): 46–54.

Timbury, M.C. (1986) *Notes on Medical Virology*, 8th ed. Edinburgh: Churchill Livingstone.

White, D.O. & Fenner, F. (1986) *Medical Virology*, 3rd ed. London: Academic Press. (An excellent Australian text suitable for medical students)

Zuckerman, A.J., Banatvala, J.E. & Pattison, J.R., ed. (1987) *Principles and Practice of Clinical Virology*. Chichester, England: John Wiley.

Immunity

Ada, G.L. & Nossal, G. (1987) The clonal-selection theory. *Sci. Am.* 257 (2): 50–57.

Bowry, T.R. (1984) *Immunology Simplified*, 2nd ed. Oxford: Oxford University Press.

Buisseret, P.D. (1982) Allergy. *Sci. Am.* 247 (2): 82–91.

Crumpton, M.J., ed. (1987) HLA in medicine. *Br. Med. Bull.* 43: i–vi, 1–245.

Dick, G., ed. (1979) *Immunological Aspects of Infectious Diseases*. Lancaster: MTP Press.

Dick, G. (1986) *Practical Immunisation*. Lancaster: MTP Press.

Edelson, R.L. & Fink, J.M. (1985) The immunological function of skin. *Sci. Am.* 252 (6): 34–41.

Goding, J.W. (1987) *Monoclonal Antibodies: Principles and Practice*, 2nd ed. London: Academic Press.

Godson, G.N. (1985) Molecular approaches to malaria vaccines. *Sci. Am.* 252 (5): 32–39.

Hilleman, M.R. (1985) Newer directions in vaccine development and utilization. *J. Infect. Dis.* 151: 407–419.

Holborow, E.J. & Reeves, W.G., ed. (1983) *Immunology in Medicine: A Comprehensive Guide to Clinical Immunology*, 2nd ed. London: Grune & Stratton.

Kennedy, R.C., Melnick, J.L. & Dreesman, G.R. (1986) Anti-idiotypes and immunity. *Sci. Am. 255* (1): 40–48.

Lachmann, P.J. & Peters, D.K., ed. (1982) *Clinical Aspects of Immunology*, 4th ed. Oxford: Blackwell Scientific.

Landsteiner, K. (1945) *The Specificity of Serological Reactions*, 2nd ed. Cambridge, Mass.: Harvard University Press. (A classic)

Leder, P. (1982) The genetics of antibody diversity. *Sci. Am. 246* (5): 72–83.

Lennox, E.S., ed. (1984) Clinical applications of monoclonal antibodies. *Br. Med. Bull. 40*: 207–306.

Lerner, R.A. (1983) Synthetic vaccines. *Sci. Am 248* (2): 48–56.

Macario, A.J.L. & Conway de Macario, E., ed. (1985) *Monoclonal Antibodies against Bacteria*, vol. 1; (1986), vol. 2. London: Academic Press.

Marrack, P. & Kappler, J. (1986) The T cell and its receptor. *Sci. Am. 254* (2): 28–37.

Milstein, C. (1980) Monoclonal antibodies. *Sci. Am. 243* (4): 56–64.

Roitt, I.M. (1984) *Essential Immunology*, 5th ed. Oxford: Blackwell Scientific.

Roitt, I.M., Brostoff, J. & Male, D.K., ed. (1985) *Immunology*. Edinburgh: Churchill Livingstone.

Rouse, B.T. & Horohov, D.W. (1986) Immunosuppression in viral infections. *Rev. Infect. Dis. 8*: 850–873.

Rose, N.R. (1981) Autoimmune disease. *Sci. Am. 244* (2): 70–81.

Tonegawa, S. (1985) The molecules of the immune system. *Sci. Am. 253* (4): 104–113.

Wilson, J.R. (1963) *Margin of Safety: The Story of Poliomyelitis Vaccine*. London: Collins.

Antimicrobial Agents

Abraham, E.P. (1981) The beta-lactam antibiotics. *Sci. Am. 244* (6): 64–74.

Ayliffe, G.A.J., Coates, D. & Hoffman, P.N. (1984) *Chemical Disinfection in Hospitals*. London: PHLS.

Baldry, P. (1976) *The Battle Against Bacteria: A Fresh Look*, 2nd ed. Cambridge: Cambridge University Press.

British National Formulary. London: British Medical Association and the Pharmaceutical Society of Great Britain. (Indispensable guide to the use of antibiotics and vaccines, revised every six months)

Datta, N., ed. (1984) Antibiotic resistance in bacteria. *Br. Med. Bull. 40*: 1–111.

Gardner, J.F. & Peel, M.M. (1986) *Introduction to Sterilization and Disinfection*. Edinburgh: Churchill Livingstone.

Garrod, L.P., Lambert, H.P. & O'Grady, F. (1981) *Antibiotic and Chemotherapy*, 5th ed. Edinburgh: Churchill Livingstone.

Greenwood, D. & O'Grady, F., ed. (1985) *The Scientific Basis of Antimicrobial Chemotherapy* (Symposium 38, Society for General Microbiology, 1985). Cambridge: Cambridge University Press.

Hare, R. (1970) *The Birth of Penicillin*. London: Allen & Unwin.

Hirsch, M.S. & Kaplan, J.C. (1987) Antiviral therapy. *Sci. Am. 256* (4): 66–75.

Kucers, A. & Bennett, N.M. (1987) *The Use of Antibiotics: A Comprehensive review with Clinical Emphasis*, 4th ed. London: Heinemann Medical.

Lorian, V., ed. (1985) *Antibiotics in Laboratory Medicine*, 2nd ed. Baltimore, Md.: Williams and Wilkins.

Mandell, G.L. et al., ed. (1985) *Anti-infective Therapy*. Chichester, England: John Wiley.

Maurer, I.M. (1985) *Hospital Hygiene*, 3rd ed. London: Edward Arnold.

Noone, P. (1979) *A Clinician's Guide to Antibiotic Therapy*, 2nd ed. Oxford: Blackwell Scientific. (Instant answers)

Pestka, S. (1983) The purification and manufacture of human interferons. *Sci. Am. 249* (2): 28−35.

Tyrrell, D.A.J. & Oxford, J.S., ed. (1985) Antiviral chemotherapy and interferon. *Br. Med. Bull. 41*: 307−405.

Wainwright, M. & Swan, H.J. (1986) C.G. Paine and the earliest surviving clinical records of penicillin therapy. *Med. Hist. 30*: 42−56.

Miscellaneous

Adler, M.W. (1984) *ABC of Sexually Transmitted Diseases*. London: British Medical Association.

Ayliffe, G.A.J., Collins B.J. & Taylor L.J. (1982) *Hospital-acquired Infection: Principles and Prevention*. Bristol: Wright/PSG.

Bagshawe, K.D., Blowers, R. & Lidwell, O.M. (1978) Isolating patients in hospital to control infection. Part I — Sources and routes of infection. Part II — Who should be isolated, and where? Part III — Design and construction of isolation accommodation. Part IV — Nursing procedures. Part V — An isolation system. *Br. Med. J. ii*: 609−613, 684−686, 744−748, 808−811, 879−881.

Beaver, P.C., Jung, R.C. & Cupp, E.W. (1984) *Clinical Parasitology*, 9th ed. Philadelphia: Lea & Febiger.

Benenson, A.S., ed. (1985) *Control of Communicable Diseases in Man*, 14th ed. Washington: American Public Health Association. (A useful pocketbook)

Bennett, J.V. & Brachman, P.S., ed. (1986) *Hospital Infections*, 2nd ed. Boston: Little, Brown.

Bruce-Chwatt, L.J. (1985) *Essential Malariology*, 2nd ed. London: Heinemann Medical.

Coid, C.R., ed. (1977) *Infections and Pregnancy*. London: Academic Press.

Conant, N.F., Smith, D.T., Baker, R.D. & Callaway, J.L. (1971) *Manual of Clinical Mycology*, 3rd ed. Philadelphia: Saunders.

Donelson, J.E. & Turner, M.J. (1985) How the trypanosome changes its coat. *Sci. Am. 252* (2): 32−39.

Emond, R.T.D., Bradley, J. M. & Galbraith, N.S. (1982) *Pocket Consultant of Infection*. London: Grant McIntyre.

English, M.P. (1980) *Medical Mycology*. London: Edward Arnold.

Evans, E.G.V. & Gentles, J.C. (1985) *Essentials of Medical Mycology*. Edinburgh: Churchill Livingstone.

Friedman, M.J. & Trager, W. (1981) The biochemistry of resistance to malaria. *Sci. Am. 244* (3): 112−120.

Hunter, T. (1984) The proteins of oncogenes. *Sci. Am. 251* (2): 60−69.

Lowbury, E.J.L., Ayliffe, G.A.J., Geddes, A.M. & Williams, J.D., ed. (1981) *Control of Hospital Infection: A Practical Handbook*, 2nd ed. London: Chapman & Hall.

Mackowiak, P.A. (1984) Microbial latency. *Rev. Infect. Dis.* 6: 649–668.

Major, R.H. (1965) *Classic Descriptions of Disease*, 3rd ed. Springfield, Ill.: Charles C. Thomas.

Manson-Bahr, P.E.C. & Bell, D.R. (1987) *Manson's Tropical Diseases*, 19th ed. London: Baillière Tindall.

Muller, R. (1975) *Worms and Disease: A Manual of Medical Helminthology*. London: Heinemann Medical.

Parker, M.T., ed. (1978) *Hospital-acquired Infections: Guidelines to Laboratory Methods*. Copenhagen: World Health Organization. (A useful summary)

Pitlik, S., Berger, S.A. & Huminer, D. (1987) Nonenteric infections acquired through contact with water. *Rev. Infect. Dis.* 9: 54–63.

Prentis, S. (1984) *Biotechnology: A New Industrial Revolution*. London: Orbis.

Prusiner, S.B. (1984) Prions. *Sci. Am.* 251 (4): 48–57.

Symposium (1981) *Adhesion and Microorganism Pathogenicity*, Ciba Foundation Symposium 80, London, England. London: Pitman Medical.

Warnock, D.W. & Richardson, M.D., ed. (1982) *Fungal Infection in the Compromised Patient*. Chichester, England: John Wiley.

Weinberg, R.A. (1983) A molecular basis of cancer. *Sci. Am.* 249 (5): 102–116.

Williams, R.E.O., Blowers, R., Garrod, L.P. & Shooter, R.A. (1966) *Hospital Infection: Causes and Prevention*, 2nd ed. London: Lloyd-Luke.

Willoughby, D.A., ed. (1987) Inflammation – mediators and mechanisms. *Br. Med. Bull.* 43: 247–477.

Index